Orthopedic Differential Diagnosis in Physical Therapy

NOTICE

Medicine is an ever-changing science. As new research and clinical experience broaden our knowledge, changes in treatment and drug therapy
are required. The author and the publisher of this work have checked
with sources believed to be reliable in their efforts to provide information
that is complete and generally in accord with the standards acccepted at
the time of publication. However, in view of the possibility of human
error or changes in medical sciences, neither the author nor the publisher
nor any other party who has been involved in the preparation or publication of this work warrants that the information contained herein is in
every respect accurate or complete, and they are not responsible for any
errors or omissions or for the results obtained from use of such information.
Readers are encouraged to confirm the information contained herein with
other sources. For example and in particular, readers are advised to check
the product information sheet included in the package of each drug they
plan to administer to be certain that the information contained in this
book is accurate and that changes have not been made in the recommended
dose or in the contraindications for administration. This recommendation
is of particular importance in connection with new or infrequently used
drugs.

Orthopedic Differential Diagnosis in Physical Therapy: A Case Study Approach

James T. S. Meadows, BScPT, FCAMT

McGraw-Hill
HEALTH PROFESSIONS DIVISION

New York St. Louis San Francisco Auckland
Bogotá Caracas Lisbon London Madrid
Mexico City Milan Montreal New Delhi San Juan
Singapore Sydney Tokyo Toronto

McGraw-Hill

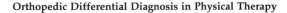

A Division of The McGraw·Hill Companies

Orthopedic Differential Diagnosis in Physical Therapy

1 2 3 4 5 6 7 8 9 0   DOCDOC   9 9

ISBN 0-07-041235-9

This book was set in Times Roman by York Graphic Services.
Project management was by York Production Services.
The editors were Stephen Zollo and Peter McCurdy;
the production supervisor was Catherine Saggese;
the cover and text designer was Robert Freese;
The index was prepared by York Graphic Services;
R.R. Donnelley & Sons was printer and binder.

This book was printed on acid-free paper.

Library of Congress Cataloging-in-Publication Data

Orthopedic Differential Diagnosis in Physical Therapy / editor, James Meadows.
     p.   cm.
    Includes bibliographical references and index.
    ISBN 0-07-041235-9
    1. Orthopedics—Diagnosis—Case studies.   2. Diagnosis,
Differential—Case studies.   3. Physical therapists.   I. Meadows,
James.
    [DNLM: 1. Physical Therapy—methods case studies.   2. Diagnosis,
Differential.   3. Physical Examination—methods.   4. Manipulation,
Orthopedic.   WB 460 D659 1999]
RD734.D54   1999
616.7'075—DC21
DNLM/DLC
for Library of Congress   98-49161
                                                                                              CIP

Contents

Preface

The aims of this book are threefold. First, to provide the undergraduate student with vicarious experiences that will temporarily fill the void that will later be filled by the student's own experiences. Second, to offer therapists, whether students or vastly experienced, the chance to challenge themselves against case histories in private to see how they do. I know that self-testing is something that few physical therapists can pass up. Third, unusual cases are exactly that, unusual. We do not individually have many opportunities to see many patients with cancers, gastric ulcers, kidney stones, hiatus hernias, and the like, so we tend to miss them because our orthopedic blinkers focus everything into orthopedic conditions. If this book does nothing more than help you realize that oddities have a way of presenting as the mundane and that we have a way of perceiving what we expect rather than what is, it will have been successful.

This is not a how-to book in the conventional sense of instruction in the techniques or examination. In general educational terms, this requirement is dealt with in school and in a plethora of books designed for exactly this purpose. However, what the student cannot gain in the classroom is experience. During clinical placements, the student is quite correctly required to rotate through the various specialties and so receives comparatively little experience in orthopedics and often none at all in orthopedic manual therapy. The schools know that when the newly graduated therapist is ready to specialize in one area, postgraduate programs are available. Unfortunately, other than clinical residencies, these classes still lack what is missing in the physical therapy school, hands-on experience. The object of this book is to try to teach how to analyze and integrate information gained from subjective and objective clinical examinations. It will help the student and practitioner of orthopedic physical therapy to differentiate patients with routine diagnoses, treatment plans, and responses to treatment from those who will be a problem to the therapist. These latter patients must be identified early so that a nonroutine approach can be taken. If physical therapy is appropriate, a unique approach can be designed for the more difficult patient. If orthopedic therapy is deemed inappropriate, the patient can be returned to the physician as quickly as possible.

To succeed in these aims, the first section of the book will consist of one clinical approach to the evaluation of the neuromusculoskeletal system. The first chapter generally describes the differential diagnostic examination and discusses the integration of the data generated from the examination. From this integration, the therapist can either generate a working diagnosis and a management plan or determine that further clinical examination is required. For example, from the differential diagnostic examination a working diagnosis might be an L4 disk extrusion with L5 spinal nerve compression with radiculopathy. From this diagnosis, a treatment plan can be made that might consist of specific exercises, traction, rest, and so on, or inappropriate pathology might be suspected and the patient returned to the physician. Alternatively, and usually more commonly, a set of signs and symptoms that do not lend themselves to a specific diagnosis are found. In this case further information is required before a specific treatment plan can be arrived at. This information is afforded by the biomechanical examination. Examples of the type of diagnosis that can be arrived at from the biomechanical examination include a right L4-5 zygapophyseal joint hypomobility, a right L3-4 torsional instability, or a left C5-6 zygapophyseal joint extension hypermobility. From this biomechanical evaluation, the therapist can initiate a specific exercise program, manual therapy, and/or stabilization treatments.

The differential diagnostic examination, designed by James Cyriax, M.D., will be, with very slight modifications, possibly the most comprehensive and rational clinical examination of the musculoskeletal system in use today. The modifications are simply additions that will increase the breadth of the diagnostic scope. The examination is based on our knowledge of the anatomy of the musculoskeletal system. The function of each subset of the system, such as the contractile tissues (muscle, tendon, and tenoperiosteal junction), the inert tissues (joint capsule, ligament, dura, bone, and bursa), the vascular system (arteries and veins), and the neurological system (peripheral and central systems) is stressed. The test stress is the function of the subset applied in as much as isolation from the other subsets as is possible.

To a large extent, the interpretation and integration of the findings will be covered in the case studies themselves, where there is immediate relevance to the clinical picture, rather than as an isolated intellectual exercise. For example, paresthesia will be discussed in general terms in Chapter 1 and mention will be made of its significance, but how the pattern of paresthesia suggests certain conditions will be discussed in detail in the discussion of a particular case.

Some of the cases in this book are given exactly as they presented; where these have been donated by colleagues, due credit is given. Other cases are composites of cases with rough edges smoothed off or added

---

*Cyriax J: *Textbook of Orthopedic Medicine,* 8th ed. London, Ballière Tindall & Cassell, 1982.

to simplify or complicate the clinical picture. The purpose of the book is to provide a learning tool, not to faithfully reproduce the clinical presentation of each patient.

Finally, the reader who hopes to find only experimentally validated techniques will be disappointed. A book that confined itself to only those assessment and treatment techniques that were criterion-validated would be about three pages long. The material presented here does contain validity, but it is mostly constructive validity. The differential diagnostic assessment techniques have been field-tested by thousands of physical therapists around the world, who seem to find them useful in that they continue to use them. This may not be a terribly scientific perspective, but it is still better than the supporting evidence for their invalidity. What the reader will get from this book is the accumulated experience of the author, his colleagues and his teachers that has been 25 years in the brewing. Take it for what it is, the accumulated clinical impressions of numerous orthopedic physical therapists.

Introduction

The Orthopedic Physical Therapist's Differential Diagnosis Examination

Increasingly, physical therapists are being called upon to act as screening professionals for orthopedic patients. More and more therapists are legally entitled to provide primary care when the apparent safety net of the physician referral is absent. As commonly as, or perhaps more commonly than primary contact, the family physician is relying on the therapist to "assess and treat" rather than follow a predetermined diagnosis and a set formula of therapy.

The subject of physical therapists making differential diagnoses is controversial. There is some genuine concern for the patient here, but there is also considerable turf protecting going on. From a patient concern perspective there is little to take issue with when the therapist makes the differential diagnoses. If the physician makes a referral and the therapist disagrees with the proffered diagnosis and sends the patient back, what harm has been done? Is the therapist capable of making a differential diagnosis, or at least recognizing red flags and sending them to the physician? In Britain a study was undertaken comparing outcomes and patient satisfaction between orthopedic physical therapists licensed to give steroid injections and orthopedic surgeons in a hospital outpatient department. The abstract gave the result as this: "An appropriately trained physiotherapist is as effective as staff grade surgeons in managing orthopedic out-patients unlikely to benefit from surgical intervention."*

There is no doubt that it is the physician's responsibility to provide as precise a medical diagnosis as possible and to communicate that diagnosis to the patient and the therapist. However, the physician's responsibility to make the diagnosis does not abrogate the therapist's responsibility to ensure that that diagnosis is correct and that the referral is appropriate. With the possible exception of postsurgical referrals from neuro- and orthopedic surgeons, it is unusual to receive a precise and accurate diagnosis from a referring physician. More commonly, the

---

*Weale AE, Bannister GC: Who should see orthopedic outpatients—physiotherapists or surgeons? Ann R Coll Surg Engl 72(Suppl 2):71, 1995.

prescription simply states "assess and treat." When a nonsurgical diagnosis is afforded, it is often of little value to the therapist as far as the determination of a treatment regimen is concerned. Such clinically valueless diagnoses include *low back pain*, *acute low back pain*, *shoulder impingement syndrome*, *rotator cuff syndrome*, *deranged knee*, *torticollis*, *back strain*, *chest wall pain*, *ankle sprain*, and so forth. These types of "diagnoses" do nothing more than regurgitate the patient's symptoms or the mechanism of injury or the area of pain. Even apparently precise diagnoses such as *tennis elbow* or the more technical *lateral epicondylitis* often do not help in determining treatment, as they are not precise enough. Take for an example *lateral epicondylitis*. Unless the exact location is known, effective treatment cannot be carried out. Is it supracondylar, epicondylar, in the tendon body, or at the myotendonous junction? Is it primary or secondary? If it is secondary, does the neck need treatment or is there a biomechanical problem at the elbow causing or contributing to the symptomatic lesion? Only a detailed examination of the patient, an in-depth analysis of the information generated from the examination, and the subsequent generation of a differential diagnosis will provide this information, which is so vital to efficient and effective treatment.

The problem is compounded by direct access. In some countries, notably Australia and the United Kingdom, and in some states and provinces in the United States and Canada, the therapist has the right of direct access to the patient without referral from the physician. In one or two of these jurisdictions in the United States, this same therapist who can see the patient without referral does not have the right to make a differential diagnosis. This is obviously a silly state of affairs. How can anybody of any discipline see patients as a primary care practitioner without making a diagnosis? To get around this stupidity, the therapists use the terms *physical therapy diagnosis* or *functional diagnosis*. So somehow, a disk prolapse ceases to exist when it is examined by a therapist but is present when assessed by a physician. It is of course impossible for the orthopedic therapist to treat any patient effectively, efficiently, or even ethically without previously examining the patient and coming to some conclusion concerning the patient's condition. It is time to realize that making a diagnosis is common to all health care professionals involved in the treatment of patients, not just physicians, and is not in and of itself practicing medicine. Regardless of what euphemisms are currently being employed to conform with state, provincial, or even national regulations regarding the right and ability of the physical therapist to make a differential diagnosis, that is exactly what we have to do in order to treat the patient appropriately.

To do this, the therapist must be able to sort through the masses of data generated during both the objective and subjective examinations to reach a provisional working diagnosis that will facilitate the formation of a rational management plan. This plan should be based on the clinical presentation of the patient and the state of the art information about the function of the body, the pathological processes that the patient is undergoing, and the therapist's experience and skill level.

The following is the abstract of an article by Weinstein* and is entirely appropriate for physical therapists in any field, but especially in orthopedic therapy.

> Clinicians must not simply decide that a patient with symptoms and a positive diagnostic test has a reason for a specific treatment, and likewise clinicians must not decide that a patient with symptoms and a negative test does not have a clinically important problem. We must also consider the sensitivity, specificity and predictive value of the diagnostic test and the individual characteristics of the patient. Treatment outcome depends on many factors. Point of service decisions vs. population based decisions are obviously different. Each patient presents to the treating practitioner on a given day, at a given time, and it is this picture upon which a plan of care is formulated.

In conclusion, the main reasons for the orthopedic physical therapist to generate a differential diagnosis are

1. To identify inappropriate referrals.
2. To identify concurrent inappropriate conditions accompanying an otherwise appropriate referral.
3. To generate a working diagnosis.
4. As a consultation measure when requested from another physical therapist from a physician and where permitted by statute from a lawyer, insurance company, or some other third party.

---

*Weinstein JN: Consensus summary of the diagnosis and treatment of lumbar disc herniation. Spine 21(Suppl 24):S75, 1996.

Acknowledgments

You do not very often get the opportunity to publicly thank those people to whom you owe a life debt. Of course, acknowledgments are not for the general readership, but for the people being thanked and for the author. Also by naming specific people, you do at least have the chance of their buying the book even if nobody else does. My apologies in advance to the readers if this list appears overly long, but I intend to take advantage of this opportunity to thank these people. Of course, you can always turn the page.

I would like to thank all of the people who have over the years helped form this version of Jim Meadows and to remind them that there is probably more blame than credit in the achievement. Having been involved in physiotherapy (or physical therapy, for my American cousins) for nearly thirty years, I have met a great number of people, mostly to advantage, who have had an impact on my professional development. Many of these people I am proud to know and number among my closest friends. There are also many people that I have never met in person but whose writings have shaped the way I think and act. Unfortunately, the sheer number of people involved prohibits my naming them all, so I hope those whom I do not include will forgive the lack of space and believe that it is not that they are not important to me. However, to those whom I have not named, and you know who you are, be assured that I do thank you.

First, James Cyriax who started my thinking about what I was actually doing. The late David Lamb who was as complete a physiotherapist as you could ever meet. Rolf Lauvik who first really showed me how effective manual therapy could be. Mike White who talked me into taking the Canadian manual therapy exams and then worked hard to make sure that I passed them. Lani Alington who continually nags and tries to improve me, usually beyond the limits of her frustration. Cliff Fowler who has a pair of the best hands in the business and who is not reluctant to call me an idiot when he feels it necessary. Erl Pettman who taught me how to teach. Diane Lee who is one of the most productive people I know and who has managed to balance a busy personal life with a rich understanding of her profession. Bob Sydenham who is clinically and politically one of the most astute physiotherapists that I have met and Gaye Sydenham who has to put up with him; I often wonder who keeps winding her spring. They have both made me more of a political animal than I ever wanted to be. David Magee who, to me, is the model that most academics should try to emulate in that he strives constantly for clinical relevance. Sharon Warren who showed me that it is possible to be a researcher and retain huge amounts of common sense. Rick Adams who, when it comes to work and our profesison, has no sense of moderation. Barrett Dorko and John Medeiros both of whom I brush up against periodically at all too-long intervals but who manage in a few hours to get me up and running again. Patty Mayer, Sue Saretski, and Gerry Bellows who keep me working and in touch with patients when I am in Calgary. Stanley Paris to whom the manual therapists in the United States owe a massive debt of gratitude and who is, for me, the epitome of effectiveness. Gail Molloy who is one of the hardest working of my colleagues and who, by unconsciously putting me to shame, can get me to do things that I do not have time for. Lance Twomey who shares the same distinction that David Magee possesses and is in every sense a gentleman and the one person I would like to be more like. Mike Rogers who has a remarkable work ethic and a very strongly developed sense of right and wrong. Richard Bourassa who has assited me on many courses and who has tolerated, to an amazing degree, my jokes at his expense. He has demonstrated to me what an ethical therapist truly is. Jim Doree who designed and runs my website, and apparently doesn't know that there is only room for physiotherapy in our lives. Mike Sutton who has the greatest natural enthusiasm and exuberance that I have ever come across and who showed me not to be concerned with what others thought, providing you believe that you are doing the right thing. Gwen Parrott who has absolutely no problem disagreeing with me and letting me know it in no uncertain terms and who constantly challenges me for the facts; and to her husband Jaime who contributes to my income via the occasional poker game in Louisville. My colleagues at the North American Institute of Orthopedic Manual Therapy including Bill Temes, Ann Porter-Hoke, Kathy Stupanski, Bill O'Grady, David Deppler, Steve Allen, Kent and Shari Kyser, Alexa Dobbs and the rest of the gang.

There are many memorably past and current students who have kept and still do keep me on my toes. In no particular order these include Rebecca Lowe, Pat Chapman, Dana Vansant, Mark Dutton, Amy Brooks, Jeff Brosseau, Chuck Hazel, Julie Gallagher, Brian Macks, Gray Cook, Shannon Doig, Mary Galatas, Randy Harms, Blaine McKie, Dawn McConkey, Colleen McDonald, Judy Black, Lorrie Maffy-Ward, Maureen Mooney, Roberto Pelosi, Myron Sorestad, Christine Wolcott, Suzanne Yakabowitch, Paul Jozefczyk, Fred Smit, Marcel Giguere, Tara Conner, Chris Soper, Audrey Bjornstad, Terry Brown, Anne Clouthier, Nathelie Savard, Heather Bryant, Jan Hodge, Joe Kelly, Gisele Le Blanc, Ralph Simpson, Korryn Wiese and many more whose faces I remember but whose names sadly are gone from my ever increasingly evasive memory.

Steve Zollo, McGraw-Hill's medical acquisitions editor who convinced me that this would an easy undertaking. Right! Anne Seitz of York Graphics whose editing ensured that the book was at least legible to the English reading person. I would also like to thank the two reviewers of an early draft of the book, Elizabeth R. Ikeda, MS, PT Assistant Professor Physical Therapy Department, University of Montana and Robert Johnson, MS, PT Loop Spine & Sports Therapy and clinical faculty at the Department of Physical Therapy, Northwestern University, whose ideas I took to heart and, for the most part, incorporated into the book assuring a better product than it would have been without their recommendations.

Finally and most importantly to my family—Sue, my wife, and Andrew and Matthew, my children. It was Sue who motivated me to write this book by saying that I could buy a new computer if I did so. Thank you all for putting up with me at any time but especially during the period I was writing this book.

PART 1

General Principles of Differential Diagnosis

CHAPTER 1

Differential Diagnosis: General Principles

The clinical differential diagnosis is always provisional and subject to change as further information from more objective studies such as blood tests and imaging becomes available or as the results of the selected treatments are noted. Spinal conditions that do not have overt neural or dural signs or symptoms are difficult to diagnose except on the provisional basis that the selected treatment has its predicted outcome. For example, back pain with somatic pain radiating into the buttock that is not accompanied by neural or dural signs or symptoms could be caused by a number of pathologies. These include a contained disk lesion, a zygapophyseal joint dysfunction or inflammation, ligamentous or muscle tearing, injury to the outer anulus fibrosis, compression or other fracture, bacterial infection, or neoplasm. Some of these pathologies are much more common than others, and by the law of probabilities alone you would probably be right more often than wrong if you generated two or three diagnoses based on frequency of incidence. Even taking into account the clinical findings, including other aspects of the history and other objective cues, the diagnosis cannot be considered as having 100% validity. The best you can do is generate a differential diagnosis in which you have the best confidence. Even imaging studies help only to confirm a clinical diagnosis, given the rate of false positives and negatives of MRIs and x-rays.

The orthopedic manual therapy examination consists of two parts, a differential diagnostic examination and a biochemical examination. Of the two, the differential diagnostic examination is the more important because it confirms that the patient is appropriate for physical therapy. The biomechanical examination is vital if specific manual therapy or specific exercise is to be administered. For the most part, the differential diagnosis is provisional, depending on further, more objective testing or, in retrospect, on the patient recovering with specific treatment. Many therapists look only for red flags on the differential diagnosis examination rather than a specific diagnosis, and although this approach is quite good for precluding inappropriate patients from treatment, it is of little value in the generation of a specific treatment plan.

An overview of the examinations would look like this:

Differential Diagnostic (Scan) Examination

- ❏ History
- ❏ Observation (inspection)
- ❏ Routine selective tissue tension tests
- ❏ Special tests
- ❏ Peripheral differential screening examination

Biomechanical Examination

- ❏ Biomechanical screening tests
- ❏ Passive physiological movements
- ❏ Passive accessory movements
- ❏ Nonligamentous articular or segmental stability tests

This book will focus on the differential diagnosis; biomechanical evaluation is too comprehensive a subject to include here, so only the principles will be covered.

The differential diagnostic examination can be divided up as follows:

- ❏ Subjective
- ❏ Observation
- ❏ Active movements
- ❏ Passive movements
- ❏ Resisted movements
- ❏ Stress
- ❏ Dural
- ❏ Dermatome
- ❏ Myotome
- ❏ Reflexes
- ❏ Special tests
  - a. Vertebral artery

            b. Upper limb tension
            c. Quadrant
            d. Phalan's
            e. Tinnel's
            f. Others

CHAPTER 2

The Subjective Examination

The history is perhaps the most important part of the clinical examination of the patient. A careful subjective examination is the tool most likely to uncover red and yellow flags. It will provide the examiner with important information regarding the patient's problem. Disabilities, symptoms, symptom behavior, irritability, and exacerbating, provoking, and relieving factors can only be ascertained from the subjective examination. A past history of similar symptoms or nonmusculoskeletal conditions can be important in arousing the examiner's suspicions that the patient's problem may not be benign in nature or musculoskeletal in origin. Past treatments and the results of these treatments may indicate the best route to follow for management and what treatments to avoid. The history will afford information regarding the patient's personality, attitude toward his or her problem, and likelihood of compliance with the therapist's instructions regarding exercises, rest, activities, and so forth.

The following section of this chapter will look at information generated from the subjective examination of the patient and possible interpretations that can be put upon it especially when combined with information garnered from the objective examinations. We will look first at questions that pertain to all regions, spinal and peripheral, and then we will discuss region-specific history taking.

The purpose of taking a history is to determine

1. Patient Profile
   ❑ Age
   ❑ Gender
   ❑ Occupation
   ❑ Leisure activities

❏ Family status
❏ Past medical history
❏ Current and past medications

2. The patient's symptomatology, including
   ❏ Onset
   ❏ Nature of symptoms
   ❏ Severity of symptoms
   ❏ Level of irritability
   ❏ Exacerbating and relieving factors
   ❏ Associated factors (diet, posture, activity, etc.)
3. The patient's level of disability
4. The stresses the patient must be able to tolerate in daily activities
5. Any other previous or current medical conditions that will impact on the assessment or treatment
6. Any current medications that might impact on the assessment or treatment
7. Any other past history of a similar type
8. Any other physical treatments for this or other similar conditions and the results of these treatments
9. Opening communication channels with the patient
10. Establishing a working relationship with the patient
11. Gaining an appreciation of the patient's likely compliance with programs
12. Gaining an appreciation of the patient's attitude toward his or her problem

The following lists the main questions that need to be asked most patients. Some are region specific. For example there is little point in asking about dizziness when the patient is attending for low back pain. The questions on the list will be discussed in detail, either in the general principles section of history taking or in the region-specific examination section of this chapter.

1. Patient Profile
❏ Age (old/young)
❏ Gender
❏ Occupation and description of duties
❏ Leisure activities and their frequency and intensity
❏ Family status
❏ Past medical history (cancer, diabetes, systemic arthritis, congenital collagen disorder)
❏ Current and past medications (steroids, NSAIDs, insulin, dizziness, provoking)
❏ Past surgeries (cancer, spinal, neurological)

2. Pain and Paresthesia

- ❏ Onset (traumatic/nontraumatic, immediate/delayed, insidious/sudden, cause/no cause)
- ❏ Location (steady/changing, local/extensive, segmental/nonsegmental, continuous/dissociated, shifting/expanding)
- ❏ Type (somatic, neurological)
- ❏ Severity (scale of 10)
- ❏ Irritability (how much stress to irritate and how much time for relief)
- ❏ Aggravating/abating factors (activities/postures, eating/diet, general/emotional stress)
- ❏ Nocturnal (aching or sudden sharp pain)
- ❏ Work related or not
- ❏ Constant, continuous, intermittent
- ❏ Episodic/nonepisodic

3. Other Symptoms and What Provokes Them

- ❏ Dizziness (type 1, 2, or 3)
- ❏ Visual disturbances (scotoma, hemi-/quadranopia, floaters, scintillations, blurring, tunnel vision)
- ❏ Taste or smell disturbances
- ❏ Dysphagia (painful/painless)
- ❏ Amnesia (traumatic/nontraumatic)
- ❏ Vomiting
- ❏ Cough changes (nonproductive to productive)
- ❏ Sputum changes (clear to yellow or green, fresh or old blood)
- ❏ Weakness
- ❏ Clumsiness
- ❏ Gait disturbances (ataxia, staggering, tripping)
- ❏ Drop attacks
- ❏ Syncope (frequency)
- ❏ Photophobia
- ❏ Phonophobia
- ❏ Hypoacusia
- ❏ Hyperacusia
- ❏ Tinnitus (high/low frequency, unilateral/bilateral, pulsatile/nonpulsatile)
- ❏ Intellectual impairment (drowsiness, concentration difficulties)
- ❏ Bladder changes (retention/incontinence, color changes, odor changes)
- ❏ Bowel changes (unable to expel, diarrhea, constipation, blood)
- ❏ Increased sweating
- ❏ Distal color changes (reddening, bluing, whitening)

❏ Changes in facial appearance (drooping, ptosis, reddening, enophthalmos, exophthalmos)
❏ Dysarthria (slurring)
❏ Dysphonia
❏ Hypoesthesia or anesthesia (unusual in the history)
❏ Hyperesthesia
❏ Indigestion
❏ Recent fever

4. Mandatory Questions
❏ Dizziness
❏ Cranial nerve symptoms
❏ Long tract symptoms
❏ Bladder, bowel, or genital dysfunction
❏ Osteoporosis
❏ Vertebral artery symptoms

5. Past Episodes and Treatments
❏ Frequency (increasing, steady, or decreasing)
❏ Symptom intensity (increasing, steady, or decreasing)
❏ Symptom location (steady or changing [spreading, shifting, or expanding])
❏ Severity (increasing, steady, or decreasing)
❏ Irritability (increasing, steady, or decreasing)
❏ Past treatment (type, helped/worsened/unchanged)

6. Other Investigations and Results
❏ X-rays
❏ MRI
❏ MRA
❏ CT scans
❏ Bone scans
❏ Scintillographs
❏ PET scans
❏ ENG
❏ EEG
❏ EKG
❏ EMG
❏ Nerve conduction studies

Patient Profile

The patient profile includes gender, age, occupation, family status, leisure activities, and past and present medical conditions and current medications.

Age

Children who are in enough pain to warrant physical therapy should always be viewed with suspicion. For the most part, children recover quickly from minor injuries. They tend not to have the chronic problems that adults suffer from, because they have not yet had the opportunity for cumulative stress or degeneration to take their toll, nor do they normally have the psychological or financial baggage that goes with adults and is capable of complicating an otherwise uncomplicated injury, so a child complaining of ongoing pain may have a more severe injury than the trauma would suggest or be suffering from a serious disease. However, now that children are being pushed harder and harder into various forms of competitive sports, we see more adult types of dysfunction in children than previously. Consequently, a detailed history must be taken not only of the immediate precursor but also of how involved the child is in sports, what if any previous injuries have occurred, and how they progressed with treatment.

The older patient is, of course, more disposed to degenerative conditions, not only of the musculoskeletal system but also of other systems. Cancer and coronary, cerebral, and brainstem infarcts may all be factors in the assessment and treatment of the older patient. The age of the patient will also give an idea of what the range of motion should be when the results of movement tests are considered. The older patient can be expected to be a little stiffer than the younger, because degeneration increasingly becomes a factor. A young person who is stiff everywhere has either very high muscle tone or possibly a systemic joint condition. A middle-aged to elderly woman is more likely to have breast cancer than a young one or a man (the median age at diagnosis is 57 years and is less than 1 per 100,000 before 25 years of age as compared to 397 per 100,000 at age 80).[1]

Gender

This will give some indication as to predisposition. Osteoporosis and gynecologic conditions are either more prevalent in or exclusive to the female; prostatitis, testicular cancer, and so forth are exclusive to the male. Lung cancer is about two and a half times more common among men than among women and has a higher incidence in those with previous pulmonary pathologies such as scleroderma and chronic obstructive pulmonary disease.[2] Breast cancer is about 146 times more common in women than men.[3]

A combination of gender and age will often sensitize the therapist more than either alone. A 30-year-old man with low back pain is less likely to have prostate cancer than is a 60-year-old. A middle-aged or elderly female is more likely to have osteoporosis because of the hormonal deficiencies of menopause.

Occupational and Leisure Activities

Although the information may give some clues about the underlying cause of the patient's problems, the need to know exactly what the patient does for a living is more important in prognostication and postrehabilitation training. When can the patient go back to work and for how long (full- or part-time)? Will modifications have to be made in the patient's job description or in the work environment? Will retraining be necessary, and if so when can it begin safely? To answer these questions, in many cases at least, a simple "What do you do for a living?" will not suffice, especially in jobs that are a little more unusual than are those normally encountered by the therapist.

Similarly, leisure activities require a detailed description as to type and intensity. Is this activity likely to have an adverse effect on the patient's progress, or could it be used as a rehabilitation tool? If the patient insists on continuing with the activity even though the therapist believes it will likely cause problems, then an accommodation must be reached. Delaying the resumption of the activity may help, especially when there is any degree of inflammation present. Reduction in its intensity may also be useful. For example, a golfer with thoracic or low back pain can be asked to not drive the ball but to play the shorter shots. This may not be what the patient wants to hear, but it at least allows him or her to pursue the activity even if in a severely modified fashion.

Family Status

Does the patient have support at home, allowing the necessary rest or time to exercise at home? Can the patient avoid adverse activities at home by having somebody else do them? Is this a period of stress at home, when little if any cooperation is to be found? Can the patient get somebody to help with the exercises if this is necessary, or will you have to modify them? What are the ages of the children, and how much care must the patient give to them? If it is necessary, the therapist must teach the patient how to modify positions for nursing or changing infants and dressing smaller children and to recruit older children to take over some of the chores.

Past and Present Medical Conditions

Most of the patient's medical history will be of no relevance to us, and when this is recognized, questioning should be discontinued on that subject, because it becomes an invasion of the patient's privacy without any clinical necessity. However, we should listen for a history of systemic arthritis, skin rashes, cancer, diabetes, coronary conditions, or cerebral strokes. Asking about cancer can be a problem. Any mention of the disease to some people generates panic, with the patients believing that you are asking because you think they have it. To avoid this, the question can be put on a questionnaire that the patient fills out before seeing the therapist. A past history of cancer should always tell the therapist to ask questions about previous screening for metastases (preferably of the physician rather than the patient unless the patient volunteers the information). There is no point in worrying the patient about something that may not be an issue, but if screenings have not been done in at least the previous 6 months, the therapist should be concerned and more than a little critical of the results of the objective examination. If cancer is a factor, ask the patient if he or she is receiving radiation therapy or has received it recently. Radiation therapy patients are often put onto systemic steroids for the duration of the therapy, and of course this will alter collagen strength.

Diabetes may cause arthropathies[3] and neuropathies[4] as well as delaying recovery. Coronary or cerebral vascular conditions should lead the therapist to be especially careful when treating cervical patients because these conditions are evidence of systemic atherosclerosis and the vertebral artery may be similarly affected. In addition, any exercise program needs to be planned with the condition in mind. Systemic arthritis, particularly rheumatoid arthritis or ankylosing spondylitis, should make the therapist cautious, especially when treating the neck. Both of these conditions are intimately linked with atlantoaxial instability and subluxation.[5-7] If a child's neck is to be treated, ask about any history of recurrent chest infections, because this can lead to Grisel's[8] syndrome with its accompanying transverse ligament laxity.

It is possible that a heart condition is producing the patient's symptoms. Heart pathology will often make itself felt through an ache down the deltoid and lateral border of the upper arm, mimicking shoulder joint pain. It is of course vital that provoking or exacerbating activities be discussed in detail.

It is also worth noting what, if anything, the patient has to say about congenital anomalies. Because almost all congenital anomalies are associated with others derived from the same affected embryological block,[9] the presence of an anomaly should be pursued. Again, this is of particular importance in the cervical region, where a cervical rib or Sprengle's deformity or polydactyly, for example, could also indicate an anomaly or anomalies of the vertebral artery.

Current Medications

Often patients forget to mention medical conditions but will tell you that they are taking a particular drug. This should lead you back to the reason for taking the medication. In addition, certain medications will affect your treatment choices. For example, it is not recommended to apply deep frictions to or give strong exercises for a tendon or ligament that has recently (say the last 3 weeks) been injected with steroid. Cortisone injections into the tissue will weaken the collagen injected and may result in rupture.[10-12] Systemic steroids will cause generalized collagen weakness, water retention, and generalized weakness and tenderness, all of which can affect the results of the examination and the outcome of the treatment. Anticoagulants are a contraindication to manipulation and deep transverse frictions. About four hundred medications are known to cause dizziness as an adverse effect. These include aspirin and other NSAIDs, systemic steroids, amminoglycosidic antibiotics, diuretics, and antianginals.[13,14] Obviously, these must be considered when assessing a patient's dizziness.

Pain and Paresthesia

Pain is the most common complaint bringing a patient into the generalist orthopedic therapist. Pain is a subjective symptom and varies not only from patient to patient for the same stimulus but from hour to hour and from context to context. A trauma that will disable one person will leave another indifferent. As a consequence, pain is not subject to objective evaluation, and the patient's description is the only source of information that the therapist has when determining its qualities. Therefore, descriptions of its type, location, behavior, intensity, and so on are extremely important in making a differential diagnosis.

Onset

Is the pain related to trauma? If so, was it immediate or delayed? An immediate onset of severe pain often indicates profound tissue damage such as ligamentous or muscular tearing or fracture. For example, the immediate onset of cervical pain following motor vehicle accidents is recognized from a number of retrospective and prospective studies to indicate a poor prognosis.[15] A delayed onset is more commonly encountered and is often caused by the inflammatory process, which takes time to make itself felt. In addition to pain, did the patient hear any noises at the time of the injury? Cracking, tearing, or popping noises could indicate sudden damage. Was there swelling, and when did it occur? Immediate, severe swelling is strongly suggestive of hemarthrosis. Significant articular trauma causing pain but no swelling could mean that there is a rent in the capsule, through which the inflammatory exudate or blood is leaking.

If the pain is not related to overt trauma, was there a particular activity that caused it? Occasionally, the patient will relate that the pain was traumatic in origin, but further questioning reveals that the trauma was very minor compared with the degree of pain and disability that the patient is experiencing. In this case, the trauma may simply be the final straw on the camel's back. You may need to search for the factors that stressed the failed area so much that a minor stress finished it off. The category into which most patients fall in general orthopedic practice is nontraumatic. The patient can relate no overstressful activity or posture that either started or provoked the problem. The cause may have been lifting a moderate load, suddenly turning the head, waking up with a "crick" in the neck, or something equally innocuous. There are more incidents of low back injury from lifting objects out of the back of the car than putting them in. Why? Probably because the lifter has driven somewhere and so predisposed the spine to injury. Life is like that: We spend our youth and young adulthood predisposing our bodies to failure from injuries that on less abused musculoskeletal systems would be insignificant. When we are a few years older, disaster strikes.

The overused term *overuse syndrome* is an example of nontraumatic pain. It suggests that simple overuse was the cause of the patient's symptoms and disabilities. In some cases, this is accurate and the term is being used as it should be, but in a substantial number of instances (I would suggest the majority), it is not an accurate descriptor. Tennis elbow is an excellent example of this. A patient attends with an epicondylar (or any other type) tennis elbow that is confirmed on clinical examination. The patient is then asked about his job. On being told that he is a carpenter and spends a large part of his day hammering nails into boards, the therapist is happy to lay the blame here and treat it as a primary tennis elbow. The fact that the patient had been doing the same job in the same way for 15 years does not enter into the equation. If *you* hammer all day, that is overuse. It is not overuse for an experienced carpenter. Perhaps if the patient had only been doing the job for 6 months, if he had just come back from a month on vacation, or if he had changed his hammer or the position he was hammering in, primary tennis elbow might have been a reasonable deduction. However, it is not a good idea to assume that the most obvious answer is the correct one. Almost certainly something had changed, if not the job then something else. Some of the factors mentioned here may obtain, or perhaps the patient's neck was dysfunctional. In the absence of a clear-cut case of *unfamiliar* overuse, the therapist needs to look for other reasons. A patient complaining of posterior thigh pain attended an orthopedic surgeon, who told her that she suffered from a torn hamstring. She said yes, she knew that, but why did it tear? He said it was because she was a runner, to which she replied, "But I run on both legs." Simplistic explanations like that offered to this young lady are the root cause of failure to improve or failure to maintain improvement. In addition, be careful of cases in which there is no apparent cause. The vast majority of these patients will be straightforward musculoskeletal problems, but it is from this group that the systemic arthritic and cancer patients will be drawn.

Pain Quality

The nature or type of pain the patient is experiencing is vital in assessing the condition. There are a number of different classifications for pain, but for the purposes of differential diagnosis the following is as good as any and better than most. Pain can be classified as neuropathic (neurological) or somatic (nonneurological). Experiments have demonstrated that simple compression of an uninjured spinal nerve or spinal nerve root (with the exception of the dorsal root ganglion) does not result in pain. The result of simple compression experimentally is paresthesia, numbness, neurological deficit, or all three, but not pain.[16,17] However, it has been demonstrated that compression or other forms of irritation of previously injured spinal nerves or nerve roots can cause pain of a very particular type. In addition, it has been postulated that intraneural or perineural edema may produce nerve root ischemia, which in turn may cause radicular symptoms.[18] This radicular pain is lancinating or shooting and less than one and a half inches in width, running down the limb or around the trunk.[19,20] As a consequence, the recognition of radicular symptoms is very easy. It is lancinating pain, paresthetic, causalgic, or numb. Any symptoms other than these cannot be ascribed to spinal nerve or root compression or inflammation. For an excellent short discourse on this subject read Bogduk and Twomey.[18]

Nonneuropathic or somatic pain is generally described as aching. It can be very severe or very mild, but it is not shooting in quality. Unfortunately this type of pain, when felt in the leg or arm, is inaccurately described as *root pain*. Based on experimental data, it is not. The nonneurological structures—the dura, the external aspect of the disk, the ligaments, periosteum, bone, and so on—are nociceptive and can generate this pain.[18,21] It does not have the electric quality commonly described when true radicular pain is experienced. The argument has been made that root pain may not be as described here and points to diabetic neuropathy and chronic root pain, as when a patient has EMG or clinical evidence that there was a neuropathy present but experiences "nonneurological" pain. However, no evidence has been presented that the pain was in fact coming from the root; it may have arisen from some other compromised somatic structure.

Typically, if the orthopedic patient is experiencing lancinating root pain, somatic pain is also present, because the compressing tissue, usually the disk, is also compressing the dural sleeve of the nerve root.[18] Somatic "sciatica" is felt either continuously or with postures such as sitting, whereas the zinging pain is very intermittent (coming on suddenly during trunk flexion, for example). At other times, the lancinating pain is typically absent. Clinically, it seems that it would be prudent to accept current experimental data and reserve the term *root pain* for those patients presenting with lancinating pain or causalgia, as this will reduce the overfrequency diagnosis of root compression and the administration of inappropriate treatments. On the other hand, it is not beneficial to the patient to misdiagnose a disk lesion that might only be compressing the dural sheath of the root or spinal nerve, or applying pressure to the undamaged nerve tissue without causing inflammation. The risk is that inappropriate treatment may damage the disk further, causing frank compression with neurological deficit. The absence of lancinating pain or other neurological symptoms does not preclude a disk herniation as the cause of the patient's disability. As always, the answer to the quandary lies with the rest of the examination. A diagnosis is not based solely on the history but on analysis of all the examination data.

Other neurological conditions causing pain have to be considered when taking a history. Thalamic pain syndromes, herpes zoster (shingles), diabetic and other neuropathies, polyneuropathies, and arachnoiditis may all be erroneously referred to the physical therapist in their early stages. The description of pain from neurological sources such as these tends to be more vivid than that of pain from orthopedic sources, even those causing spinal nerve or root compression. Descriptors include *stabbing, knifelike, a storm or shock, burning, bandlike, flesh tearing,* and *indescribable.* It is believed that the reason for this difference in descriptors between neurological and somatic causes may be that dysesthesia confuses the patient, who does not know how to describe this totally unfamiliar sensation.[22]

Visceral referral of pain to the skin is believed to occur as a result of the synapsing of primary somatic sensory neurons and visceral sensory neurons onto common secondary neurons of the dorsal horn of the spinal cord.[23] Because of the distribution of nociceptors and pain fibers, visceral pain is generally felt to be different from musculoskeletal pain. With the exception of the parietal linings of the cavities (pleural, peritoneal, and pericardial), nociceptors are sparingly distributed in the viscera and fast pain fibers are for all intents and purposes absent.[24] As a consequence, the fast pain associated with the musculoskeletal system is not common in visceral disorders unless the cavity linings are involved, as they may be with advanced disease. Visceral noncavity pain is frequently described as *deep, diffuse,* and *wavelike*[25] but also often in the same way as musculoskeletal pain. Consequently, it becomes difficult to rely on the quality of pain to discriminate between pain arising from the viscera and that coming from a musculoskeletal problem. It is therefore very important that no definite conclusion be reached one way or the other until further information is obtained. This information may well be forthcoming as the history progresses. The patient who relates that the pain is associated with diet, eating, or the position assumed while eating is probably telling you that a gastric disorder exists. Cholycystitis or gastric or duodenal ulcers may all present in this manner. However, remember that the patient is sitting when eating, so make sure that you ask about the chair and whether sitting in this chair or one like it when not eating causes the same problem.

Chest or shoulder pain on generalized exertion such as running for a bus or walking upstairs or nonphysical stress may likely be caused by cardiac problems. On the other hand, pleural pain from adhesions or pleuritis can be extremely difficult to differentiate from a thoracic spine or rib dysfunction, because the structure is innervated by fast pain fibers and so can produce a musculoskeletal type of pain. The pleura is also attached to the ribs, which complicates the objective examination picture, as trunk motion will probably reproduce the patient's pain.

Location

Because of the multiplicity of the levels innervating most tissues and the number of tissues that might be the source, the location of pain is usually of little value in the exact localization of the source of the pain. However, the site of the pain may be useful in obtaining an idea of the embryological levels from which the affected tissue is derived. Neither radicular nor somatic pains are consistent in their areas of spread. The referred areas of both neurological and somatic sources of pain vary between individuals as well as within the same individual, and the latter seemingly is a function of the intensity of the stimulus. However, neurological symptom sites are a better indication of source than are somatic pain sites.

The degree of radiation is directly related to three factors:

❏ Stimulus intensity (the higher the intensity the more referral)
❏ Stimulus centrality (the more central the more radiation)
❏ Stimulus superficiality (the more superficial the less radiation)

Consequently, the greater the degree of radiation the more likely is the chance that the problem is acute and/or proximal, but, even with the diagnostic limitations placed on us by the vagaries of pain, useful information can often be gained from the location of pain. Very local pain is very likely to be from a structure under the pain area, and referred pain that is not diffuse may indicate the spinal segment from which it is derived. It is the therapist's job to judge how reliable the pain site is likely to be in a particular case and to integrate that information with other data generated from the history and objective examinations to produce a working hypothesis about the pain's source.

Grieve[26] made the following conclusions on pain quality:

1. All root pain is referred pain, but not all referred pain is root pain.
2. Severe referred pain is not necessarily caused by root compromise from inflammation or other forms of irritation.

3. Referred pain caused by root involvement is not necessarily severe.

4. Simple root compression does not cause pain and may not cause neurological deficit.

5. The imprecise terminology concerning referred pain at present reflects traditional assumptions (often unproven) about its cause rather than its true nature.

6. The topography and nature of referred pain in any one patient is inadequate as a single factor in differential diagnosis of both the tissue involved and the segmental level.

I would add one more to the list. Lancinating (radicular) pain is caused by nerve root or dorsal ganglion involvement and is produced by more than simple compression.

Be careful of dissociated pains. Upper lumbar pain associated with shoulder pain is very difficult to reconcile with a single musculoskeletal disorder but easy to associate with a visceral disease irritating the diaphragm. Gall bladder, liver, basal lung, spleen, esophageal, and stomach conditions can all cause shoulder pain. In general, abdominal visceral disease tends to cause low back and/or pelvic pain, and intrathoracic problems tend to cause shoulder pain.

Isolated anterior thoracic and abdominal pain may be caused by musculoskeletal problems, but there is a very real possibility that the pain may be visceral in source. Spinal conditions will usually cause local pain in addition to any referred pain; therefore, any isolated anterior pain is an oddity and should be treated with suspicion. On the other hand, visceral referral can easily be posterior, mimicking spinal musculoskeletal disorders. Perhaps the most urgent condition that causes trunk pain that may be inappropriately referred is a dissecting aortic aneurysm. The pain is often felt only in the lumbar and groin regions, sometimes referring pain into the testicle just before the artery ruptures.

Goodman and Snyder's *Differential Diagnosis in Physical Therapy*[24] gives excellent diagrams of which organ refers to where. However, the role of the therapist in the identification of visceral problems lays not in identifying which organ is causing the pain but in determining that the pain is not musculoskeletal in origin. However, the following are the main viscera, their segmental innervation level[27] and most likely cutaneous referral area.[24,28,29]

The pharynx is innervated by the maxillary branch of the trigeminal, the glossopharyngeal, and the vagus nerves and the superior cervical ganglion, giving its most common pain areas as the throat and ear, which are not usually mistaken for symptoms of a musculoskeletal problem.

The sensory supply of the esophagus comes from the vagus nerve and the upper five sympathetic ganglia. This gives the pattern of referral as the anterior neck if the superior part of the esophagus is involved, substernal if the lesion affects the middle levels, and from the xiphoid around the chest to the lower posterior midthoracic region.

Tracheobronchial lesions are felt in the throat and anterior upper chest near the suprasternal notch. The vagal nerve and medial branches of the sympathetic nerves from the upper five thoracic ganglia supply the trachea and bronchi.

The vagus nerve and the 2-5 thoracic sympathetic ganglia together with the cervical sympathetic trunk supply the lung, but this tissue is essentially painless unless the parietal pleura is affected. The mediastinal and central diaphragmatic parietal pleura are innervated by the phrenic nerve; the costal and intercostal nerves supply the lateral diaphragmatic pleura. The pattern of pain radiation can include the neck and upper trapezius if the apical pleura is involved. If the costal pleura is affected, the pain can be felt anteriorly, posteriorly, or laterally at the level of the lesion. If the basal pleura is affected and irritates the diaphragm, shoulder pain can result. If metastases spread cranially from the apical pleural, the lower brachial plexus and inferior cervical (stellate) ganglion can be affected, resulting in Pancoast's syndrome.

The heart is autonomically supplied by the cervical and upper thoracic sympathetic ganglia and from the vagus and recurrent laryngeal nerves. Because of common segmental levels in the thorax and neck (including the cervicotrigeminal nucleus), referred pain from cardiac conditions may be felt in the anterior or posterior chest, the throat, jaw, teeth, and even, inexplicably, the abdomen. The common area of reference is the left deltoid area and the left inner arm and hand, although the right shoulder may be affected.

The diaphragm is supplied by the phrenic nerve (cervical 3, 4, and 5) for its motor innervation but also carries fibers from cervical 4 to supply sensation to the more central parts of the muscle. The lower six intercostal nerves supply the peripheral diaphragm. Central diaphragmatic pain is generally felt through the fourth cervical root at the shoulder, and peripheral lesions may cause pain in the thoracoabdominal junction area anteriorly, posteriorly, or laterally, depending on the site of the lesion.

The peritoneum encloses all of the abdominal and pelvic organs and is the largest serous membrane in the body. The visceral peritoneum receives the same autonomic supply as the organ it is associated with and is insensible to pressure, cutting, chemicals, or heat. The diaphragmatic parietal peritoneum is supplied in the same manner as the diaphragm; that is, the central part is supplied by the fourth cervical segment and the peripheral part by the lower thoracic intercostal nerves. The remainder of the parietal peritoneum is supplied by the overlying skin and trunk musculature. With this in mind, the pain distribution of the specific organs is actually the pain distribution of the organ's peritoneum.

The stomach and duodenum refer pain to the upper abdomen just below the xiphoid, with radiation to the posterior trunk level in the case of lesion between the sixth thoracic and the tenth thoracic levels. If the diaphragmatic peritoneum is affected, the pain can be felt in the right shoulder and upper trapezius.

The small intestine pathology may produce umbilical pain and, if severe, may cause mid to low lumbar region pain.

The large intestine can produce pain that is felt in the lower abdomen and sacrum.

Liver and gall bladder disease is usually felt in the right upper quadrant or epigastrum, with referral potential to the right shoulder, midthoracic, and right inferior scapular regions.

Midline or left to midline pain may be pancreatic in origin and may radiate to the lumbar region or, if the diaphragmatic peritoneum is affected, to the left shoulder.

The appendix is generally felt in the right abdominal lower quadrant with referral into the epigastrum, the right groin and hip, and occasionally the right testicle.

Spleen pain may be felt in the right shoulder if it affects the diaphragmatic peritoneum of the left upper quadrant, epigastric, or umbilical region.

The prostate in older men is one of the more sinister causes of low back pain. Usually bladder problems in the form of hesitancy followed by retention are the normal onset of prostatitis from any cause, but occasionally the onset may be low back pelvic and hip pain.

The kidney and ureters, unlike most of the abdominal viscera, do appear, at least in part, to be pain sensitive, with laceration, puncture, and pressure pain signals being transmitted by the sympathetic supply from the lower thoracic and upper lumbar plexi. As a consequence, kidney pain can be extreme and very musculoskeletal in its quality. The pain is mainly felt in the posterior flank but can refer around the trunk to the lower abdominal quadrant and then to the ipsilateral groin and testicle and, if the diaphragm or its pleura is affected, to the ipsilateral shoulder.

The bladder and urethra are felt primarily anteriorly in the suprapubic and lower abdomen with referral to the lumbar region.

Gynecologic conditions including pelvic inflammatory disease, cancer of the uterus, and so on tend to cause abdominal pain with radiation into the anterior and or medial thigh(s) more than posterior trunk pain.

With all of these visceral conditions, the pain distribution patterns by themselves will not make the diagnosis. Pay attention to the quality of the pain descriptors—*cramplike, vice-type, gnawing, wavelike, diffuse and ill-defined,* and so on. Also, listen and look for evidence of dysfunction of the viscera itself such as nausea, vomiting, jaundice, changes in coughing habits, changes in sputum appearance, and so forth. Additionally, look for sympathetic signs or symptoms such as increased sweating or nausea. The dysfunction of the viscera may also show up in the way the pain behaves. Pain onset or relief after eating or onset before eating would suggest a gastrointestinal source.

Cutaneous areas are associated with the viscera via their nerve supply. Head[30] gave the following:

Heart	T1-5
Bronchi and lung	T2-4
Esophagus	T5-6

Stomach	T6-10
Liver and gall bladder	T7-9
Spleen	T6-10
Kidney	T10-L1
Ureter	T11-12

Pain Behavior

Is the pain constant, continuous, or intermittent? Is it felt only during the day, or does it disturb sleep? Does it feel better or worse at any particular time of the day? Is it related to particular activities or postures? How much activity or time in a given posture does it take to evoke the pain, and how long does the pain take to recede when the area is rested? The answers to these questions can often give information concerning the pain's source, its acuteness, and irritability.

Constant pain is generally accepted as suggestive of chemical irritation, bone cancer, or some visceral lesions. The determination that the pain is constant is made by understanding that at rest neither the patient nor the therapist can find any position that reduces the pain; that is, rest does not ease the pain. With most musculoskeletal inflammatory conditions it is easy to exacerbate the pain with testing, so it cannot accurately be described as constant because it does change, but for clinical purposes, the term *constant pain* is a good one. However, the main criterion is that short-term relief of stress does not reduce the pain.

If the therapist is unable to exacerbate the pain by selective tissue tension testing, this suggests that the source of the pain does not lie in a tissue vulnerable to such testing. This site may be in the viscera or in bone, which does not have a ligament or muscle lying close enough to pull on the painful area during testing. Inability to increase the constant pain with normal testing procedures is not a good sign. If bony point tenderness is associated with this inability, it is possible that the patient has serious bone disease.

Regardless of where you think the source of the pain lies, the presence of constant pain requires either referral back to the physician, if serious disease is suspected, or, if a nonserious musculoskeletal condition is present, anti-inflammatory treatments rather than biomechanical ones. Aggressive treatment that exacerbates the patient's constant pain tends to aggravate the condition, but ice, rest, pain-free exercises, and electrophysical agents tend to reduce the pain if its source is musculoskeletal.

Intermittent pain is pain that during a particular episode is either completely absent or present according to the presence of stress factors. This is mechanical pain (assuming its source is the musculoskeletal system) and is generally benign, although there have been some notable exceptions to this (see the cases). The mechanical stressing of a nociceptive structure causes this pain behavior. All things being equal, pain of this type generally bodes well for fairly aggressive therapy, including manual therapy and exercises.

Continuous pain is pain that is always there but varies in intensity over the short and long term, a more or less intense level of background pain that is exacerbated or relieved by posture, activity, or time of day. This type of behavior suggests a certain level of chemical pain associated with a level of mechanical pain. The therapist must determine just how irritable this condition may be, and this can best be done by estimating how severe the background pain is, how easily it is exacerbated, how long it lasts, and how easily is it relieved. The more severe the background pain, the more chemical involvement (inflammation) there is. The more easily the pain is exacerbated, the more irritable and the longer it lasts, and the more difficult it is to relieve, the more inflamed it is. A patient with this type of pain can be more of a treatment problem than a patient who complains of constant pain because the treatment for the latter is pretty much preset. It is easy to misjudge and apply too aggressive a treatment and flare the patient.

The following table may help to distinguish the type of pain encountered, always remembering the complexity of the nature of pain in its dependence on context, on the individual, and on the source and level of stimulation. However, also remember that pure chemical or pure mechanical pains are rarities and some degree of overlap is usually present.

Chemical Pain	Mechanical Pain
• Constant or continuous nocturnal • Morning stiffness lasting more than 2 hours • Unaffected by rest • Night pain may disturb sleep	• Intermittent • Morning stiffness lasting less than a few minutes and relieved with rest and appropriate activity • Eased by rest • Sleep without waking from pain

The presence of episodic pain over a long period reduces the risk that the patient is suffering from some serious pathology but also reduces the chances of an excellent outcome. Episodic pain often follows a very definite provocation. An example is where a worker once or twice a year has to do an unfamiliar job. Each time that job is done, the pain reintroduces itself. This type of episodic behavior is an excellent diagnostic indicator, giving the cause of the patient's symptoms and usually a solution to the problem—even if that is only counseling the patient that it will end with cessation of the job (although not always true, this is a good bet). Less useful is pain that recurs periodically without adequate provocation or on an activity that the patient can carry out successfully numerous consecutive times but on occasion produces symptoms and dysfunction. These completely unpredictable episodes afford very little diagnostic, prognostic, or therapeutic information. Often the underlying cause is instability, in which case the patient will often tell the therapist that providing an exercise or activity program is maintained, there is no problem, but stopping it for a few days results in recurrence of the pain. Careful questioning of the progress of each episode compared with previous ones will often give information on the general progress of the condition. A typical history given by patients is an original onset of low back pain 5 years previously; this was treated successfully and quickly (two or three sessions) with chiropractic. The pain recurred perhaps a year later with some definite provocation such as driving a long distance. Chiropractic again helped. The pain recurred again with minor provocation (perhaps mowing the grass) 6 months later. This time chiropractic took a dozen treatments and did not completely eliminate the patient's symptoms. A month or so later the back pain recurred with no apparent provocation, chiropractic did not afford any relief, and now you have the patient in your clinic. This is a case of increasing instability in the condition and probably in the spinal segment, and as such it becomes increasingly difficult to manage.

Is the pain expanding, shifting, or remaining stable? Shifting pain suggests that whatever the cause of the pain is, it is not growing but moving. An unstable disk herniation may do this. Expanding pain, though, is indicative of a growing lesion such as bone cancer or infection.[31] An example of expanding pain would be pain that starts in the right low back, then spreads to the buttock and down the leg; the pain might then also be felt spreading to the other limb.

Is the condition progressing? This was partly addressed earlier when episodic pain was discussed. Assessing pain to see if the condition is worsening is mainly based on three factors. First, is the quality of the pain changing? Lancinating pain that changes to somatic pain is evidence of decreasing pressure on neurological tissues and so would generally be considered an improvement. Second, is the pain centralizing or peripheralizing? Centralizing pain would suggest that the intensity of the stimulus has decreased or that it has shifted to a tissue that is less able to refer pain. On the other hand, the centralization could be apparent. Hypoesthesia or anesthesia may have replaced the pain; the objective examination will determine which has occurred. Peripheralization of the pain is generally not a good symptom because it tends to indicate that there is an increase in stimulus intensity or that a structure more able to refer pain is now involved or involved to a greater extent.[32] Disk herniations often behave this way, starting off as small herniations and progressing to the point of extrusion. Related to centralization and peripheralization is the concept of shifting and expanding pain. The patient who relates that the pain started in the low back (for example), worsened, then spread to the right buttock then down the leg, and finally across to the other leg is describing expanding pain. This is an enlarging lesion. It may be an increasing herniation, or it may be something less benign such as an infection or a growing neoplasm.[31] The opposite of this would be the patient who tells you that the pain started in the lumbar spine and then shifted to the right buttock. This would suggest something moving rather than enlarging and is a better prognostic indicator. Third, is the severity of the pain lessening? If it is, we can assume that the pain stimulus is abating. However, by itself this may not be an indication of an improving condition. The decrease in pain may simply be the result of good compliance with the instruction to rest the area. On the resumption of normal or even increased activities, the pain returns. Both function impairment and pain must decrease for optimal resolution of the patient's condition.

Severity and Disability

The severity of pain can be very difficult to establish. The therapist cannot feel the patient's pains, nor is there a valid or reliable way to objectively quantify pain. Consequently, the therapist must rely on the patient's own assessment of how bad the pain is. Because pain is very personal, the amount of tissue damage cannot be determined with any degree of confidence if severity is the only measure used by the therapist. Some patients are extremely stoic, others are not, and although severe pain is severe pain, as far as the patient is concerned, the patient's inability to tolerate pain may obscure the degree of stimulus causing the pain. The standard method of assessing pain levels is to ask the patient to put the current pain on a scale of 1 to 10 where 10 is the worst pain that this problem has produced or that the patient has ever felt. Another method that can be used, either in isolation or complementary to the pain scale, is to ask about disability. However, care must be taken here also. A compulsive workaholic will continue to work even in the most severe pain but will give up leisure activities.

Of course, knowledge of the patient's level of disability is vital in and of itself. This and pain are what have brought the patient in to see you. The therapist needs to be fully aware of the demands patients make on their bodies, but heavy workers may actually be easier to deal with in this respect than are sedentary workers. The patient with moderate low back pain working as a carpenter on a building site may be able to get by nicely by having a laborer do the lifting and heavier work whereas the sedentary worker may not be able to sit for prolonged periods even with ergonomic modifications. The issue of disability is obviously important to the therapist and the patient from a rehabilitation and retraining perspective, but it offers little information for diagnostic purposes other than what has already been discussed concerning disk herniations, claudication, and stenosis.

Paresthesia

This is a more reliable indicator of source. Paresthesia (defined as a pins and needles sensation) is felt when a neuropathy is present.[33] The most common neuropathy that the orthopedic therapist will come across is compression from a disk herniation, but other more serious causes will probably be encountered during a career. Patterns of paresthesia will afford information about where the lesion lies. The following is a rough indication of the level of the lesion from the distribution of the paresthesia:

Peripheral	Peripheral nerve
Segmental	Spinal nerve or root
Bilateral	Spinal cord
Quadrilateral	Spinal cord
Hemilateral	Brainstem or cortex
Facial	Trigeminal
Perioral	Brainstem or thalamus
Stocking-glove	Neurological or psychiatric, or vascular disease

Most distributions of paresthesia that the general orthopedic therapist will encounter will be segmental, arising from compression or ischemia of the nerve root or spinal nerve. Although this distribution of paresthesia often indicates strong compression and a real problem for the patient, it usually does not suggest dangerous pathology.

Possible spinal cord and neurovascular distributions are potentially health or life threatening if inappropriate treatment is given, and it is for these that the therapist must be alert. Hemilateral paresthesia in orthopedic patients suggests that one or both spinothalamic tracts are compromised, usually in the brainstem and maybe as part of the lateral medullary (Wallenberg's) syndrome, possibly caused by vertebral artery problems.[34,35] Perioral paresthesia is quite well understood to be a symptom of vertebrobasilar ischemia.[36,37] Although the exact mechanism is not understood, it is believed that the disturbance lies in the centromedian part of the trigeminothalamic tract in the thalamus itself.[38] This is one of the few tracts that is represented bilaterally and receives sensation from the mouth, gums, and teeth, so a lesion on one side would give bilateral symptoms. Facial paresthesia may indicate a deficit in the trigeminal nerve. This must be carefully distinguished from dysesthesia, in which pinprick testing provokes paresthesia as well as hypersensitivity. The latter case might indicate trigeminal facilitation from a craniovertebral or temporomandibular joint dysfunction; the former may be caused by vertebrobasilar ischemia. In any event, the presence of paresthesia, provoked or unprovoked, demands cranial nerve testing and vertebrobasilar system testing. Specific patterns of paresthesia will be discussed in the regional sections and in the case studies.

Aggravating and Abating Factors

What, if anything, makes the symptoms worse or better? Ideally, the therapist is looking for intermittent pain of an episodic nature that is aggravated by a particular mechanical stress and relieved by the avoidance of that stress. This case is very unlikely to be caused by anything other than a benign musculoskeletal system dysfunction. With acute inflammation, the patient cannot find a position of ease, so nothing relieves the pain. If nothing mechanical makes the pain worse, chances are the problem lies in the viscera or in some part of the musculoskeletal system that is not vulnerable to mechanical stress. Bone distant from muscle attachment is a good candidate, and early neoplastic disease affecting these regions often presents as such a musculoskeletal condition. In any event, constant pain that is not made worse by mechanical stress is potentially a symptom of severe disease. In those patients who relate symptom changes that are associated with altering mechanical stress, a better outlook is afforded. Lumbar pain that is aggravated by walking or other extension activities or postures is less likely to be caused by disk herniation than is pain that is aggravated by sitting or other flexion activities and postures. The effects of central spinal stenosis may well cause pain on walking set distances that is eased by flexion, pain caused by walking set distances that is not relieved by flexion but by time may be due to intermittent claudication. Pain related to eating or dietary intake is almost certainly not caused by musculoskeletal problems regardless of where the pain may be felt. General physical or emotional stress causing chest or arm pain must be suspected to be from cardiac origin.

Night pain can be a major issue. It is of two main types: Sudden sharp pains that wake the patient, usually as he or she turns in bed, is the more benign type and, if it accompanies sacroiliac area pain, often indicates sacroiliitis. The more sinister type is the ache that often gives the patient trouble getting to sleep and then wakes him or her after a few hours. This type of pain usually indicates inflammation or increasing pressure. Most patients with this will have straightforward inflammatory problems, but a small percentage will prove to have cancer. However, from experience, my own and others, and from reading cases in the literature, the relentless progressive nocturnal pain that is often taught as being symptomatic of cancer is not its normal presentation. This type of presentation tends to occur in advanced cancer, especially metastases, but in the early case, night pain may be only minimal or may not even be a feature. The point is that the absence of night pain does not exclude serious pathology as cause of the symptoms.

Other Symptoms

Listen for symptoms that are atypical, especially if they are of recent onset. Cranial nerve symptoms are often difficult for the patient to sense and/or relate, so direct questioning might be necessary. The presence of cranial nerve symptoms will demand a cranial nerve examination, which may clarify the urgency and/or the inappropriateness of the problem. If signs and symptoms are present, a brainstem lesion must be suspected and follow-up testing of the long tracts is required. The potential presence of a brainstem lesion demands that the patient be immediately referred to a physician before any further treatment is undertaken. The presence of cranial nerve signs and symptoms could indicate brainstem concussion, petechial hemorrhaging, neoplastic disease, neurological disease, or vertebrobasilar compromise. Obviously, some of these conditions are more urgent than others but the physician should be made aware of your concerns. These signs and symptoms together with testing procedures will be discussed in the examination of the cervical region.

Potential spinal cord and cauda equina symptoms must be carefully evaluated, and if they prove to be from these structures, the patient must be referred to the physician. Bilateral or quadrilateral paresthesia with or without trunk symptoms is probably the most common complaint in patients suffering minor (if that word can be used in this connection) spinal cord compression or ischemia. Hemilateral paresthesia may indicate cerebral or brainstem compromise. Any patient complaining of a distribution of paresthesia that does not conform to a segmental or peripheral nerve origin must be objectively evaluated for signs of compromise. The therapist may start the ball rolling with clinical neurological testing of the cranial nerves and/or long tracts. However, this should only be carried out if the therapist believes that there is no risk to the patient; that is, there is no possibility of ligamentous rupture, further neurovascular damage, craniovertebral dislocation, or further migration of discal material. In practice, the mere presence of such symptoms should be sufficient to refer the patient to the physician.

Cauda equina compression is usually associated with severe bilateral sciatic pain and paresthesia, although some case reports have documented clinically significant compression without the patient reporting any pain. An almost pathognomic symptom is perineal paresthesia with or without hypoesthesia or anesthesia, which indicates fourth sacral nerve palsy. Listen for symptoms of bladder, bowel, or genital dysfunction. These include urinary retention or incontinence, lack of expulsive bowel function, impotence, frigidity, and penile deviation. Any of these symptoms should cause you to refer the patient out.

Potential motor disturbances include ataxia, drop attacks, clumsiness, and weakness. The patient does not always recognize them for what they are. For example, a colleague told me of a patient who felt that he had magnets in his pockets that were causing him to be attracted to furniture. As silly as that sounds, it merits evaluation. What this patient ultimately turned out to be describing was lateral ataxia; he was in the middle of a cerebellar infarct. My father had trouble holding a folded newspaper under his arm when walking; it kept dropping to the floor. He was having transient ischemic cerebral attacks.

> Dizziness, diplopia (vertical or horizontal), dysarthria, bifacial numbness, ataxia, and weakness or numbness of part or all of one or both sides of the body (i.e., a disturbance of the long motor or sensory tracts bilaterally) are the hallmarks of vertebral-basilar involvement.[39]

Drop attacks occur when the patient suddenly and without any warning falls, almost invariably forward, while remaining conscious. The fall is extremely rapid and not in the least like a faint. The causes of this are numerous and include vestibular dysfunction, brain tumor, diseases of the cerebellum and posterior tract, and less commonly vertebrobasilar ischemia.[39] Tripping over minor objects or even nonexistent objects may indicate foot drop from any of its causes.

Post-traumatic amnesia is an integral part of concussion. It is usually consistent in its effect, being around the time of the trauma for a greater or lesser period depending on the severity of the concussion. In fact, amnesia is a better method of establishing that the patient was concussed than is asking about being knocked unconscious because the period of unconsciousness can be so brief that the patient is unaware that it occurred. The length of time covered by the amnesia can be used to evaluate the severity of the concussion.[39] Other forms of amnesia are less benign in nature and may indicate neurological disease processes or more serious degrees of traumatic brain injury. Short- and long-term memory loss must be reported to the physician for evaluation. Other forms of intellectual impairment include drowsiness, concentration problems, comprehension difficulties, and so forth. These will be discussed in more detail in the region-specific examination of the neck.

If the patient is complaining of coldness in the hands, ask about color changes. Blueness may indicate venous congestion, whiteness sympathetic disturbance, and redness certain systemic arthritides or infection.

A feeling of heat in an area may be caused by inflammation or may be causalgia. If the feeling is causalgia, the sensation will run down the limb or around the thorax and is burning, and painful in nature. If the heat sensation is inflammatory in origin, it will be around the joint or over its superficial aspects.

Patients who say they feel unstable or that their head is going to drop off if they move may be right on the money. I have heard reports that post-traumatic patients have died on moving their heads when asked to do so by the physician. These people had undisplaced fractures of the dens that became displaced on relaxing their protective guarding. A less serious complaint is that the spine feels unstable, feels as if it is moving about, or consistently clicks. Often on subsequent testing, the feeling proves to be correct, and there is a segmental instability present.

On a systemic level ask about changes in sweating, coughing, the product of coughing, unexplained weight loss, recent fever, changes in bladder or bowel habits and/or the products of those functions, recurrent infections, indigestion, and dysphagia. Any alterations in these may indicate the presence of a systemic disease or cancer, and if the physician is not aware of these changes, he or she should be made aware. Again, it is possible to capture this information on a questionnaire filled in by the patient on the first visit. Of course, not all of these questions need to be asked of every patient, just those with unusual presentations.

Mandatory Questions

These are region specific and will be discussed in more detail in their pertinent section. They are questions that must be answered by the patient either spontaneously or on direct questioning. They relate to serious pathologies such as vertebrobasilar compromise, spinal cord involvement, and cauda equina compression that the therapist could easily make much worse with inappropriate treatment.

Previous Treatments and Results

If the condition that the patient is attending for has been experienced in the past, valuable information can be gained from the history. Are the pain's quality, location, behavior, and irritability similar to sensations in previous episodes? By assessing the answers we can obtain an idea about whether the problem is generally improving, worsening, or staying much the same. The purpose of the question, "Have you had any other treatment including chiropractic, other physical therapy, osteopathy, acupuncture, medication, or anything else?" is to see if you can learn from other practitioners' experiences. Often, however, the patient can mislead you. I have a friend and colleague who is an excellent manual therapist, probably one of the best in the world, near whom I used to live. Occasionally I would get patients that he had seen either for that condition or for another. The question, "Have you had other treatments and if so what?" would often be answered "Yes, from Mr. X, but he only put hot packs on me." Knowing the therapist, I also knew that this was not something that he would do. I therefore engaged in a little more prodding.

"Did he touch you?"

"Yes."

"Did he click your joint?"

"Yes."

"Did he use any electrical treatments?"

"Yes."

"Did he give you exercises?"

"Yes."

Patients often do not recall what actually happened, and you need to ask further and more direct questions when the patient's answers do not seem likely.

Other Investigations

I do not look at the results of imaging tests until after I have examined the patient. There are two reasons for this. First, the imaging results tend to bias my interpretation of the results of the clinical examination. If the x-ray says degeneration is present, I usually find it clinically. Second, if the imaging results or the image itself agree with my clinical diagnosis, I am considerably more confident of my conclusion. On the other hand, the specificity and sensitivity of many tests are not fully understood yet. We know that x-rays fail to demonstrate about 30% of spinal fractures on first reading but usually show them on a subsequent reading, when a better idea of the diagnosis is present.[40,41] About 30% of lumbar MRIs demonstrate disk prolapse on asymptomatic patients.[42] It is well understood that in the lumbar spine there is an inverse relationship between the presence of radiographic degeneration and pain. Degeneration worsens as the patient ages but the incidence of significant pain decreases. The peak age for lumbar pain is considerably lower than the peak age for degeneration.

After examining the patient, a therapist will often request the physician to order imaging for a specific problem that is being postulated by the therapist from information gained from the examination. This is the better method. The radiologists have a better chance of seeing the lesion on the image if they know what they are looking for before looking for it. Unfortunately, nowadays, imaging and other lab tests are being used to diagnose the problem rather than confirm the clinical diagnosis. When these tests turn out to be negative, the patient is very often labeled as hysterical or a secondary gainer.

Potential Systemic Indicators from the History

❑ Initial onset at over 45 years of age
❑ Nocturnal pain
❑ Pain that causes writhing
❑ Constitutional signs or symptoms (nausea, vomiting, diarrhea, fever)
❑ Previous history of cancer
❑ Back and abdominal pain at same level
❑ Pain unrelieved by recumbency
❑ Unvarying pain
❑ Severe and persistent pain with pain-free back movement
❑ Severe back and lower limb weakness without pain
❑ Back pain associated with eating or diet

Notes

1. Cameron RB (ed): *Practical Oncology,* p 417. Norwalk, CT, Appleton & Lange, 1994.

2. Cameron RB (ed): *Practical Oncology,* pp 189–190. Norwalk, CT, Appleton & Lange, 1994.

3. Schumacher Jr HR (ed): *Primer on the Rheumatic Diseases,* 10th ed., pp 191, 243. Atlanta, Arthritis Foundation, 1993.

4. Weiner WJ, Goetz, CG: *Neurology for the Non-Neurologist,* 3d ed., pp 166–167, 1994.

5. Sharp J, Purser DW: Spontaneous atlantoaxial dislocation in ankylosing spondylitis and rheumatoid arthritis. *Ann Rheum Dis* 20:47, 1961.

6. Stevens JC et al: Atlantoaxial subluxation and cervial myelopathy in rheumatoid arthritis. Q J Med 40:391, 1971.

7. Boyle AC: The rheumatoid neck. Proc R Soc Med 64:1161, 1971.

8. Park WW et al: The pharyngovetebral veins: an anatomic rationale for Grisel's syndrome. J Bone Joint Surg Am 66:568, 1984.

9. Beals RK et al: Anomalies associated with vertebral malformations. Spine 18:1329, 1993.

10. Wiggins ME et al: Healing characteristics of a type 1 collagenous structure treated with corticosteroids. Am J Sports Med 22:279, 1994.

11. Oxlund H: The influence of a local injection of cortisol on the mechanical properties of tendons and ligaments and the indirect effect on the skin. Acta Orthop Scand 51:231, 1980.

12. Walsh WR et al: Effects of a delayed steroid injection on ligament healing using a rabbit medial collateral ligament model. Biomaterials 16:905, 1995.

13. Sevy RW: Drugs as a cause of dizziness and vertigo, in *Dizziness and Vertigo,* AJ Finestone (ed). Boston, John Wright, pp 81–97, 1982.

14. Ballantyne J, Ajodhia J: Iatrogenic dizziness, in *Vertigo,* MR Dix, JD Hood (eds). Chichester, UK, John Wiley, 1984.

15. Sturzzenegger M et al: The effect of accident mechanisms and initial findings on the long-term course of whiplash injury. J Neurol 242:443, 1995.

16. McNab I: The mechanism of spondylogenic pain, in *Cervical Pain,* C Hisch, Y Zotterman (eds). Oxford, UK, Permagon, pp 89–95, 1972.

17. Howe JF et al: Mechanosensitivity of the dorsal root ganglia and chronically injured axons: a physiological basis for the radicular pain of nerve root compression. Pain 3:25, 1977.

18. Bogduk N, Twomey LT: *Clinical Anatomy of the Lumbar Spine,* 2d ed., pp 151–159, 1991.

19. Smyth MJ, Wright V: Sciatica and the intervertebral disc. An experimental study. J Bone Joint Surg Am 40:1401, 1959.

20. McCulloch JA, Waddell G: Variation in of the lumbosacral myotomes with bony segmental anomalies. J Bone Joint Surg Br 62:475, 1980.

21. El Mahdi MA et al: The spinal nerve root innervation, and a new concept of the clinicopathological interrelations in back pain and sciatica. Neurochirugia 24:137, 1981.

22. Adams RD et al: *Principles of Neurology,* 6th ed. (CD-ROM version). New York, McGraw-Hill, 1998.

23. Wilson-Pauwels L et al: *Autonomic Nerves,* pp 42–43. Hamilton, BC Decker, 1997.

24. Goodman CC, Snyder TE: *Differential Diagnosis in Physical Therapy,* 2d ed., pp 6–7. Philadelphia, WB Saunders, 1995.

25. Holleb AI et al (eds): *Textbook of Clinical Oncology,* p 555. Atlanta, American Cancer Society, 1991.

26. Grieve GP: Referred pain and other clinical features, in *Grieve's Modern Manual Therapy,* 2d ed., JD Boyling, N Palastanga (eds). Edinburgh, Churchill Livingstone, 1994.

27. Williams PL, Warwick R: *Gray's Anatomy,* 36th ed. Edinburgh, Churchill Livingstone, 1980.

28. Cameron RB: *Practical Oncology,* p. Norwalk, CT, Appleton & Lange, 1994.

29. Holleb AI et al (eds): *Textbook of Clinical Oncology,* p. Atlanta, American Cancer Society, 1991.

30. Head H: *Studies in Neurology,* p 653. London, Oxford Medical Publications, 1920.

31. Cyriax J: *Textbook of Orthopedic Medicine,* 8th ed. London, Balliere Tindall & Cassell, 1982.

32. McKenzie RA: *The Lumbar Spine: Mechanical Diagnosis and Therapy.* Waikanae, NZ, Spinal Publications Ltd., 1981.

33. Weiner WJ, Goetz, CG: *Neurology for the Non-Neurologist,* 3d. ed., p 155. Philadelphia, JB Lippincott, 1994.

34. George B, Laurian C: *The Vertebral Artery: Pathology and Surgery.* New York, Springer-Verlag, 1987.

35. Adams RD et al: *Principles of Neurology,* 6th ed. (CD-ROM version). New York, McGraw-Hill, 1998.

36. Ausman JI et al: Posterior circulation revascularization. Superficial temporal artery to superior cerebellar artery anastomosis. J Neurosurg 56:766, 1982.

37. Pessin MS et al: Basilar artery stenosis: middle and distal segments. Neurol Clin 37:1742, 1987.

38. Kandal ER, Swartze JH: *Principles of Neural Science,* 2d ed., pp 567–569. New York, Elsevier.

39. Adams RD et al: *Principles of Neurology,* 6th ed., Part 4 (CD-ROM version). New York, McGraw-Hill, 1998.

40. Dalinka MK et al: The radiographic evaluation of spinal trauma. Emerg Med Clin North Am 3:475.

41. Reid DC et al: Etiology and clinical course of missed spinal fractures. J Trauma 27:980.

42. Hu SS et al: Disorders, diseases and injuries of the spine, in *Current Diagnosis and Treatment in Orthopedics,* HB Skinner (ed). Norwalk CT, Appleton & Lange, 1995.

CHAPTER 3

Observation

A more detailed discussion of what to look for in each region will be found in the region-specific examination sections. In general, the observed phenomenon should be readily apparent; if you cannot see it within a very few seconds, it is probably not significant for this part of the examination. Look for the following:

Gait
    Antalgic limp
    Vertical limp
    Lateral limp
    Neurological gaits
        Ataxia (wide-based or lateral)
        Trendelenberg
        High stepping
        Foot drop
        Others
    Reduced or absent arm swing
    Reduced or absent trunk rotation
Static
    Posture
        Obvious postural anteroposterior deviations
          (hyperlordosis/hyperkyphosis)
        Obvious postural transverse deviations (lateral shifts)
        Obvious postural rotatory deviations (rotoscoliosis)
        Torticollis
        Lateral lean
    Atrophy
    Hypertrophy

Surgical scars
Skin creases (anterior and posterior)
Vertebral wedging
Vertebral ledging

Edema
Bruising
Congenital anomalies
    Sprengel's
    Klippel-Feil syndrome
    Poly-, syn-, or adactyly
    Dwarfism
    Down's syndrome
    Birthmarks
    For a more complete list see page 000
General appearance
    Pupil aniscoria
    Ptosis
    Horner's signs
    Grayness or yellowness
    Nystagmus
    Facial drooping
    Strabismus
    Cyanosis
Speech, language, voice
    Dysphasia
    Dysarthria
    Dysphonia

Gait

There are a number of problems with assessing gait. There are too many areas to observe at one time. Often there is not enough space available to allow the patient to get up to normal walking speeds. The patient is conscious that he or she is being watched, and artificial gait may be executed.

What aspect of the patient's body you observe depends on what you are looking for. Remember that you are not in a gait lab but in a clinic trying to make sure that the patient has been appropriately referred and that you will give the correct treatment. Gait is a very secondary issue at this point in the examination and takes on more importance when assessing nonroutine patients with nonorthopedic manual therapy conditions such as neurological disease, amputation, diabetes, and so on. The types of gait deviation discussed in this section are those more commonly seen in neurological conditions and those used to assess possible causes of the orthopedic problem.

In an antalgic limp there is a shortened stride length of the affected limb with the foot usually turned outward. Of course, this is not always the case. With an Achilles tendonitis, for example, patients will walk on their toes to avoid stretching the injured area. Similarly, with a knee injury that causes a flexion posture, toe walking is necessary to get the foot to the ground. A lateral limp is recognized by watching the patient's shoulders during gait. The shoulders tend to drop down to one side as the patient steps onto that leg. This may indicate a short leg on that side. A vertical limp can best be seen by watching the head bob up and down more than is usual. This frequently suggests a long leg on that side, as the body vaults over it. The Trendelenberg limp is a lateral limp and again can best be observed by looking at the shoulders. However, it is different from the lateral limp caused by leg length discrepancy in that the limp occurs once the patient is on the leg at midstance rather than at heel strike. Generally a Trendelenberg gait suggests weakness of the hip abductors of the weight-bearing leg for whatever reason. Ataxia takes many forms; the most significant for the orthopedic therapist are lateral and wide-based ataxia. Lateral ataxia may be caused by vertebrobasilar ischemia (among other neurological conditions); wide-based ataxia is frequently caused by vestibular disorders. A high-stepping gait is often caused by neurological diseases that reduce proprioception, perhaps the most notorious of which is neurosyphilis with a tabetic gait. However, one patient I saw had a unilateral high-stepping gait that had lasted for 15 years and disappeared almost immediately with some simple exercises. Go figure! Foot drop is often heard before it is seen and is a result of paresis or paralysis of the dorsiflexors caused by peripheral or spinal nerve palsy or a stroke.

Static

Posture

Usually what is meant by posture is the position taken up by the subject in quiet standing, the lordoses and kyphoses. Of course, posture actually means much more than this and is basically any weight-bearing static position—sitting, standing, bending, and leaning. If we take it as it is usually meant, static quiet standing, then a number of considerations have to be given. If we are going to assess posture have we an adequate yardstick to measure our patient against. Certainly, optimal or ideal postures have been advanced; perhaps Florence Kendall has been the most influential in this area.[1,2] Axial extension, in which the subject attempts to line up, as much as possible, the vertebrae so as to minimize shearing forces, muscle activity, and ligamentous stress is the most usual definition of good posture, but is this a good gold standard? EMG studies have consistently demonstrated that a freely adopted posture requires minimum and consistent muscle activity between subjects.[3-7] Have a look at the general population and at yourself. How many people do you see maintaining this posture? It might be *optimal,* but it is certainly not *normal* in the statistical or clinical senses. Even if you do subscribe to this ideal, is there a normal variation and is this normal variation the same for all body types? The examination of posture, which on the surface seems straightforward, is anything but.

To complicate this further, it is extremely unlikely that the patients whose posture you are observing are in their habitual state. They are in pain, they are dysfunctional, and any alteration in posture may well be occurring to relieve some of their pain. It is not reasonable to assume that a posture is habitual until you have returned the patient to his or her habitual condition. It would be better to note the patient's posture and look for changes as the patient's condition improves. In addition, be a little more active in your assessment of posture; ask patients to move through the range of postures from axial extension to axial flexion. If they are able to do so, you can presume that they are doing so, at least every now and then, and that at least they do not have a fixed postural deficit. Later, once the immediate problem that has brought the patient to you has been addressed, the postural assessment can be done with the knowledge that it has more relevance. These results can be compared with your initial results. If there has been a dramatic change, it is reasonable to assume that the initial posture was more probably a result of the patient's symptoms rather than their cause. Even if you believe that there is a postural deficit, are the patient's symptoms being caused or aggravated by that deficit? Although there is a postural dysfunction, it may be completely irrelevant to that patient.

Lateral shifting is a form of postural deficit but is more likely to be directly related to the patient's complaints. Robin McKenzie popularized the significance of the lateral shift. McKenzie maintains that about 50% of patients with low back pain exhibit a lateral shift and gives a number of reasons for this, including congenital anomaly, remote mechanical cause, alteration of nucleus position, and abnormal joint configuration.[8] It is worth bearing in mind when figures such as this are used that the author's case load may be entirely different from yours, so do not get too upset when you find yourself at variance with such an author. If you find a lateral shift, is there an element of rotation involved (this is a rotoscoliosis) or does the spine just reach out laterally without any obvious rotation? The former may well be part of a congenital or developmental scoliosis. Equally it may be caused by a zygopophyseal joint dysfunction or a disk lesion; the rest of the exam will indicate which. The straight shift is more likely to be caused by mechanical dysfunctions. If it corrects easily and has a normal end feel, the cause is likely to be remote. If spasm intervenes, a disk lesion or an acute zygapophyseal joint problem may be the cause. Spasm and referred pain, particularly if radicular in nature, are likely to be caused by a disk herniation compressing either the dural sleeve and/or the spinal nerve root. Resistance in the form of a springy end feel may indicate some form of transverse discal instability and may be fairly easily corrected. A lateral lean is recognized by the whole body leaning to one side from the legs, not just from the pelvis as in the case of the lateral shift. The usual cause is an ipsilateral short leg.

Torticollis means "twisted neck." It may be painful or pain-free, fixed or correctable. The most common torticollis seen by the orthopedic therapist is fixed and painful, and it requires treatment. Painless and correctable torticollises are often the result of visual disturbances (diplopia in particular) and hearing problems[9] but may be caused by hysteria.

Infantile torticollis may be caused by a number of things including difficult labor, breech deliveries, caesarian deliveries, sternomastoid tumors, or simple postural and muscle shortening. The vast majority of cases respond to simple stretching and positioning, with only a very low percentage requiring surgery. Most benign infantile torticollises are congenital.[10] Be more careful of acquired torticollis, as this could be the result of some more serious disease process. Childhood torticollis usually affects children between the ages of 2 and 10. In some there is an orthopedic cause, but in a substantial number the cause may be infection with inflammation of the cervical glands irritating the sternomastoid, neurological disease, or neoplasm. Palpate the submandibular area for tenderness and enlargement of the glands, and if one or both are found return the patient to the physician. Similarly, if no very obvious biomechanical dysfunction is apparent with testing, again refer out. Adolescent torticollis is the most common type, usually affecting children between the ages of 9 and 14.[11] This is a very painful condition and noncorrectable on testing. There is often a biomechanical dysfunction in the upper part of the neck. If this is left untreated, the acute pain and range disturbance lasts about 10 days. If treated, it lasts about a week and a half! With careful treatment (I use heat, manual cervical traction, a soft collar, and lots of reclining), about 80% of the pain will disappear in less than 24 hours. If an adolescent presents with torticollis that has lasted much more than 10 days or that is not improving, there is an increased possibility of a more sinister underlying pathology.[12] Adult torticollises are usually caused by straightforward mechanical problems, although occasionally a presumptive disk protrusion large enough to cause mechanical problems but big enough to cause neural signs will give a springy end feel and be very difficult to treat.

Muscle Atrophy and Hypertrophy

Profound atrophy in the absence of other obvious long-standing neurological signs is generally suggestive of lower motor neuron disease or peripheral nerve palsy. Fasciculation often goes along with atrophy.

Lower motor neuron palsies tend to produce coarse fasciculation; upper motor neuron problems produce fine atrophy.[13] Upper motor neuron conditions tend to take much longer to produce atrophy, and nerve root compression produces only very slight atrophy because of the multisegmental nature of innervation to most muscles. Atrophy can also occur because of inhibition from painful joint lesions. Quadriceps wasting with meniscal injuries is an example.

Consider the distribution of the wasting. Does it conform to a peripheral nerve distribution or to a spinal segment, or is it multisegmental or nonsegmental? The last two are particularly worrisome, as they could indicate an upper or lower motor neuron disease. Atrophy is of particular significance if it occurs in the intrinsic muscles of the hand or hands. It may be the first indication of a lower motor neuron disease because low cervical disk lesions rarely produce palsies of these muscles.[11] Unilateral atrophy of the hand intrinsics may occur as part of thoracic outlet syndrome or Pancoast's syndrome, which are caused by trauma, breast, or apical lung cancer disrupting the sympathetic transmission at the stellate ganglion and the lower brachial plexus. Atrophy of the sternomastoid or, more usually, the trapezius muscles suggests an eleventh cranial nerve palsy, which in turn may be caused by a neuroma, occipital metastases, or fracture. This certainly demands a cranial nerve examination. If other cranial nerve signs are evident, a brainstem injury or ischemia is possible. If the atrophy is isolated, consideration must be given to a lesion of the nerve itself. If the atrophy follows trauma, an occipital fracture should be ruled out, in which case, the nerve may have been stretched by the mechanics of the injury. If there is no trauma, a neuroma or metastatic cancer of the occiput are possibilities.

Isolated hypertrophy could be caused by overuse in a muscle or muscles trying to support an unstable region. This is particularly common in the tibialis posterior and anterior as they try to support an unstable foot. Of course, the hypertrophy may be more apparent than real, as it is in Duchenne's muscular dystrophy.[14]

Surgical Scars and Creases

Surgical scars will redirect the patient's attention to previous medical conditions and their treatment, thereby jogging the memory. Most scars are not relevant to the patient's complaints, but some, even though far removed from the symptomatic region, will be. These are scars from cancer surgery. Obviously, if you are treating the low back and the patient exhibits surgical scars, this will have a bearing on the patient's condition, but more from a treatment perspective than a diagnostic one.

Skin creases offer information on hypermobility and instability, especially when these appear on movement. They are most commonly seen in the cervicothoracic junction and in the lumbar spine on extension.

They are usually unilateral or if bilateral are seen at different levels, and they generally depict extension hypermobility or rotatory instability. Low abdominal anterior creases can only be seen if the underpants are lowered in front. This crease is almost pathognomic of spondylolithesis. Be aware, though, that the mere presence of a crease does not necessarily mean that instability is present, and even if it does, it does not help us determine if the instability or hypermobility is clinically relevant.

Local Bony Changes

A local kyphus is wedging. It generally occurs with a compression fracture of the body of the vertebra. Often the patient cannot remember the injury, as it may have occurred in childhood and be nothing more than a vague memory of low back pain. If the kyphus is painful to palpation, percussion, and the application of a low-frequency tuning fork, be careful. If there was no overt trauma, this may be a pathological fracture caused by osteoporosis, bone cancer, or some other bone disease. Ledging is a little different. Here the therapist can run a finger down the spinous process and come to one that sticks out as it does with the wedged vertebra, but on continuing down the spine, the other spinous processes are found to be level. This would suggest the presence of a degenerative type of spondylolithesis in which the entire vertebra has shifted forward on those below. When there is a defect in the pars articularis, this ledge may not be seen, because the neural arch is left behind and remains level with the spinous processes below. A retrospondylolisthesis would appear in the opposite way, with the dip coming underneath and continuing down the spine.

Bruising and Swelling

These are not commonly seen in spinal trauma but are significant when they do occur. Bruising over the mastoid is called *Battle's sign* and frequently indicates fractures of the temporal or occipital bones. Raccoon mask bruising is bilateral black eyes similar to the features on a raccoon's face and is a companion of facial fractures.[15] Bruising over the erector spinae in the thoracic or lumbar spine may indicate tearing of these muscles, most usually by direct impact. Shoulder injuries resulting in bruising running down the arm generally indicate a capsular tear or that a major muscle, such as the pectoralis major, biceps, or brachialis, is torn in its belly. Bruising with ankle inversion injuries can often indicate how severe the damage is. Extreme bruising may be caused by a fracture. Bruising on the medial side of the ankle with inversion injuries means that considerable inversion has occurred, allowing compression of the medial tissues. Generally the more extensive the bruising is, the more severe the injury.

There are many types of swelling, and some are difficult to see, especially those around the spine and the shoulder. In the neck after trauma you may see swelling in the clavicular triangle or you may have to palpate for it. In my experience, these patients take a good deal longer to recover. Because it is so deep, the shoulder rarely demonstrates swelling after trauma, but when it does, recovery is difficult. Lumbar and thoracic edema are extremely rare and difficult to judge, but in keeping with the motto "If it's unusual, it must have an unusual etiology," be careful. Swelling of the buttock is not a good sign, especially in the absence of severe trauma. It may indicate infection, neoplastic disease, fracture, and so on. If there is swelling, ask the patient how long after the trauma it came on. If it was immediate, you are probably looking at a hemarthrosis; if delayed, simple effusion. If an entire region is edematous, the cause is reduced venous return. If this followed trauma, it may simply be disuse and a dependent position. If there was no trauma, other, more serious causes could include congestive cardiac failure and deep vein thrombosis.

Congenital Anomalies

Congenital anomalies are important to recognize because in addition to their direct effect on the diagnosis and treatment, they can also indicate other more serious deficits. The following tables are made from information from an article that looked at subjects with known vertebral malformations for associated anomalies. It was more the rule than otherwise that the presence of a vertebral malformation was associated with other anomalies, usually from the same embryological block. It is important because although the presence of say, syndactyly, might not affect the patient's neck, the problem may be associated with vertebral artery anomalies.

Name of Defect	Clinical Features
Generalized	
Osteogenesis imperfecta	Fragile soft bones easily fractured or deformed, joint laxity
Diaphysial aclasis (multiple exostosis)	Cartilage-capped metaphysial exostosis with deficient remodeling and stunted growth
Achondroplasia	Defective long bone growth with short limbs, dwarfing, and a large head
Osteopetrosis	Hard dense bone with increased risk of fracture
Gargoylism (Hurler's syndrome)	Dwarfism with kyphosis caused by deformed vertebrae, mental deficiency, large liver and spleen

Craniocleido dystosis | Impaired ossification of the skull with deficient clavicles

Craniocleido dystosis	Impaired ossification of the skull with deficient clavicles
Arthrogryposis multiplex congenita (amyoplasia congenita)	Defective development of the muscles resulting in stiff deformed joints.
Pseudohypertrophic muscular dystrophy	Progressive muscular weakness between the ages of 3 to 6 years
Fibroplasia ossificans progressiva	Extopic ossification in the trunk and limbs, short big toe
Familial hypohosphatemia	Congenital rickets (bone weakness)
Cystinosis (renal tubular rickets)	Rarified bones with deformity
Neurofibromatosis (Recklinghausen's syndrome)	Café au lait spots, cutaneous fibromata, and cranial or peripheral nerve palsies
Hemophilia	Prolonged clotting times, leading to hemarthrosis and soft tissue bleeding
Gaucher's disease	Cystlike appearance of bones with large liver and spleen
Down's syndrome	Mental and physical impairment, micro- or adensia

Central Nervous System Trunk and Spine

Klippel-Feil syndrome	Short stiff neck and low hairline caused by fused or deformed cervical vertebrae
Sprengel's deformity	Unilateral (usually) tethered and high-scapular, no-neck appearance
Cervical rib	Usually asymptomatic but may result in vascular or neurological thoracic outlet syndrome
Hemivertebra	Unilateral vertebral defect leading to scoliosis
Spina bifida (spinal dysraphism)	Spina bifida occulta, menigocele, or myelocele may be asymptomatic or lead to leg deformities and incontinence because of neurological involvement; may be associated with hydrocephalus.
Arnold-Chiari malformation	Elongation of the cerebellum and medulla into the spinal canal with the potential development of central neurological signs with neck extension or manipulation in adulthood.
Congenital intracranial arteriovenous fistulas and hemangioma	Varying in size, and can occur anywhere in the cranium; if large enough, will cause pressure signs and symptoms; may enlarge or rupture, causing childhood or adult symptoms, usually between the ages of 10 and 31, but can be delayed to 50 years; may suffer from pulsatile tinnitus
Dissecting aortic aneurysm	Severe interscapular and/or chest and/or lumbar pain

Limbs

Congenital amputation	Part or all of a limb missing
Phocomelia	Aplasia of the proximal part of the limb with the distal part present
Constriction rings	Limb or digit constriction as if by a purse string; may be associated with syndactyly

(continued)

Absence of radius	Hand deviated laterally because of lack of support
Absence of proximal arm muscles	Trapezius, deltoid, sternomastoid, and/or pectoralis major
Madelung's deformity (dyschondrosteosis)	Ulna head dislocated from the radius, which is bowed
Syndactyly	Fused or webbing of two or more fingers
Polydactyly	More than five digits
Extrodactyly	Lobster-claw hand
Congenital dislocation of the hip	Neonatal dislocation with possible flattened femoral head in adulthood
Coxa vara	Defective femoral neck ossification with reduced neck angle
Congenital short femur	Foot small and everted; lateral two digits together with their metacarpals possibly absent
Club foot	Foot inverted and plantaflexed or everted and dorsiflexed
Curled toe	Lateral angulation of one or more toes

In a review of 218 subjects with known vertebral malformations Beals et al.[16] found that most malformations were associated with other anomalies (386 vertebral and 322 other anomalies), with 61% of the subjects showing multiple anomalies. The systems affected were

❏ Musculoskeletal
❏ Neurological
❏ Genitourinary
❏ Otolaryngeal
❏ Gastointestinal
❏ Cardiac
❏ Pulmonary

The study found a prevalence of thoracic and lumbar anomalies (55.5% and 21% respectively) with the cervical spine having about 15% and the sacrum about 8%, giving an average of 1.77 anomalies per patient.

Anomalies Associated with Vertebral Malformation

Frequency of Diagnosis	Number of Patients
Cranial nerve palsy	24 (11%)
Upper limb hypoplasia	21 (10%)
Club feet	20 (10%)
Lower limb hypoplasia	19 (9%)
Dislocated hip	18 (8%)

Sprengel's deformity	18	(8%)
Hemifacial microsomia	18	(8%)
Renal anomaly	17	(8%)
Cardiac anomaly	16	(6%)
Neurogenic incontinence	15	(7%)
Inguinal hernia	14	(6%)
Lower motor neuron lesion of lower limb	11	(5%)
Seizures	5	(2%)

Source: From RK Beals et al: Anomalies associated with vertebral malformations. Spine 18:1329, 1993.

General Appearance

Pupils *Aniscoria* is the term for asymmetrical pupils, either in side-to-side or in shape. The pupils should be within 15% of the same size as each other and round, and they should react equally to light, convergence, and surprise.[17]

Constriction of the pupils is a parasympathetic function in relation to increasing light levels. The constrictor muscles are controlled by the Edinger-Westphal nucleus (part of the third cranial nucleus) via the oculomotor nerve; the dilator muscles are sympathetically innervated by fibers from the superior cervical ganglion. The control of pupil diameter is a coordinated effort between the sympathetic and parasympathetic systems, with the parasympathetic system dominant so that under ambient light and environmental levels, the pupils tend to constrict.

If there is a sympathetic paralysis, the parasympathetic tone is unopposed and the constrictor muscles close the pupil. Light reaction may absent, sluggish, or oscillating. Pathologies causing Horner's syndrome are the most common cause of this condition that the OMT is likely to encounter. Constriction of the pupils also occurs during convergence of the eyes via Brodman's area in the frontal and the Edinger-Westphal nucleus lobe, although the exact mechanism is not well understood.

Dilation of the pupils occurs, either as a result of reduced parasympathetic tone in reducing light conditions or from increasing sympathetic tone in threat conditions. Abnormal dilation of the pupil is caused by unopposed sympathetic tone; generally because of oculomotor paralysis or paresis. In these cases, the pupil fails to respond normally to the absence or reduction of light in the initial part of the consensual reflex test or if the flashlight is moved away from the eyes. Pupil dilation with ptosis is almost pathognomic of oculomotor lesions.

Addie's pupil is a tonic pupil whose size depends on its last light environment. It does not react normally to light reflex testing but will change its shape over time in different light conditions and once changed maintains its diameter. It responds better during converges than it does to light stimulation, although still abnormally slowly, and to near target testing. It is often associated with symmetrical or asymmetrical deep tendon hyporeflexia and appears to be a mild benign polyneuropathy. It has no significance for the orthopedic therapist.

The Argyle-Robertson pupil is an irregular pupil that does not constrict to light but does constrict on convergence or near vision. It is specific to neurosyphilis. The near vision and light reflex discrepancy with regular pupils is found with conditions other than syphilis.

Ptosis Ptosis is pathological depression of the superior eyelid such that it covers part of the pupil. The muscles responsible for opening the eye and maintaining it opened position are the levator palpebrae and Muller's muscle. The levator palpabrae is innervated by the third cranial nerve (oculomotor), because this nerve causes elevation of the eyeball. It is efficient then that the same impulses that result in orbit elevation also cause superior eyelid elevation. The small, sympathetically innervated Muller's muscles are attached to the inferior and superior tarsals (fibrocartilaginous plates in the eyelids). When the muscle contracts, it pulls on the plate and causes the eyelid to raise.

Paralysis or paresis of one or both of these muscles causes ptosis. If an oculomotor paresis/paralysis is present, the ptosis is generally not capable of correction by effort, because the levator palpabrae is the larger of the two muscles. If a sympathetic paralysis is present (Horner's syndrome) the patient is usually able to elevate the eyelid on command and the ptosis is most noticeable at rest. Because sympathetic paralysis leads to miosis and oculomotor to mydriasis, looking for these as associated signs will further help differentiate the source of the ptosis.[17]

From an orthopedic perspective, ptosis may mean a neurovascular compromise. If the thalamus, reticular formation or the descending sympathetic nerve are affected, Horner's syndrome results and the ptosis will be accompanied by miosis, facial reddening, anhidrosis, and enophthalmos, as well as other neighborhood signs. Other possible sites for damage that could cause Horner's syndrome are the thoracic outflow, the inferior or the superior cervical ganglion, or anywhere along the sympathetic chain in the neck. If the third nerve is impaired the ptosis will be associated with pupil dilation and extraocular paresis or paralysis.

Horner's Signs[17] These are caused by sympathetic paralysis or paresis caused by a lesion affecting one of the following structures:

❑ Thalamus
❑ Reticular formation
❑ Descending sympathetic nerve

- ❏ Cervicothoracic outflow
- ❏ Inferior cervical ganglion
- ❏ Middle cervical ganglion
- ❏ Superior cervical ganglion

The most serious lesions are preganglionic (rostral to the inferior cervical ganglion), but for the therapist there is no way of clinically determining if a lesion is pre- or postganglionic, so all patients presenting with Horner's syndrome must be considered as suffering from serious pathology until proven otherwise. The physician can determine whether this is pre- or postganglionic by infusing the eye with cocaine and amphetamine solutions and watching for dilation.

The clinical signs of Horner's syndrome are

- ❏ Ptosis (small because of paralysis of Muller's muscle)
- ❏ Anhydrosis (lack of sweating)
- ❏ Miosis (constricted pupil)
- ❏ Facial flushing
- ❏ Apparent enopthalmos (retraction of the eyeball)

There are a number of causes, including

- ❏ Cervical lymph node inflammation or tumor
- ❏ Posterior fossa tumors
- ❏ Trauma to one of the cervical ganglion
- ❏ Dissection of the carotid artery
- ❏ Apical lung cancer invading the lower brachial plexus and ganglion (Pancoast's syndrome)
- ❏ Breast cancer invading the lower brachial plexus and ganglion (Pancoast's syndrome)
- ❏ Syringomyelia and syringobulbia
- ❏ Trauma of the cervicothoracic outflow
- ❏ Vertebrobasilar compromise lateral medullary (Wallenberg's) syndrome
- ❏ Idiopathic
- ❏ Hereditary (the iris is usually a different color blue from the other side)

Nystagmus[17,18] Nystagmus is nonvolitional rhythmic motion of the eyes and is sorted into two main types, jerk and nonjerk (an alternative method is spontaneous, gaze evoked, and gaze suppressed). In jerk nystagmus, the more common form, there is a fast component (saccades) in one direction and a slow recovery to midline. Nonjerk nystagmus is pendular, in that is there is no fast component and generally an equal displacement on each side of midline. Nonjerk nystagmus may be congenital, part of albinism, and is frequently associated with visual problems so that the eyes move to find the most sensitive spot on the fovea. Jerk nystagmus is caused by disturbances in the cerebellum or the vestibular system, including the labyrinth, nuclei, neural projections, and mechanoreceptors in the cervical spine. A subdivision of jerk nystagmus is central and peripheral. Central nystagmus is nystagmus of central neurological origin and is the more serious of the two, being caused by brainstem ischemia, neurological disease, and posterior fossa tumors. Jerk nystagmus is named after the direction of the fast component and can be lateral (the most common), vertical (upbeat and downbeat), converging, retracting, a combination of these, or seesaw, where one eye moves up and the other down. Central nystagmus has characteristics that differentiate it from peripheral nystagmus, whose commonest cause is labyrinthine dysfunction. The following table lists some of the characteristics that are easier to identify on clinical examination.

Central	Peripheral
Brainstem neighborhood signs, possibly Wallenberg's syndrome if VBI (Vertebrobasilar ischemia)	± sensorineural or conduction hypoacusia/tinnitus depending on the cause
Vertigo intensity mild to moderate	Vertigo intensity mild to severe
Vertigo duration long (may be indefinite)	Vertigo duration short (0–2 min)
Vertigo and oscillopsia possibly related to the nystagmus and not head movement	Vertigo and oscillopsia related to head movement
Horizonal or vertical nystagmus and without a torsional element, but possibly purely torsional	Usually horizontal, always has a torsional element combined with the linear displacement
Positional nystagmus usually static and direction changing	Positional nystagmus usually paroxysmal and may be direction fixed or changing
Gaze evoked	Gaze suppressed after short period (<1 week)

There are numerous causes of nystagmus, most of which are relatively benign, but the orthopedic therapist usually does not have the knowledge, training, skills, or tools required to determine if a particular case falls into this category, so, in the event of meeting a previously undiagnosed case of nystagmus, it is prudent to refer the patient to a physician for further investigation.

The following table looks at the various types of nystagmus and its causes.

Type	Characteristics	Causes
1. Spontaneous	• Not dependent on gaze of head position although may be worsened, eased, or altered by gaze direction	
Congenital	• Spontaneous • Fixation dependent • May be monocular (latent) • High-frequency (2 to 6 bps) • May be pendular	• Congenital
Pendular	• Nonjerk • High-frequency	• Congenital • Multiple sclerosis • Retinopathies
Periodic alternating (PAN)	• Periodically changes direction with change of head or eye position • Cycles	• Congenital • Brainstem ischemia (VBI) • Multiple sclerosis • Syphilis • Syringobulbia • Trauma
Peripheral	• Combined torsional-horizontal but mainly horizontal • Inhibited by fixation • Obeys Alexander's Law	• Peripheral vestibular dysfunction • Cervical dysfunction
Central	• Pure vertical, horizontal, torsional or combined • Not dependent on fixation • Gaze directed into direction increases frequency • Gaze directed away from direction changes direction	• Eighth nucleus • Cerebellar atrophy • VBI • Arnold-Chiari • Multiple sclerosis • Medullary tumors and infarcts
2. Gaze evoked	• Unable to maintain stable eye deviation away from central position and corrective saccades reset gaze position • Always in direction of the gaze	
Symmetrical	• Equal left-right amplitude	• Medication (phenobarbital, phenytoin, diazepam, alcohol) • Myasthenia gravis • Multiple sclerosis • Cerebellar atrophy
Asymmetrical	• Unequal left-right amplitude • May be combined with peripheral spontaneous nystagmus with eighth neuromas	• Cerebellopontine tumors • Acoustic neuromas • Recovery from gaze paralysis

(continued)

Rebound	• Changes direction with fatigue or resetting of primary position	• Cerebellar disease and atrophy
Dissociated	• Overshoots the abducted position • The nonaffected eye adducts more slowly than the affected abducts	• Medial longitudinal fasciculus lesions, demyelinating diseases (bilateral), VBI (unilateral) • Myasthenia gravis (worsens as gaze is maintained)
3. Positional Peripheral paroxysmal	• Provoked by head positioning • Provoked by Hallpike-Dix maneuver • Associated with vertigo • Commonly has a 3 to 10-s latency period • Onset of high frequency but rapidly dissipates and rarely lasts >30 s • Often disappears with repeated testing • Combined torsional-horizontal • Usually provoked in one direction only, with recovery producing opposite direction nystagmus	• Head injury • Labyrinthitis • Internal auditory artery insufficiency (VBI)
Central paroxysmal	• Does not have latency period • Does not disappear with repeated testing • Lasts >30 s • Provoked by many directions of movement, and direction of nystagmus may change with direction of test • Often vertical • May or may not be associated with vertigo	• Brainstem lesions • Cerebellar lesions
Static	• Remains as long as the position is held • May fluctuate in frequency and amplitude • May be unidirectional or change with position • May be apparent after paroxysmal positional nystagmus has disappeared • Comes on with slow and fast positioning	• Peripheral vestibular disorders (most common causes) • Central lesions (nonsuppressible with fixation)

Facial and Eye Asymmetry[17,19] Look at the eye position. Strabismus (squint) may either be paralytic or nonparalytic. Nonparalytic strabismus is a nonneurological condition that occurs in childhood and persists if not corrected, it affects the nondominant eye. Paralytic strabismus occurs when one or more extraocular muscles are paralyzed or paretic and the unopposed pull of the antagonists cause malpositioning of the eye. The tracking tests discussed in the section on cranial nerve testing will determine which is which. Paralytic strabismus is associated with brainstem function compromise and needs to be referred back to the physician.

Facial droop is caused by an upper motor neuron lesion above the facial nucleus or a facial nerve palsy. If the muscles above the eye are involved, the droop is a peripheral palsy such as a Bell's palsy; if they are not, the lesion lies above the nucleus because there is a partial decussation of the corticobulbar tract fibers.[20]

Color Changes Grayness often indicates systemic disease and makes the patient look ill. Yellowness may be caused by jaundice, especially if the conjunctiva are also yellow. Causes of jaundice include bile duct stenosis, gallstones, pancreatic stones, pancreatitis, hepatitis, liver cancer, pancreatic cancer, gallbladder cancer, and hemolytic anemia—all conditions that require that the patient be further assessed by a physician. Facial flushing may be part of Horner's syndrome and can accompany carotid artery disease.

Speech, Language, and Voice Changes[21]

Listen for

- Dysphasia
- Dysarthria
- Dysphonia

In dysphasia the ability to say a word is unaffected but the ability to use the word appropriately is lost. Other than middle cerebral artery strokes, the most serious condition causing dysarthria that the therapist will likely come across is vertebrobasilar ischemia. Wernike's area is vascularized by the temporal branch of the posterior cerebral artery, the terminating branch of the basilar cerebral artery, so an embolus could cause dysphasia. Obvious strokes will never get to the therapist, so the signs and symptoms will be transient and may only show up on turning or extending the head. Consequently, dysphasia may only become apparent on testing the neck or vertebral artery or while applying treatment, and then only if the patient is talking. Listen for word substitutions, word omissions, and neologisms (new words that do not exist). The patient may talk around the subject to avoid a word that cannot be brought to mind. Aphasia, the complete loss of the spoken word, is caused by an infarct in Broca's area, which is supplied by the middle cerebral artery, a branch of the internal carotid.

In dysarthria, the correct word is chosen but is pronounced incorrectly. In cerebellar dysfunction, which may be the result of vertebrobasilar ischemia, the speech is slow and slurred, and it looks as if the patient has to work hard to articulate. A similar sound is heard if control of the mechanics of speech, the tongue and pharynx, is affected in medullary problems, again possibly because of vertebrobasilar problems.

Dysphonia is a voice aberration in which words are pronounced and used correctly, but the voice is usually low and rasping, sounding like laryngitis but without the pain. Dysphonia is caused by paresis or paralysis of the laryngeal muscle, which may result from ischemia of the vagal nucleus, which is supplied by the vertebral artery.

Notes

1. Kendall HO et al: *Posture and Pain.* Baltimore, Williams and Wilkins, 1952.

2. Kendall HO, Kendall FP, Wadsworth GE: *Muscles: Testing and Function,* 2d ed. Baltimore, Williams and Wilkins, 1971.

3. Lundervold AJS. *Electromyographic Investigations of Positions and Manner of Working in Typewriting.* Oslo, W. Broggers, Boktrykkeri A/S, 1951.

4. Carlsoo S: The static muscle load in different work positions: an electromyographic study. Ergonomics 4:193, 1961.

5. Basmajian JV, DeLuca CJ: *Muscles Alive: Their Functions Revealed by Electromyography,* 5th ed., pp 252–264, 1985.

6. Portnoy H, Morrin F: Electromyographic study of postural muscles in various positions and movements. Am J Physiol 186:122, 1956.

7. Murray MP et al: Normal postural stability and steadiness: a quantitative assessment. J Bone Joint Surg Am 57:510, 1975.

8. McKenzie RA: *The Lumbar Spine: Mechanical Diagnosis and Therapy,* pp 35–36, Waikanae, NZ, Spinal Publications, 1981

9. Adams RD, et al: *Principles of Neurology,* 6th ed. (CD-ROM version). New York, McGraw-Hill, 1998

10. Cheng JC, Au AW: Infantile torticollis: a review of 624 cases. J Pediatr Orthop 14:802, 1994.

11. Cyriax J: *Textbook of Orthopedic Medicine,* 8th ed. Balliere Tindall & Cassell, London, 1982.

12. Stern PJ et al: Cervical spine osteoblastoma presenting as mechanical pain: a case report. JCCA 38:146, 1994.

13. Gilman S, Winans Newman S: *Manter and Gatz's Essentials of Clinical Neurology and Neurophysiology,* 7th ed., pp 59–62. Philadelphia, FA Davis, 1987.

14. Adams RD et al: *Principles of Neurology,* 6th ed., Part 5 (CD-ROM version). New York, McGraw-Hill, 1998.

15. Adams RD et al: *Principles of Neurology,* 6th ed., Part 4 (CD-ROM version). New York, McGraw-Hill, 1998.

16. Beals RK et al: Anomalies associated with vertebral malformations. Spine 18:1329, 1993.

17. Weiner WJ, Goetz CG: *Neurology for the Non-neurologist,* 3d ed., pp 315–318. Philadelphia, JB Lippincott, 1994.

18. Herdman SJ (ed). *Vestibular Rehabilitation,* pp 58, 115–164, 213–229, 251–257. Philadelphia, FA Davis, 1994.

19. Adams RD et al: *Principles of Neurology,* 6th ed., Part 2 (CD-ROM version). New York, McGraw-Hill, 1998.

20. Wilson-Pauwels L et al: *Cranial Nerves,* pp 82–95. Toronto, BC Decker, 1988.

21. Adams RD et al: *Principles of Neurology,* 6th ed., Parts 1 and 2 (CD-ROM version). New York, McGraw-Hill, 1998.

CHAPTER 4

The Musculoskeletal Examination

The differential examination that will be outlined in this book is a modification of James Cyriax's and is based on his concepts of selective tissue tension testing.[1] For the most part, the Cyriax examination is based on anatomy and pathology. The examination works on the principle of isolating the function of a tissue, as much as possible, and making it perform its action in that isolation. For example, having the patient perform an isometric contraction would test for a tear in a muscle belly or for a tendonitis. The nature of the contraction would minimize joint movement and the stress put through noncontractile tissues. However, it is apparent that some stress would be present in these noncontracting tissues, and compression and translation would still occur to some extent. As a consequence, the examiner must understand that no single test is capable of generating a diagnosis. Rather, it is the integration and analysis of all of the data, both positive and negative, that allows the therapist to come to a rational determination of the patient's problem.

Cyriax divided the musculoskeletal system into four parts:

❏ Inert tissues (capsule, ligaments, bone, bursa, fascia, dura, nerve tissue)
❏ Contractile tissues (muscle, tendon, tenoperiosteal junctions, near muscle bone, compressed bursa)
❏ Neurological tissues (afferent, efferent, and inhibitory functions)
❏ Vascular tissues (arteries and veins)

These are tested with

❏ Active movements (contractile and inert tissues)
❏ Passive tests (inert tissues)
❏ Resisted movements (contractile tissues)
❏ Myotome, dermatome, and reflex tests (neurological function)
❏ Repeated or sustained contractions (vascularization)

*Items 1 through 3 are discussed in this chapter. Item 4 is the subject of Chapter 5. Item 5 are special tests for vascular sufficiency which were discussed in Chapter 10.

Active Movements

Active motion testing nondifferentially tests the contractile and inert tissues of the musculoskeletal system and also the motor aspect of the neurological system in cases of profound weakness and patient motivation and anxiety. It does this by demonstrating the following:

❏ Range of motion
❏ Pattern of restriction
❏ Quality of movement
❏ Onset and type of symptoms
❏ The patient's willingness to move

Typically, the movements tested are the major movements (the cardinal movements), flexion, extension, rotation, abduction, adduction, and side flexion. The combined movements (quadrants) are generally not tested initially in the differential diagnostic examination for good reason. If the cardinal movements are positive in that they reproduce symptoms or demonstrate reduced movements, the combined tests usually add little if any further information and become redundant and potentially a source of confusion. For example, if cervical extension, right side flexion, and right rotation reproduce pain, then I can be very confident that the right posterior quadrant test that combines these movements will also reproduce the patient's symptoms.

There are situations where the combined movement tests become very useful if not indispensable. The spinal quadrants are

❏ Right Anterior: flexion, right side flexion, right rotation
❏ Left Anterior: flexion, left side flexion, left rotation
❏ Right Posterior: extension, right side flexion, right rotation
❏ Left Posterior: extension, left side flexion, left rotation

These quadrant tests can help differentiate the cause of lancinating pain. Here we know that the pain is caused by neurological tissue insult but we cannot be sure what is causing the insult. If the problem is stenosis on an inflamed spinal nerve, the pain should be reproduced with extension and/or unilateral extension to that side with the posterior quadrant tests. If a small disk bulge is compressing an inflamed spinal nerve, flexion or unilateral flexion away from the side (contralateral anterior quadrant test) may well produce the symptoms. A large herniation would probably cause lancinating pain with both the contralateral anterior and the ipsilateral posterior quadrant tests.

The quadrant tests may also demonstrate pain and restricted movement when the cardinal tests do not because the quadrant tests are at the full extreme of range. Usually, you cannot attain this with cardinal movements. To demonstrate, try this exercise. Extend your head as far as possible; now side flex it. You have just extended it past full range because the initial full range was symmetrical; that is, both sides of the segment underwent the same movement. You cannot simultaneously flex or extend both zygapophyseal joints. One joint or side of the segment has to unflex or unextend for the other to reach its full excursion of motion. The same happens in the periphery, at least in those joints that have fewer than three degrees of motion. Unless the conjunct rotation (see Chapter 9 "The Biomechanical Evaluation") is included in the movement, the motion being tested cannot reach its full range. The quadrant test includes that rotation. In sum, the quadrant test is a more functional test than is the cardinal motion test and is better at determining the functional ability of the patient.

The active range of motion is normally a little less than the passive range, and these two ranges should be compared. Is there severe, moderate, mild, or no restriction? The last should be assessed very critically because what is often taken for full range is slightly limited or slightly increased. In addition, in the spine in particular, remember that you are assessing multiple joints, and if one is hypomobile, there is an excellent chance that one or more of the others have been hypermobilized and are compensating and giving a false impression of full range. Painful hypermobility and/or instability can also fool you. The motion may automatically stop before the affected tissues become symptomatic, again giving an impression of full range rather than excessive range. If the range is restricted, what is the pattern of the restriction, capsular or noncapsular?

Recently, Cyriax's capsular patterns have been called to question, at least in the knee.[2] These patterns were often based on rheumatoid arthritic patients during quiescent periods and sometimes on acute systemic or post-traumatic arthritis.[3] This makes interpreting the pattern of restriction difficult. He did not always use every motion available at a given joint. The shoulder is a prime example of this because flexion and extension were ignored. It is also difficult to judge sometimes how he measured the restriction and from which neutral point. The hip demonstrates this clearly. Cyriax's pattern is gross limitation of flexion, abduction, and medial rotation, relatively slight limitation of extension, and minimal if any loss of lateral rotation and adduction. However, if you fix the ischium rather than the ilium, thereby better restricting the pelvis's ability to rotate anteriorly as you extend the femur, a different pattern is found. Now extension and medial rotation are the most limited movements. In the early case, the pattern is again often different, with extension and medial rotation being limited but painless and flexion, especially when combined with adduction and medial rotation, being painful. Perhaps a better way of determining the presence of an arthrosis or arthritis is to look for two movements that are not coupled to produce combined movements to be restricted and or painful. For example, in the wrist, flexion and extension should be affected rather than just extension and radial deviation, because these movements couple physiologically. Alternatively, flexion and radial deviation may indicate a capsular pattern of limitation. The end feels should be hard capsular, spasm, or a combination of both in different ranges.

Noncapsular restrictions are caused by nonarthritic or nonarthrotic conditions. We may not be able to be certain about what a capsular pattern is, but it seems likely that we can know what a noncapsular pattern should look like. When only one motion is restricted, it is safe to say that this cannot be caused by a lesion affecting the entire joint as a capsular pattern must. If only two movements are functionally coupled—that is, normal functional physiological movement employs these movements—the restriction is probably noncapsular. If the movement toward the close pack position is not at least painful, the pattern of restriction is probably noncapsular. There should be a capsular or spasm end feel (depending on the acuteness of the arthritis) at the end of at least one range. It is clear from this that any determination from the active movement tests that there is a capsular pattern present is extremely tentative and has to be confirmed with passive movement testing and the appreciation of the end feels.

The quality of motion is an important observation to make. Is it a smooth, practiced motion, or are there glitches? Painful arcs are evidence of abnormal motion and may be avoided by deviating the limb or trunk out of the optimal path of motion. Neck and trunk deviation also occur because of mechanical blocks, and these will be discussed in the region-specific examination sections. Recovery from a motion should be the same as the motion itself. An example in which this is not the case is in the lumbar spine, when after trunk flexion, patients have to walk themselves up their thighs with their hands to come back to erect standing. Abnormal recovery movement patterns often indicate instabilities. The inability to manage smooth, coordinated motion may be one of the first indicators of cerebellar problems from whatever cause. This finding demands a fairly detailed neurological examination of the patient, including cranial nerve and cerebellar tests. When you are watching spinal movements, the trunk may appear to move fairly normally, but does the spine? Look for segmental motion as well as trunk motion.

In some cases, active movement will not reproduce symptoms. The patient may have learned when to stop the movement before the pain starts, or the cardinal movements (uncombined movements) may not be sufficiently sensitive to reproduce the pain. In the more usual case, in which the cardinal movements do reproduce symptoms, what are they, when do they start in the range, and do they get worse as the patient pushes further into the range? The reproduction of lancinating pain or paresthesia with active movement indicates that a neurological tissue is being compressed, tractioned, or irritated in some other way. Generally, if this is allowed to continue, the patient stands little chance of quick recovery, so steps must be taken to limit these occurrences. The further distally referred pain is experienced, the more intractable the condition is likely to be and, again, the less often the patient reproduces this pain, the better.

Is there a painful arc in the range? If this occurs with trunk flexion, a small disk protrusion may be catching the spinal nerve at this part of the range. This is frequently associated with a painful arc in the straight leg raise, especially if the size of the bulge is not weight dependent to any great degree.

Passive Tests (Inert Tissues)

These include

❑ Physiological movements
❑ Ligamentous stress tests
❑ Nonspecific stress tests such as axial compression and traction
❑ Dural tests
❑ Upper limb neural tension/provocation tests

Inert tissues are those that do not have an inherent ability to contract or to transmit blood or neurological impulses include the joint surfaces, bone, joint capsule, ligament, bursa, and dura. Inert tissues are tested with full-range passive movements. These movements include physiological movements, ligament stress tests, dural mobility tests (straight leg raise, prone knee flexion or femoral nerve stretch, scapular retraction), spinal compression and traction, and vertebral posteroanterior pressures. Of course, passive movements will also apply stress to noninert tissues such as the muscle-tendon unit, blood vessels, nerves, spinal cord, and even, to a small extent, the medulla. This attribute is sometimes exploited when testing some of these structures. Vertebral artery testing is based on active or passive positioning of the neck and upper limb tension testing, which, among other things, tests the mobility and tension tolerance of those tissues composing the brachial plexus and its continuations into the arm and hand. For the main part any effect on the noninert tissues is considered complicating and is unwanted, but it cannot be eliminated entirely, so the therapist must again use judgment when interpreting the results of the passive movement tests.

❏ End feel
❏ Pain and other symptoms
❏ Range of motion
❏ Pattern of restriction
❏ Association between the onset of symptoms and the onset of tissue resistance

From these and their integration within themselves and with the rest of the examination, a fairly accurate picture of the state of the inert tissues can be built up.

End Feel

This is defined as the sensation imparted to the examiner at the end of the available range of motion. It affords information about the restrictor of the movement. Is it normal or abnormal, and if abnormal what is it? I believe that the end feel is a more valid way of assessing movement, especially with spinal segmental motion, for which objective measurement is all but impossible. The assessment of end feel rather than range of motion precludes the many problems associated with measuring actual motion and comparing it to normative data. The main problem is with the normative data. From what population was the sample taken? Were they men or women, old, young, or middle aged? Were they endomorphs, mesomorphs, or ectomorphs, or were they a mixture of ages, sexes, and body types? What size was the sample (was it large enough)? Was the normal figure arrived at the average, or was a range of normal values obtained, and if a range was given, what was it? What was the standard deviation? Is the patient whose range of motion you have just tested in the same population as that from which the sample was drawn? Is the difference in range enough to measure? In large joints with a gross loss of range, the answer to this last question is yes, but if the range of motion loss is small or the joint has a very small range of motion (the spinal joints spring to mind), goniometric error may prevent you from measuring the difference. In orthopedic manual therapy, the range of motion loss is usually very small, frequently less than five degrees. If the spine is being assessed biomechanically, then we are looking at segmental ranges of motion that are commonly less than five degrees. A restriction of 50% of range means that the therapist has to be able to pick up motion differences of less than three degrees. Now some (or maybe all) physical therapists may be able to do this, but I cannot, so I have to assess movement differently. I believe that the properly trained therapist can recognize the differences in end feel in both normal and dysfunctional joints. Does the joint feel stiff, jammed, reactive, squishy, devoid of end feel? These are all everyday terms for end feels, and most therapists can tell the difference with practice.

The following table presents a list of end feels, modified from Cyriax, together with their major identifying characteristics and a normal example of each.

End Feel	Characteristics	Normal Example
Capsular	Stretchable to a variable extent	Wrist flexion (soft) Wrist extension (medium) Knee extension (hard)
Bony	Abrupt and unyielding	Elbow extension in pronation
Elastic	Recoil	Ankle dorsiflexion with the knee extended
Springy	Rebound	No normal example in physiological movements, but compression testing of the cervical spine produces it
Boggy	Squishy	No normal example
Soft-tissue interposition	No resistance	Knee flexion; elbow flexion is capsular unless the elbow flexors are massively developed
Pathomechanical	Jammed	No normal example
Spasm	Reactive response in the opposite direction to the movement	No normal example
Empty	Limited only by severe pain and the examiner's reluctance to continue the test	No normal example

The following table lists the end feels and their implications both normal and abnormal.

End Feel	Possible Implication
Normal capsular	Normal range of motion
Hard capsular (stiff)	Pericapsular tissue hypomobility caused by arthrosis, adhesions, or scarring; requires some type of stretching, usually joint mobilizations
Soft capsular (loose)	Nonirritable hypermobility or instability; requires mechanical stress reduction with rest and/or mobilization techniques and/or orthoses
Bone in elbow extension	Normal range of motion with elbow extension in pronation or juxtapositioning from osteophytosis, fracture fragment angulation in any other range; no further movement obtainable
Boggy (squishy and limited)	Hemarthrosis; requires aspiration
Early spasm (reactive early in the range)	Treat the source of the spasm not the spasm itself; often caused by arthritis, grade 2 muscle tear, fracture near a muscle insertion, dural sleeve, or other meningeal compression and/or inflammation
Late spasm (reactive at the end of the expected range)	Caused by irritable hypermobility; avoid irritating the overstretched tissues and remove stress with mobilization and/or orthoses
Soft tissue interposition (squishy and unlimited)	Normally found only on knee flexion; other causes are massive development of muscles or obesity; no treatment
Elastic (recoil)	Muscle tone; usually muscle can be stretched through, but the gastrocnemius is designed not to allow the capsule to be reached, so ankle dorsiflexion with the knee extended should give this muscle tone end feel. In other cases of this end feel suspect hypertonicity. This may be caused by segmental facilitation.
Springy (rebound)	This is not normal with physiological movements and is present with internal derangements such as meniscal injuries and loose bodies.
Pathomechanical (jammed)	Always abnormal; it can be very hard like bone or more springy like the internal derangement. It indicates a biomechanical dysfunction requiring manipulation or nonrhythmic mobilizations.
Empty	No end feel is reached. The therapist stops the test because of the extreme pain and distress the patient is exhibiting. This is almost always caused by serious pathology in structures that are incapable of provoking spasm.

I can remember learning to appreciate end feels, or at least trying to. I can also remember thinking that the instructor was talking out of the top of his head because everything I felt, felt the same. I eventually came to realize that the first resistance that is met on passively moving a joint is muscle, and if this is not stretched sufficiently, the underlying end feel cannot be appreciated. To obtain the end feel of the ultimate, rather than the initial, restrictor in joints with minimal movement loss, the force applied has to be sufficient to stretch the muscle enough to reach the restrictor. With more dramatic range loss, this is not a problem because the range does not reach the point where muscle is capable of acting as a passive barrier. Consequently, spasm, severe arthrosis, subluxation, fibrosis, and any other cause of severe tissue shortening can be felt without applying the same magnitude of force necessary in normal or minimally reduced ranges.

A question that always arises is whether the therapist should apply overpressure in the presence of pain. Often the teaching is to not do this because it might damage the patient further. However, almost all relevant end feels will be experienced in the painful range. The empty end feel can only be felt in the painful range, and the same is true for early spasm. Consequently, if the end feel is not sought in the painful range, there is no point in performing any passive movements on the patient because no relevant information will be forthcoming.

In addition to evaluating the restrictor of the movement, the acuteness of the condition can be assessed. By comparing the onset of tissue resistance to the onset of pain, a pseudo-quantifiable estimate of acuteness can be reached.

Pain/Resistance Relationship	Acuteness	Possible Pathology
Pain and no resistance	Empty end feel	Usually serious pathology
Constant pain	Hyperacute	Very acute arthritis, system arthritic flare-up, overt fracture, cancer, visceral problems
Pain felt before resistance	Acute (mainly inflammation)	Typical after injury, acute traumatic traumatic arthritis
Pain with resistance	Subacute (chemomechanical)	Subacute traumatic arthritis
Pain felt after resistance	Chronic or nonacute (mechanochemical)	Usual coupling seen, usually mechanical dysfunction
Resistance without pain	Stiff (mechanical)	It is unusual to have a patient present this way as the main complaint, but during treatment, the coupling can go from pain after resistance to resistance and no pain.

Range of Motion and Pattern of Restriction

In addition to assessing the end feel, the examiner using a passive movement test should also look at the angular displacement that the joint undergoes during testing. This will afford an idea of the range of motion (given the limitations already discussed) and the pattern of restriction.

The passive range of motion should also be compared to the active range. Normally the passive range is a little greater than the active. If it is greatly increased, the possibilities are that the patient is

❑ Overanxious
❑ Amplifying
❑ Fabricating

If the movement at a joint is restricted, assess the pattern of restriction. This can be more easily done with passive movements than with active ones because the patient's anxiety or gain issues are minimized. Is the restriction capsular or noncapsular? In light of some of the concerns regarding the validity of capsular patterns, care should be taken when coming to the conclusion that there is one present, and a more flexible approach to the definition of capsular patterns should be taken (see "Active Movements").

However, for those of you who would be more comfortable with established patterns (and only the knee has been demonstrated experimentally to be suspect), the following lists the capsular patterns as described by Cyriax.

Region or Joint	Capsular Pattern of Restriction
Neck	Side flexion and rotation equally limited bilaterally; flexion full or nearly full, and extension limited
Sternoclavicular	Pain at the extremes of shoulder range
Acromioclavicular	Pain at the extremes of shoulder range
*Glenohumeral	Lateral rotation most limited, abduction next limited, and medial rotation least limited
Elbow	More limitation of flexion than extension, with pronation and supination only being affected in more severe arthritis
Inferior radioulnar	Full ranges with pains at extremes
First carpometacarpal	Limitation of extension and abduction, full flexion
Interphalangeal	Flexion more than extension
*Thoracic	Almost impossible to determine except in gross arthritis
*Lumbar	Almost impossible to determine except in gross arthritis

*These patterns as given are those described by Cyriax. I do not agree completely with these and the differences will be described when that part of the body is discussed.

Sacroiliac	Pain when stress falls on the joint
Symphysis pubis and sacrococcygeal	Pain when stress falls on the joint
Hip	Gross limitation of flexion, abduction, and medial rotation, slight limitation of extension, and minimal or no limitation of adduction and lateral rotation
Knee	Gross limitation of knee flexion, slight limitation of extension, with rotation remaining unaffected except in gross arthritis
Superior tibiofibular	Pain when biceps contraction stresses the upper joint
Inferior tibiofibular	Pain when mortise is stressed
Ankle	Plantaflexion more than dorsiflexion if the muscles are of normal length
Talocalcaneal	Limitation of varus (inversion) until in gross arthritis it fixes in valgus
Midtarsal	Limitation of dorsiflexion, plantaflexion, adduction, and medial rotation with abduction and full-range lateral rotation
First metatarsophalangeal	Gross limitation of extension and slight limitation of flexion
Other metatarsophalangeals	Variable; usually tend to fix in extension with the interphalangeal joints flexed (claw toes)

By assessing the end feel, its association with the symptoms, and the range of motion, the examiner can make a provisional determination of the range of motion and the acuteness and seriousness of the condition. The proviso will be the remainder of the examination.

A potentially serious sign is the patient with continuous or constant pain who has full-range pain-free movement. It is reasonable to expect that musculoskeletal conditions causing constant or continuous pain will have significant signs. Various types of bone cancer have been reported to appear in this way, and visceral conditions will for the most part be unaffected by physical stress.

Ligament Stress Tests

Partial or complete rupture of the ligaments or gradual overstretching of ligaments is a cause of one type of instability, the ligamentous instability. The second type of instability, articular or segmental instability, for the peripheral and spinal joints, respectively, is discussed in Chapter 2. Ligaments prevent movements that should not take place at all, such as abduction of the extended knee, or limit movements that should occur, such as inversion of the foot. Insufficiency of a ligament leads to instability of the joint. How fast this instability occurs depends on the presence and thickness of secondary restraints and the stress that the joint is made to tolerate. Another factor to consider is whether the instability is clinical or functional; that is, does it interfere with the patient's function, or is it simply a clinical finding? The implications for treatment are different for each. Determining which is the case can be difficult. The following are the criteria that may be considered provisional indications for beginning a course of stabilization therapy:

❑   Sudden, moderate to severe trauma
❑   Episodic pains
❑   Unpredictable behavior of the problem to treatment or everyday stresses
❑   Symptom-related clicks or clunks
❑   Symptom-related feeling of instability
❑   Hypermobility
❑   Recurrent subluxations
❑   Locking
❑   Giving way

The initiation of stability therapy depends in part on finding the instability but more importantly on having one or more of these characteristics present. Instability is not always detectable clinically.

Ligament stress tests are carried out by fixing one bone to which the ligament is attached and moving the other bone away from it such that the connecting ligament is stretched maximally. Obviously, to avoid doing further damage, the stress must be gradually progressive until a positive test is obtained or until the therapist is satisfied that the test is negative. There is no set time to hold the stress. Some teach that the stress must be held for 5, 10, or 30 seconds so that creep can be taken out. Creep cannot be taken out in this length of time.[4] Even if it could, is the period suggested in a thick ligament or a thin ligament, in an adult or a child, in a woman or a man, in an ectomorph or an endomorph, in an athlete or a nonathlete? Each of these people would have a different thickness for the same ligament, so each would demand a different period of stressing. It is better to hold the stress until a normal end feel is felt, at which point you have taken out the crimp, which is about all you can expect to do in less than 15 minutes.

A positive ligamentous stress test is one in which there is

❑   Pain
❑   Excessive movement
❑   A softer end feel than should be present

Positive tests can be classified as follows:

Grade	Characteristics
1, minimal tear	Pain with no excessive movement and normal capsular end feel
2, partial tear	Pain with moderate excessive movement and abnormally soft capsular end feel
3, complete tear	No pain with severely excessive movement and very soft capsular end feel

The classification system can be confused with an old grade 2 tear that is no longer irritable but still allows excessive movement. This can appear to be a grade 3 tear. Careful evaluation of the history and end feel must be made to determine which it is.

In the peripheral joints, the need for ligamentous stress testing is obvious. In the spine, it is less so. The transverse ligament and alar ligament are two ligaments that are routinely tested; the iliolumbar ligament is less commonly evaluated. These tests are discussed in their relevant chapter. The differential diagnostic stress tests in the spine and pelvis are

- ❑ Transverse ligament
- ❑ Alar ligament
- ❑ Compression
- ❑ Traction
- ❑ Anteroposterior
- ❑ Torsional (rotational)
- ❑ Sacroiliac primary (compression and gapping)

Compression and traction may both be used as stress tests in all areas of the spine. Compression will stress the disk, the vertebral body, and the end plate. Unfortunately, acute zygapophyseal joint problems will also become painful when this stress is applied to the region in which they lie. Traction has been postulated to stress the anulus fibrosis, the zygapophyseal joint capsules, the long ligaments, and the interspinous ligaments. Pain is the positive for traction as a stress test; relief of pain may be used as an indicator of relief of stress from disk or stenotic compression.

Posteroanterior pressures over the vertebrae are also a form of stress test, although not a very good one because they do produce a good deal of physiological motion. It is therefore difficult to say with any degree of certainty that any reproduced pain is due to ligamentous damage.

Pressure over L3, for example, will produce an anterior shear at L3-4 but a posterior shear effect at L4-5. At the same time L2 will extend while L4 flexes, both resulting in extension at L2-3 and L3-4. If the inferior vertebra of the segment to be tested with a posteroanterior pressure can be stabilized, the test becomes more useful as a stress test because it produces a purer anterior shear and extends only one segment. General torsion can be tested in the lumbar spine by stabilizing T12 and pulling directly back on the anterior superior iliac spine. This results in contralateral axial rotation of the spine. If this reproduces pain, each segment can be tested individually by stabilizing the superior bone and pulling through the innominate. In all of these tests, the therapist looks for excessive movement, spasm end feel, and pain. However, because there are many causes of these signs and symptoms other than instability, the diagnosis is very provisional, and biomechanical segmental stability tests should be carried out and correlated with the patient's history.

The sacroiliac joints are stress tested, but for inflammation rather than instability. Commonly called *anterior gapping* and *posterior compression,* the tests seek to reproduce the patient's sacroiliac pain. If the results are positive, inflammation is suggested.

Dural (Neuromeningeal) Mobility Tests[1,5,6]

The dura is tested both centrally and peripherally. The dural sheath is not stretch sensitive but does seem to be sensitive to compression and is certainly very sensitive to inflammation; meningitis demonstrates that very nicely. The dural sleeve is innervated by the sinuvertebral (recurrent meningeal) nerve from its own level and the adjacent levels. Consequently, the pain experienced when this tissue is producing pain is multisegmental rather than segmental and has no defined boundaries in the way a dermatome does. For example, when the straight leg raise test produces dural pain, it may be positive for pain felt in the leg, the back, or the buttock, or all three. Of course, the dural sleeve cannot be tested in isolation, because the neural tissue contained within it must also move to some degree. The pain produced by the dura is somatic, that is, an ache, not the lancinating pain or paresthesia of neurological tissue. If paresthesia or lancinating pain is felt, then tissues other than or in addition to the dura are being irritated and the condition must be considered more serious. The dural tests are

Test	Dural Sleeve Tested
Neck flexion (central)	Nonspecific
Coughing (central)	Nonspecific
Inspiration (peripheral)	Thoracic levels
Scapular retraction (peripheral)	First thoracic

Trunk flexion (central)	Nonspecific
Trunk extension (central)	L2-3
Slump (central and peripheral)	Nonspecific
Straight leg raise and adjunct tests (peripheral)	L4-S2
Prone knee flexion (femoral nerve) (peripheral)	L2-3

Neck flexion moves the dura centrally by elongating the spinal column. Consequently, it cannot be assigned a particular level or levels because it moves the entire spinal dura. Coughing raises the intrathecal pressure and again can only be considered as nonspecific. Trunk flexion is akin to cervical flexion but can be isolated from the neck by having the patient keep the neck in a neutral position or extension. In fact this is not necessary, because the dysfunctional point will identify its region of location by the site of the pain. Trunk extension moves the femoral nerve dural sleeve. Because this nerve passes anterior to the hip, it can be distinguished from pain from the lumbar joints by having the patient bend from the waist rather than from the hips. The slump test moves the dura both centrally and peripherally, depending on the sequence in which the test is carried out, and moves all of the spinal dura. The straight leg raise moves the fourth lumbar through the second sacral dural sleeves and is peripheral. Prone knee flexion tests the mobility of the femoral nerve dura by pulling it during knee extension.

The region-specific tests are discussed in Section 3.

Resisted Movements (Contractile Tissues)

The contractile tissues mainly comprise the muscles, tendons, tenoperiosteal junctions, and underlying bone. However, other structures may be substantially affected by the contraction of the muscles and become painful when this occurs. Holding sometimes honorary memberships in the contractile tissue club because of this are bursae and bone in particular. The contractile tissues are tested by isometric contraction. Despite what was to my mind a somewhat flawed (there was no evidence that the type of muscle injury susceptible to selective tissue tension testing had occurred) showing of the contrary,[7] there is no reason to doubt the original observations made by Cyriax concerning the response of injured contractile units. Lesions of the contractile and noncontractile tissues that would show up positive for pain or weakness on isometric testing include the following:

❏ Grade 1 through 3 tears of the belly or tendon
❏ Tendonitis (often considered as a grade 1 tear)
❏ Tenoperiostiitis
❏ Bursitis
❏ Fractures near a tendon insertion
❏ Acute arthritis, particularly rheumatoid and infective arthritis
❏ Bone cancer near a tendon insertion

Cyriax advocated that these tests be carried out in the resting position of the joint to minimize articular stress during the test and false positives. However, a more efficient procedure is to carry out the isometric contraction in the stretched position of the muscle if that position is attainable. When this positioning is combined with a maximum force contraction, the contractile tissue has been stressed as fully as possible. This saves retesting all of the negative tests in the resting position, but Cyriax was correct in his feelings of false positives. Any significant inflammation of the joint or irritation of the joint capsule will be painful when tested using this technique. Perhaps the best marriage of specificity and efficiency occurs when a minimal progressing to maximal contraction is carried out in the stretched position. If this does not prove to be positive, nothing further needs to be done in the assessment for contractile lesions. However, if there is pain or weakness, the contraction is repeated from minimal to maximal in the resting position of the muscle. From these two tests, the placement of the "positiveness" of the test on a spectrum can be made. When a minimal contraction in the rest position of the muscle of the muscle is painful, the test can be considered strongly positive for a contractile lesion. However, if it takes a maximal contraction in the stretched position to reproduce pain, the test is weakly positive for a contractile lesion and other explanations are as likely or more likely.

There are two variables to be considered when carrying out contractile tests, pain, and weakness. Extensibility, although important for other reasons, will play no role in assessing for contractile lesions. Each test will generate information about these leading to four variables:

❏ Painless and strong
❏ Painless and weak
❏ Painful and strong
❏ Painful and weak

A test resulting in a maximum contraction that in the stretched position was painless and strong would suggest that there is little if anything wrong with the contractile tissues being tested. A finding of painless and weak on testing might suggest a neurological palsy, segmental facilitation, a grade 3 (complete) tear in which there was no tissue to irritate, deconditioning, and painless inhibition from an articular problem (quadriceps inhibition from a meniscus tear would be one example). A painful and strong contraction could indicate the presence of a minor contractile lesion such as a tendonitis, a grade 1 tear, or a bursitis. The final combination is the most worrisome, because it can be a grade 2 tear but may also be acute arthritis, bone cancer, or a fracture. Finding painful weakness demands a very careful examination of the patient.

Notes

1. Cyriax J: *Textbook of Orthopedic Medicine,* 8th ed. London, Balliere Tindall & Cassell, 1982.

2. Haynes KW et al: An examination of Cyriax's passive motion tests with patients having osteoarthritis of the knee. Phys Ther 74:697, 1994.

3. Cyriax J: Personal communication, 1972.

4. Bogduk N, Twomey LT: *Clinical Anatomy of the Lumbar Spine,* 2d ed., pp 53 – 64, Churchill Livingstone, Edinburgh, 1991.

5. Slater H et al: The dynamic central nervous system: examination and assessment using tension tests, in JD Boyling, N Palastanga (ed): *Grieve's Modern Manual Therapy,* 2d ed. Edinburgh, Churchill Livingstone, 587, 1994.

6. Butler DS: *Mobilization of the Nervous System.* Edinburgh, Churchill Livingstone, 1991.

7. Franklin ME et al: Assessment of exercise induced minor muscle lesions: the accuracy of Cyriax's diagnosis by selective tissue tension paradigm. J Orthop Sports Phys Ther 24:122, 1996.

CHAPTER 5

The Neurological Tests

The neurological tests include the function of the

- ❏ Central nervous system (cortex, cerebellum, brainstem, and spinal cord)
- ❏ Spinal nerve and root (afferent and efferent functions)
- ❏ Peripheral nerve (afferent and efferent functions)

They do this by investigating the integrity of the myotome (key muscles), dermatome, and reflexes.

The standard neurological tests in the differential diagnostic examination look at strength, fatigability, sensation, deep tendon reflexes, and the inhibition of those and other reflexes by the central nervous system. It is worth noting that one surgical study comparing neurophysiological tests (including dermatomic evoked potentials) with the level of disk lesion found on surgery concluded that "neurophysiology is not useful to diagnose the exact level of a nerve root lesion, but may reveal whether it is present."[1]

Myotome Tests

The efferent system is tested with resisted movement tests to muscles that are most representative of the motor innervation from a given spinal segment. We use the word *myotome* incorrectly in this regard because it is actually an embryological term that means "a muscle or group of muscles innervated exclusively from one segment." There are very few of those muscles in the body. With the possible exceptions of the multifidus, the rotatores, and the suboccipital muscles, multiple segments supply all others. The term *key muscle* is more precise, but *myotome* is in such common misusage that it will almost certainly continue.

Evaluating the strength and fatigability of the muscles innervated primarily from its segment tests the myotome. A key muscle, that is, one that is most representative of the supply from a particular segment, is selected, and it is made to undertake a maximum contraction. To ensure that the contraction is maximal, the therapist must break the contraction; if this is not done, there is no guarantee that the patient has made maximum effort and that you are assessing the full power of the muscle. If the muscle is felt to be weak, two follow-up tests are carried out. Another muscle innervated mainly from the same segment, the alternate, is assessed for strength. If a segmental distribution is established, the possibility that this is a nerve root paresis is strengthened. Repeated contractions or a sustained contraction then assess fatigability. There is no experimental evidence for it, but the combined clinical experience of numerous Canadian and American orthopedic therapists over many years suggests that spinal nerve paresis causes abnormally fast fatiguing of the affected muscles. If a segmental distribution of abnormally fatigable weakness is found, spinal nerve or nerve root paresis is assumed. Hoppenfeld stated that "repetitive muscle testing against resistance helps determine whether the muscle fatigues easily, implying weakness and neurologic involvement."[2]

This assumption will be reinforced if a segmental distribution of hypoesthesia and/or deep tendon hyporeflexia is later found. If nonfatigable segmentally distributed weakness is discovered, other signs of segmental facilitation are sought. Segmental facilitation and its effects will be discussed later. Alternatively, a nonfatigable segmental weakness may be caused by an old root palsy that has not fully recovered its strength.

If paralysis rather than paresis is found, a diagnosis of spinal nerve palsy should not be made regardless of the distribution of the paralysis. Because multiple segments innervate muscles, paralysis is not an effect of compression of a single spinal nerve or root and the culprit must be looked for elsewhere. Because these culprits include serious neoplastic and neurological diseases and severe injuries to the brachial plexus, the therapist should eliminate the peripheral nerve as a possible cause and then refer the patient back to the physician.

Dermatome Tests

Because of the overlap of the segmental innervation of the skin,[3] only a small area within what we think of as the dermatome is exclusively or almost exclusively supplied by a given segment. This is the autogenous area and is composed of a small region, usually at or near the distal portion of the dermatome. This area varies not only between individuals but also within the same individual from day to day and possibly from hour to hour. The inter- and intrasubject variation is confined mainly to the size of the area rather than to its location. Grieve put it well when he said that

> the experimentally-observed size of an isolated dermatome is a variable quantity, and at any one moment is more of an index of the efficiency of sensory transmission in the same and neighbouring segments of the spinal cord, than an anatomically fixed cutaneous territory.[4]

The determination of skin sensitivity is a major key in the puzzle of neurological tissue involvement. There are many causes of sensory changes in the skin and many different types of change (and many different definitions depending on whom you read). These include

- ❏ Hypoesthesia: decreased light touch, pain, or heat sensation
- ❏ Anesthesia: complete loss of light touch, pain, or heat sensation
- ❏ Dysesthesia: the substitution of one sensation (usually pain) for another
- ❏ Hyperesthesia: increased nonnociceptive sensation
- ❏ Allodynia: the sensation of pain with a nonnoxious stimulus

Each of these can occur with a multitude of insults or disease processes. The pathologies include ischemia, infarction, compression, traction, neuromas, CNS neoplasms, and neuritis.[5] The tissues that can lead to sensory changes if so affected include the

- ❏ Spinal nerve, posterior root, or posterior root ganglion
- ❏ Spinal cord (anterior and lateral spinothalamic tracts)
- ❏ Cauda equina
- ❏ Peripheral nerve
- ❏ Brainstem (spinothalamic tracts and trigeminal nucleus)
- ❏ Thalamus
- ❏ Internal capsule
- ❏ Posterior sensory cortical gyrus

In orthopedic manual therapy, the most common lesion that we see affecting sensation is compression of the spinal nerve or root by a disk herniation, so the most common presentation that we see is one reflecting that pathology. Because there is so much overlap in the dermatome, compression usually results in hypoesthesia rather than anesthesia in the bulk of the dermatome but anesthesia or near anesthesia in the autogenous area. The amount of sensory loss depends on the degree of pressure exerted on the neural tissue, if compression is the cause, the amount of ischemia if that is the cause, and the length or amount of contact with the nucleus, if this is a factor. Large-scale anesthesia is not a sign of spinal nerve insult for the same reason that paralysis is not: There is too much overlap to allow anything other than autogenous area anesthesia.

How you test depends greatly on what you are looking for. If a spinothalamic tract problem is suspected or has to be eliminated, the limbs must be tested with both light touch and pinprick (temperature sensation does not need to be tested separately because it is carried through the lateral spinothalamic tract together with pain). If a spinal nerve or nerve root compression is being tested for, though, there is no need to test both, because we are simply interested in whether or not sensation impulses can pass through these tissues to reach the conscious level. Pinprick is generally regarded by neurologists as more sensitive than light touch for testing hypoesthesia because there is greater dermatomal overlap with vibration and light touch than there is for pain and temperature.[6] If light touch is to be employed for sensation testing, stroking the skin with the fingers does not do it. This is the least sensitive method for sensation testing because it is easily felt even in hypoesthesia. Better is the use of a monofilament, but still useful in orthopedic patients are the neurological brush or soft tissue paper.

If segmental hypoesthesia to pinprick is being tested for, it is best if the dermatome being tested is compared to the same dermatome on the other side of the body. The patient is asked if this is the same as that, this and that being the pinwheel sweep on the affected and unaffected limbs or sides of the trunk. Disposable pinwheels are best because these easily maintain the same amount of pressure and the entire dermatome can be tested in one sweep of the wheel. If light touch is tested, then patients are asked to close their eyes and indicate whenever they feel the dab of the instrument or tissue paper. The areas of reduced or absent sensation are mapped out for the autogenous area, and then the presumed dermatome is tested with pinprick to map out the whole of the hypoesthetic area.

As with paresis, the distribution of the sensory changes must be carefully evaluated. Does it conform to a segmental pattern, is it hemilateral, bilateral, or quadrilateral? The following are typical distributions and the tissues that cause those distributions.

❑ Segmental: spinal nerve or dorsal root
❑ Hemilateral: brainstem, thalamus, internal capsule, or cerebrum
❑ Bilateral: spinal cord, bilateral spinal nerve, or root
❑ Quadrilateral: spinal cord

Deep Tendon Reflexes

The value of reflex testing was discovered in 1875 by Erb, who used clinical observation and his knowledge of neurophysiology to develop the principles of deep tendon reflex testing.[7] Any muscle with a spindle has the potential to be reflexive when its intrafusal fibers are suddenly stretched. Striking the tendon or the belly of the muscle sharply with a reflex hammer will test the afferent and efferent function of the peripheral nerve, spinal nerve, and cord pathways. It also tests the ability of the central nervous system to inhibit the reflex. Although it is useful to grade the response in neurology, this is not as important in orthopedic manual therapy. For our purposes the reflex can be classified much more simply as

- ❏ Areflexic
- ❏ Hyporeflexic
- ❏ Brisk
- ❏ Hyperreflexic

Generalized hyporeflexia or even areflexia can have many causes including neurological disease, particularly affecting the cerebellum, chromosomal metabolic conditions, anxiety, hypothyroidism, and schizophrenia.[8] Peripheral neuropathy, spinal nerve or spinal root compression, and cauda equina syndrome may cause nongeneralized hyporeflexia. Orthopedic therapists more commonly run into the latter group. Again, it is important to test more than one reflex if there is a possibility that the reflex is reduced or absent. This will allow the therapist to establish if the reduced reflex is part of a segmental or peripheral nerve pattern. If the reflexes are reduced or absent in a generalized distribution, one of these causes may be at play, but the cause may also simply be that patient's makeup. If the patient is not suffering from any symptoms other than pain, that assumption may be made. However, if there are complaints of symptoms that appear to be generated from the central nervous system or if any other central nervous system signs are found, the patient should be referred to the physician.

True hyperreflexia will have some degree of reverberation (clonus within it) that will distinguish it from an overly brisk reflex. However, the reverberation cannot be felt in most positive tests because of the way the reflex is tested. Unless the stretch is maintained during the test, the clonus will not, of course, occur and the reflex will simply look brisk. The exception to this is the Achilles tendon reflex. Here, the tester does hold the ankle in some amount of dorsiflexion during the test and clonus can be elicited. My suggestion is that if a reflex or reflexes appear brisk, redo the test but this time maintain a stretch. In addition, look for recruitment of other muscles during the reflex contraction of the target. A simple increase in briskness may be caused by segmental facilitation, some psychiatric conditions, hyperthyroidism, and high muscle tone.

Having determined that there is a change in the reflex, look at the distribution pattern of the change and any coexistent neurological signs. Are the changes segmental, bilateral, hemilateral, or quadrilateral? If all reflexes are absent or reduced, consider that this may be part of systemic condition, neurological disease, or simply the patient's makeup. Segmental hyporeflexia could be part of a spinal nerve palsy. Hemilateral hyperreflexia may be a sign of a brainstem or cerebral lesion. Quadrilateral hyperreflexia may be caused by spinal cord compression, multiple sclerosis, or some other neurological disease. Quadrilateral or hemilateral hyporeflexia may be caused by cerebellar disease. Other signs and symptoms are important in putting the reflexes into perspective. If there is reduced or absent reflexes, are there also weakness, hypotonia, and/or sensory changes? Hyperreflexia should be associated with a Babinski response to the extensor-plantar test, clonus, and/or spasticity. If there is spinal cord compression, there should also be some paresthesia, and if there is disk prolapse, there should be pain and articular signs to support the diagnosis. As with all else we do, each test that proves positive should be part of an overall picture that generates the provisional clinical diagnosis. No single test will provide this.

Notes

1. Tullberg T, Svanborg E, Isaccsson J, Grane P: Spine 18:837, 1993.

2. Hoppenfeld S: *Orthopedic Neurology: A Diagnostic Guide to Neurologic Levels,* pp 1 – 3. Philadelphia, JB Lippincott, 1977.

3. Denny-Brown D et al: The tract of Lissauer in relation to sensory transmission in the dorsal horn of the spinal cord of the macaque. J Comp Neurol 151:175, 1973.

4. Grieve GP: Thoracic musculoskeletal problems, in JD Boyling, N Palastanga (eds). *Grieve's Modern Manual Therapy,* 2d ed. Edinburgh, Churchill Livingstone, 1994.

5. Adams RD et al: *Principles of Neurology,* 6th ed., Part 2 (CD-ROM version). New York, McGraw-Hill, 1998.

6. Jaradeh S: Cauda equina syndrome: a neurologist's perspective. Reg Anesth 18:474, 1993.

7. Louis ED, Kaufmann P: Erb's explanation for the tendon reflexes. Links between science and the clinic.

8. Adams RD et al: *Principle's of Neurology,* 6th ed., Part 5 (CD-ROM version). New York, McGraw-Hill, 1998.

CHAPTER 6

The Special Tests

Special tests are nonroutine tests that are carried out only when there is an indication to do so either from something in the history or previous objective examination or from deciding on a particular treatment that requires some kind of pretest before it is carried out. For example, the presence of paresthesia in the arm may lead you to carry out an upper limb tension (provocation) test, or you may decide to mobilize a cervical segment, in which case, vertebrobasilar sufficiency testing would be appropriate.

Among the special tests in this differential diagnostic examination are

- ❏ Dizziness/vertebrobasilar sufficiency tests
- ❏ Equilibrium tests
- ❏ Vestibular screening tests
- ❏ Cranial nerve tests
- ❏ Selective long tract tests
- ❏ Spinal quadrant tests
- ❏ H & I tests
- ❏ Upper limb tension (provocation) tests
- ❏ Vascular tests
- ❏ Fracture tests
- ❏ Local specialized tests (Tinnel's, Finklestein's, Phalen's, etc.)

There are numerous tests for both the spinal and peripheral joints for various pathologies and symptoms—so many, in fact, that the clinician can get lost among the many different ways of doing the same test and the conflicting interpretations placed upon positive tests. David Magee has written an excellent book that reviews almost every special orthopedic text known.[1] In principle, it is best if a particular test is only carried out when there is a specific indication for it. In addition, do not do more than one test for each suspected condition because duplication is inefficient and can be confusing. The following table integrates the test with its indication. Most of the tests listed in the table will be dealt with in more detail in the discussions region-specific examinations.

Test	Indication	Test Protocol
Dizziness/ vertebral artery sufficiency	Complaints of dizziness, after trauma Before manipulation or mobilization Before any treatment likely to stress the vertebral artery	Carotid pulses, reproduction and differentiation tests Cranial nerve tests
Equilibrium	Complaints of dizziness or disequilibrium Observed disequilibrium or ataxia	Rhomberg's test, sharpened Rhomberg's test, single-leg stance, eyes closed and single-leg stance
Vestibular screens	Complaints of dizziness after trauma	Hallpike-Dix (once the vertebral artery is cleared)
Cranial nerve tests	Complaints of dizziness after trauma Central neurological symptoms or signs	Confrontation Consensual Tracking/convergence Facial sensation Jaw reflex Jaw clonus Smile/frown Body/head tilting Finger rustling/hum Uvular/phonation Resisted shoulder elevation Tongue protrusion
Selected long tract	Positive cranial nerve tests Long tract symptoms or signs	Strength Pain sensation Light touch sensation Proprioception Spasticity Vibration Graphagnosis
Spinal quadrant	Radicular symptoms Full-range and/or pain-free spinal movements	Flexion right rotation/side flexion Flexion left rotation/side flexion Extension right rotation/side flexion Extension left rotation/side flexion

H & I	Indications of segmental instability	Quadrant tests done with care on sequencing the side flexion and rotation in each quadrant
Upper limb tension provocation	Upper limb paresthesia Upper limb pain when the obvious cause cannot be found When a double crush syndrome is suspected	Applied constant length phenomenon in which the position of the elbow and wrist determine which main brachial nerve is moving, tensing, and/or being provoked
Vascular	Intermittent claudication symptoms Complaints of coldness or color changes in the periphery	Pulses Sustained or repeated exercises/contractions
Fracture	Sudden onset of post-traumatic pain Noises heard during trauma Failure to recover Angulation	Compression Shearing Percussion Tuning fork application Ultrasound
Localized specialized	Suspected specific pathology such as nerve compression, DeQuervain's syndrome, carpal tunnel syndrome	As the test dictates

Spinal Quadrant Tests

These are combined movement tests and can be used in any part of the spine. The patient is instructed to flex, side flex, and rotate to the same side in both directions, and to extend, side flex, and rotate to the same side in both directions. This test is particularly useful when the cardinal movements of flexion, extension, side flexion, and rotation are full range and pain free. Only the quadrants can take the zygapophyseal joints to their extreme ranges, and if only this part of the range is dysfunctional only this movement may reproduce the patient's pain.

Spinal quadrant tests are also useful in cases exhibiting neurological pain (lancinating or causalgia). Although the tester knows what tissue is causing the symptoms, he or she may not know what structure or tissue is aggravating the inflamed or scarred neural tissue or how severe the problem is. If we assume right leg pain, for example, the following patterns of quadrant pain may indicate disk prolapse, extrusion, or lateral stenosis.

If only the anterior quadrant reproduces the pain, the problem is unlikely to be caused by stenosis, because flexion tends to open the intervertebral foramen. An extrusion or large prolapse is more likely to be problematic into flexion and extension rather than just flexion. Therefore, an anterior quadrant position provoking lancinating pain is probably the result of a disk prolapse.

If only the posterior quadrant is positive for neurological pain, the most likely cause is lateral stenosis closing on an irritated spinal nerve or nerve root as it closes the foramen. If both quadrants cause neurological pain, there is either a very large prolapse or an extrusion.

Peripheral Differential Screening Examination

The purpose of a screening examination is to focus the examiner's attention on a particular area or movement, not to make a specific diagnosis. Furthermore, screening tests can only screen in, they cannot screen out, because even the best screening tests are not as comprehensive as a full examination. This must be remembered, or patients may be considered clear when in fact they are not. A screening examination must be quick and as comprehensive as possible without making the examination so long that it is just as quick to carry out the full examination. On the other hand, some of the quicker screens are not comprehensive enough and are not worth doing. A good screening examination, then, is comprehensive enough to give the examiner fair confidence that little has been missed and can be carried out fast enough to make doing it worthwhile.

There are various ways of screening for this part of the examination. The most common screening examination for the upper limb is to have the patient attempt to clench the hands behind the upper back. This is done by having the patient actively elevating and laterally rotating one arm and extending and medially rotating the other so that they meet (or nearly meet) each other at the level of the scapula. The movement is then reversed. This test certainly meets one criterion, because it is fast, but it is not very comprehensive because it does not test elbow extension or wrist motion. For the lower limb, the most usual way of screening is to have the patient squat. Again, this is very fast, but it does not test hip or knee extension, nor does it test ankle plantaflexion or eversion of the foot. In both the upper and lower limb screening tests, the examiner can have only the most modest confidence that the test has included most pathologies. A better test, although it takes a little longer, is to have the patient take the joint being tested through its full active range in each of the major movements; the therapist then applies overpressure, and then resists recovery of the movement, producing an isometric contraction. This gives the therapist an idea of the function of the neurological, inert, and contractile tissues. It does miss the stress tests, but no screening test is 100% inclusive. The test takes about a minute per limb, so it is longer than the other screening tests, but its inclusivity more than makes up for that.

A bigger question than how to do the test is what you are going to do with the results. For example, a patient presents with neck pain and your examination determines that there is a biomechanical dysfunction present that you are going to treat with manual therapy and exercises. You have included the peripheral screening tests in the examination, and these tell you that the patient has an asymptomatic restriction of lateral rotation of the right shoulder. Now what? OK, you do what the screening examination demands, a full examination of the shoulder, and you find that there is a specific restriction of lateral rotation of the glenohumeral joint, probably caused by post-traumatic adhesions or scarring. Are you going to treat this or ignore it? If you treat it, you run the risk of producing symptoms where none existed before. The counterargument is that not treating the hypomobility leaves the patient with increased predisposition to shoulder problems. There is no evidence to support this hypothesis, and there is little defense against a lawsuit under these circumstances. I would suggest that the screening examination not be carried out unless you are looking for something specific. An example of this would be when a tennis elbow has been diagnosed but there is no adequate explanation as to cause. Now screening the upper quadrant for a causal or contributing factor makes sense and with adequate explanation to the patient and sometimes to the physician, treating the demonstrated problem is legitimate.

Note

1.   Magee D: *Orthopedic Physical Assessment.* Philadelphia,
       WB Saunders, 1992.

CHAPTER 7

Cancer and the Orthopedic Therapist

The following is a broad and very shallow overview of cancer; for more information numerous oncology texts are available, two of which are predominantly used in this text.[1,2] It is not necessary for the therapist to understand the details of cancer or of its treatment. What is needed is a general knowledge of its incidence and its presentation to the orthopedic therapist; that is, what red flags it flies.

In addition to the more specific findings from the usual neurological and orthopedic examination that would alert the therapist to the need for referral to a physician, the following may show up in the general chat with the patient:

❏ Change in bladder or bowel habits
❏ A sore that does not heal
❏ Unusual bleeding or discharge
❏ Thickening or a lump in the breast or elsewhere
❏ Prolonged indigestion or difficulty in swallowing
❏ Obvious changes in a wart or mole
❏ Nagging cough or hoarseness

Incidence of Cancer[3]

In the United States, after heart disease (34%), cancer is the second leading cause of death (23%). One out of three people will at some point in their lives develop a life-threatening malignancy. Although the incidences of stomach and uterine cancers have decreased over the last 30 years, the incidences of other types have remained steady or even increased (lung cancer has increased by 160%). The 5-year survival rate for all cancers is now 50%.

Site	Male (%)	Female (%)
Skin (melanoma)	3	3
Oral	3	2
Lung	17	12
Breast	Negligible	32
Stomach	3	
Pancreas	2	2
Colon and rectum	13	13
Prostate	28	—
Urinary	9	4
Ovarian	—	4
Uterine	—	8
Leukemia and lymphomas	8	6
Others	14	14

The following table is adapted from the American Cancer Society's book[4] and is intended to make you a little more familiar than you might be at present with terminology for various cancers.

Originating Tissue	Benign	Malignant
Squamous cells	Squamous cell papilloma	Squamous cell carcinoma
Basal cells		Basal cell carcinoma
Glandular or ductal epithelium	Adenoma	Adenocarcinoma
	Cystadenoma	Cystadenocarcinoma
Transitional cells	Transitional cell papilloma	Transitional cell carcinoma
Bile duct	Bile duct adenoma	Bile duct carcinoma
Liver	Hepatocellular adenoma	Hepatocellular carcinoma
Skin	Nevus	Malignant melanoma
Sweat glands	Sweat gland adenoma	Sweat gland carcinoma
Sebaceous glands	Sebaceous gland adenoma	Sebaceous gland carcinoma
Renal epithelium	Renal tubular adenoma	Renal cell carcinoma
Testes and ovaries		Embryonal carcinoma
		Yolk sac carcinoma

Blood/lymph		Leukemia
		Lymphoma
		Hodgkin's disease
		Multiple myeloma
Nerve sheath	Neurilemmoma	Malignant peripheral nerve sheath tumor
Nerve cells	Ganglioneuroma	Neuroblastoma
Retinal cells		Retinoblastoma
Connective tissue		
Fibrous tissue	Fibromatosis	Fibrosarcoma
Fat	Lipoma	Liposarcoma
Bone	Osteoma	Osteogenic carcinoma
Cartilage	Chondroma	Chondrosarcoma
Muscle		
Smooth muscle	Leiomyoma	Leiomyosarcoma
Striated muscle	Rhabdomyoma	Rhabdomyosarcoma
Blood vessels	Hemangioma	Angiosarcoma
Lymph vessels	Lymphangioma	Kaposi's sarcoma
Synovium		Synovial sarcoma
Mesothelium		Malignant mesothelioma
Meninges	Meningioma	Malignant meningioma
Uncertain origin		Ewing's tumor

Cancer Pain Syndromes

The incidence of pain with cancer varies with the authority, but somewhere between 30%[5] and 90%[6] of all cancer patients experience pain at some point in their illness. Pain may occur as a direct effect of the tumor or as a result of the treatment, or it may be unrelated to the disease or the therapy.

Somatic pain is usually poorly localized and is described as a dull aching that, when it arises from the musculoskeletal or cutaneous system, is well localized. However, visceral pain is poorly localized and is often referred to the dermatome derived from the viscera's segment. Pleural, peritoneal, and pericardial pain can be very similar to musculoskeletal pain.

Neurological pain is felt as radicular or causalgic, and is often accompanied by paresthesia and dysesthesia. Somatic pain responds to normal analgesics, but neurological pain does not. This type of pain responds better to anticonvulsant and antidepressants.[6]

The three major causes of pain associated with cancer are

❑ Direct tumor involvement
❑ Iatrogenic
❑ Unrelated

Direct tumor involvement accounts for about 62% of pain in outpatient cancer patients and results from metastatic bone disease, nerve compression/infiltration, or hollow viscus involvement. Bone invasion is the most common cause of pain. The pain is believed to be caused by both the osteoclastic and osteoblastic activity from prostaglandin synthesis. Pain may also arise from pathological fractures, local nociceptor activation, and compression of nerves and vascular structures. About 25% of pain in outpatient patients results from radiotherapy, chemotherapy, or surgery, and about 10% of outpatient patients have pain unrelated to their cancer or their therapy.

Orthopedic Clinical Presentation of Neoplastic Disease

The presentations listed here may be found on the orthopedic examination and may indicate the presence of a neoplastic disorder.[7-11] However, it should be noted that in the majority of cases, these clinical features are of benign origin. Many neoplastic conditions will not demonstrate any of these features and will appear just like a run-of-the-mill biomechanical dysfunction. If a mechanical lesion does not respond rapidly to a mechanical treatment, the therapist needs to reconsider the differential diagnosis.

❏ Constant unrelenting or continuous pain (always some degree of background pain but varies in intensity)
❏ Nocturnal pain
❏ Waves of pain
❏ Severe spasm
❏ Expanding pain
❏ Empty end feel
❏ Signs worse than the symptoms
❏ Upper limb radicular pain with coughing
❏ First or second lumbar root palsy
❏ Two or more cervical or three or more lumbar roots affected
❏ Bilateral neurological signs
❏ Weakness and/or atrophy of the hand intrinsic muscles
❏ Nontraumatic lower thoracic pain in the elderly
❏ Forbidden area pain
❏ Horner's or Pancoast's syndrome
❏ Nontraumatic central nervous system (including cranial nerve) signs or symptoms
❏ Bone point tenderness, especially in the absence of articular signs

❑ Signs of the buttock
  a. Limited trunk flexion
  b. Limited hip flexion
  c. Limited straight leg raise
  d. Noncapsular pattern of restriction at the hip
  e. Painful weakness of hip extension
  f. Swollen buttock
  g. Empty end feel on flexion

Paraneoplastic Syndromes[12]

These result from the indirect effect of the tumor or its metastases and are remote symptom complexes. It is suspected that they are caused by an autoimmune mechanism. The neurological syndromes (cerebral, cerebellar, spinal cord, peripheral neuropathies, and autonomic) are associated with lung, ovarian, renal, breast, and gastrointestinal cancer, lymphoma, and Hodgkin's disease. Cardiovascular syndromes tend to result from cutaneous, urogenital, metabolic, and gastrointestinal cancers. Of those syndromes most relevant to the therapist, peripheral neuropathies are the most common and present in the usual way, with atrophy, weakness, areflexia, hypoesthesia or anesthesia, parasthesia, proprioception loss, and paralysis.

Neurological Syndromes

Cerebral syndromes are mainly associated with lung cancer and Hodgkin's disease, with the patient suffering dementia, cranial nerve deficits, seizures, depression, motor poliomyelitis, optic neuritis with bilateral scotomas, and decreased acuity.

Cerebellar paraneoplastic syndromes are mainly caused by lung, cervix, ovary, prostate, and colorectal cancer. The syndrome includes bilateral ataxia, nystagmus, dysarthria, and dementia.

Spinal cord syndromes should not be a problem for the orthopedic therapist because they involve rapid and progressive upper and lower motor neuron and sensory affects. Lung and renal cancer and lymphoma cause them.

Peripheral neuropathies are the most common neurological paraneoplastic syndromes and the ones most likely to get through to the orthopedic therapist because they most mimic orthopedic conditions with neurological involvement. They are associated with breast, lung, gastrointestinal, and thoracic cancers and lymphoma. Paresthesia, pain, areflexia, atrophy, weakness, proprioception and sensory loss, and paralysis may all be part of the syndrome.

Autonomic Neuropathies

These are caused by small cell lung carcinoma. Axonal and neuronal degeneration occurs and presents with orthostatic hypotension, neurogenic bladder, and altered peristalsis.

Neuromuscular Syndromes

These cause myasthenia gravis or similar diseases. They are associated with thymoma and cause weakness and excessive fatigability, although one condition (Eaton-Lambert syndrome) actually caused the patient's strength to increase with repeated testing. Because the hip and thigh muscles are weak and the areas are painful, the patient may end up in the therapist's office.

Other Syndromes

These include cardiovascular, cutaneous, urologic, reproductive, gastrointestinal, and metabolic diseases.

Bone Metastases

Pathology Almost all malignant cancers have the potential for metastasizing to bone, with 50% to 80% of breast, lung, kidney, prostate, gastrointestinal, and thyroid cancers producing metastases. These metastases are usually not life-threatening unless they affect the upper cervical spine, but they are painful and liable to allow fractures to occur as a result of what would otherwise be nonthreatening stresses. The incidence of bone metastasis has increased as improved therapy has increased survival rates in cancer patients. Pain is often caused by pathological fractures, but joint pain and direct bone pain from the presence of the tumor are also factors. Purely osteoblastic lesions may be asymptomatic until fracturing occurs.

Clinical Presentation A metastasis may be the first symptom of cancer, predating signs or symptoms from the primary tumor. Swelling may be seen if the joint is superficial or the patient is thin; there is usually point tenderness, decreased ROM (Range of Motion), spasm, painful weakness, parasthesia, and paresis if the fracture affects neurological tissue, and this can include spinal cord signs and symptoms. The pain is generally related to increased activity but is also relentless in nature, being present at rest and frequently worse at night. The effects of a paraneoplastic syndrome may be perceived and/or systemic effects such as weight loss, fever, malaise, and so forth may be present.

Investigations

X-Rays: These should be taken in at least two planes, including oblique views of the spine if it is involved. However, often more than 50% of the bone density must be lost before the x-ray demonstrates the presence of the metastasis.

Bone Scans: Technetium-90m is effective for demonstration of bone metastases but has a 10% false positive rate.

MRI/CT Scan: This is required only in the presence of neurological signs from spinal problems.

Management

Peripheral fractures are treated with rest; internal and external fixation with immobilization times 2 or 3 times longer than are conventional because of the slowness of bone healing when radiation therapy is being administered. Periarticular fractures are generally treated by joint replacement. Impending fractures (more than 50% cortex destruction or cortical lesions larger than 2.5 cm or 1 inch) may be fixed for prophylaxis. Spinal compression fractures are stable but painful and do not require surgical intervention. Cervical fractures are frequently unstable and, if so, require surgery.

Skull Base Metastases Pain precedes neurological signs by weeks. Plain radiographs are usually useless, with MRI and CT scans being more helpful.

Jugular Foramen Syndrome This is marked by occipital pain with reference to the vertex and the ipsilateral shoulder and arm. Head movement reproduces pain, and there is occipital tenderness over the occipital condyle. There is variable cranial nerve (those that exit through the occiput) involvement, which may include dysphonia, dysarthria, dysphasia, neck rotation and shoulder elevation weakness, ptosis, and Horner's syndrome.

Clivus Metastasis The symptom is vertex headache increased with neck flexion. Cranial nerves 6 through 12 are involved. Initially the signs and symptoms are felt and observed unilaterally, but they progress to become bilateral.

Sphenoid Sinus Bifrontal headaches with radiation to both to temporal regions and intermittent retro-orbital pain are experienced. There is often nasal stuffiness and fullness of the head, associated with diplopia and bilateral sixth cranial nerve palsy.

Vertebral Body Pain is early and precedes neurological signs, and if the cause is not detected early, irreversible neurological deficits such as paraplegia or quadriplegia may develop. In more than 85% of cord compression patients, metastases are present, and in 10% of patients with cord compression the only complaint was of pain.

Dens Fracture Pain results from the fracture itself and/or the secondary subluxation. There is often resultant cord or brainstem compression. The pain is felt to radiate over the occiput and into the vertex, and is exacerbated by neck flexion. Progressive sensory and motor signs are found initially in the upper limbs and are associated with autonomic changes. Manipulation and mobilization are extremely dangerous. MRI is the most useful imaging technique.

C7-T1 Metastases This is a common site for lung and breast cancer and lymphoma. The spread may be via the vascular system or more directly from involvement of the brachial plexus or the paravertebral space. The pain is usually localized to the adjacent paraspinal region and is characteristically a dull aching, constant pain radiating bilaterally to both shoulders. Percussion tenderness is generally present over the spinous process of the involved vertebra. If there is nerve root compression, there is radicular pain, usually unilaterally, in the C7, C8, and T1 distributions. Neurological findings include numbness and paresthesia in these distributions with weakness of the intrinsic muscles, triceps, and wrist flexors. Horner's syndrome may be present if the paraspinal ganglion has been affected. CT scanning is the best imaging technique.

Lumbar Metastases This mainly affects L1. The symptom is usually a dull, aching midback pain radiating to the SI area and iliac crest that may be unilateral or bilateral. That the pain is exacerbated by lying or sitting and relieved by standing is characteristic. Movement increases the pain, particularly movement from lying to standing. L1 or L2 motor or sensory palsy should always make the therapist concerned because disk lesions at these levels are rare.

Sacral Metastases Aching pain felt in the sacrum, coccyx, and/or low back is characteristic. The pain is worsened by lying or sitting and relieved by walking. There may be neurological signs, which include perianal sensory deficit and bowel, bladder, and genital dysfunction. The greater sciatic notch area may be tender, and there may be sciatic radicular pain if there is compression of the nerve. CT scanning is the imaging technique of choice.

Neurological Metastases

Tumor infiltration and sudden or progressive compression caused by pathological fractures give rise to the signs and symptoms. The tissues affected include the peripheral nerve, root, plexus, spinal cord, and meninges, and the pain can be somatic or radicular.

Peripheral Nerve Typically, the patient complains of constant causalgia, dysesthesia, and hypoesthesia. There is commonly radicular pain.

The most common area affected is the intercostal nerve from infiltration by a rib tumor. CT scanning images the condition best.

Brachial Plexus The lower plexus is the most common site (C7-T1), although breast cancer and lymphoma may well involve the C5-6 roots. Pain patterns will vary with the levels involved and may reach paraspinally down to the T4 region from the upper plexus and infrascapularly from the lower. Pain typically precedes motor signs, and these precede sensory ones. Spread along the nerve root to the cord is common, and 50% of these patients will eventually present cord signs and symptoms. Horner's syndrome may be present. CT scan is the best imaging technique.

Lumbosacral Plexus The most common infiltration occurs from gynecologic, genitourinary, and colon cancers. Pain was the presenting symptom in 90% of these patients; with weakness, in 60%, second; and numbness in 40%. Two types of pain are typical: local pain in the sacrum, SI joint, low back, or groin, and radicular pain in the lateral, anterior, and posterior leg. CT scanning is the best imaging technique, although MRI has not been fully evaluated for its sensitivity.

Leptomeningeal This is infiltration of the cerebrospinal fluid with or without neurological invasion. About 40% of these patients present with pain of one or two types—constant headaches with or without neck stiffness or low back and buttock pain. The pain results from traction on the tumor-infiltrated nerves and meninges. Lumbar puncture demonstrates the CSF changes, and myelography images the nodes on the nerves. Multilevel neurological signs and symptoms strongly suggest this condition.

Epidural Cord Compression Severe neck and back pain, which occurs from either local bone or root compression, is characteristic and is the presenting symptom in 95% of these patients. The pain is of two types:

1. Local pain over the involved vertebral body or radicular pain in the root, distributed unilaterally in the cervical and lumbar regions, bilaterally in the thoracic spine.
2. Neurological symptoms that will vary with the level of the lesion; 85% of patients with neurological signs have accompanying vertebral body lesions.

Multiple Myeloma

This condition composes 14.5% of all hematologic malignancies and 1.1% of all malignancies—4.6/100,000 males and 3.1/100,000 in females with 3.5 and 2.4 deaths per 100,000, respectively.

Pathology This is a plasma cell carcinoma (PCN) or plasma cell dyscrasia (PCD) that has multiple foci and mainly affects the bone, bone marrow, and extraosseous sites. The proliferation of monoclonal plasma cells results in osteclastic activity and consequent fractures and bone pain.

Risk Factor

- ❏ Age: Median age at diagnosis is 68, with <1/100,000 under age 40 and 28.2/100,000 by age 80.
- ❏ Sex: Males are at 1.5 times greater risk.
- ❏ Race: Blacks are at 1.8 times greater risk.
- ❏ Genetic: First-degree relatives are at greater risk.
- ❏ Previous Pathology: Patients with systemic inflammatory diseases such as RA, systemic lupus, and scleroderma are at greater risk.
- ❏ Occupation: Workers in printing, plastics, leather, woodworking, rubber, and petrochemical, and those exposed to arsenic, asbestos, and lead have increased risk.

Clinical Presentation Some patients are asymptomatic, and the condition is discovered incidentally during a workup for an unrelated condition. Most present with a combination of local and systemic signs and symptoms.

1. Local.   These result from bone lesions. Severe intractable pain, particularly low back pain, tenderness, and swelling occur in the majority of patients. Bone pain (60%), fractures (20%), and spinal cord compression signs and symptoms from vertebral compression fractures (15%) are also seen.

2. Systemic.   Anemia, hypercalcemia, fatigue, weakness, renal insufficiency, Reynaud's syndrome, intellectual dysfunction, headaches, mucosal bleeding, urinary tract infection, and mixed sensory/motor peripheral neuropathy are the usual indications.

Prostate Cancer

This is the most common male malignancy and the second leading cause of death from cancer, 85.5/100,000 occurring in males with 23.5 deaths per 100,000. The incidence is higher in Northwestern Europe and North America, lower in Scandinavia and the Orient.

Risk Factors

- ❏ Age: The median age for diagnosis is 70 years, and 70% of males over 90 years have a focus.
- ❏ Race: Blacks are at 1.5 times greater risk than whites, with a lower onset age.

❑ Genetic: The risk is slightly higher in first-degree relatives.
❑ Diet: High-fat diets are implicated.
❑ Previous Genitourinary Infections: Increased sexual activity is a risk factor, possibly because of venereal disease.

Clinical Presentation Early cancer may have no signs or symptoms.

1. Local.   Bladder irritation with hesitancy, nocturia, retention, frequency, and uncommonly hematuria.

2. Systemic.   Back and hip pain, fatigue, malaise, and weight loss. No paraneoplastic syndromes are associated with prostate cancer. Any elderly patient presenting with unusual back pain should have the prostate examined by the physician before any treatment is initiated.

Screening Programs Rectal examinations and prostate serum antigen (PSA) testing are recommended between ages 50 and 70 routinely, or from age 40 in those patients with a family history.

CNS Malignancy

These compose 1.7% of all cancers, with incidences of 7.5/100,000 males and 5.1/100,000 females, with 4.9 and 3.3 deaths per 100,000 respectively.

Risk Factors

❑ Age: Children are at higher risk.
❑ Sex: Males are 1.47 times at risk.
❑ Race: Caucasians are 1.5 times more at risk than blacks.
❑ Previous CNS Pathology: None.

Clinical Presentation

1. Local.   These manifestations depend on the locality of the tumor and include seizures, weakness, sensory changes, headache, nausea and vomiting, personality changes, and intellectual changes; gait disturbances such as ataxia, with cranial nerve dysfunction (because the brainstem is affected), and hemiplegia, decreased consciousness levels, hemianopia, and decorticate and decerebrate posturing.

Lung Cancer

This is the second most common malignant cancer in men, the third most common in women (after breast cancer), and the leading cause of death from cancer in both sexes. The incidence is 83/100,000 in men and 35/100,000 in women, resulting in 74 and 26 deaths per 100,000 respectively.

Risk Factors

❏ Age: Risk increases with age, with the incidence going from 1/100,000 at 30 years to 330/100,000 at 70 to 74. The average age at diagnosis is 60 years.

❏ Sex: Males are at 2.4 times greater risk than women, chiefly because of cigarette smoking habits.

❏ Race: Blacks 1.4 times more likely than whites to develop lung cancer.

❏ Genetic: First-degree relatives are 2.4 times more likely to develop lung cancer.

❏ Diet: Diets deficient in vitamins A and E and beta-carotene have been demonstrated to increase the risk of lung cancer.

❏ Smoking: This accounts for 85% of all lung cancers, with the risk being directly proportional to the amount smoked. Cigarette, cigar, and pipe smoking each have a decreasing risk. On stopping smoking, the risk decreases after 5 to 6 years and approaches that of nonsmokers after 15 years. Passive smoking increases the risk in nonsmokers by 2 to 3 times and accounts for 25% of cancers in nonsmokers.

❏ Previous Pulmonary Pathology: Other benign lung conditions seriously increase the risk of lung cancer—9% of COPD patients will develop lung cancer within 10 years.

❏ Environmental: Air pollution and occupational exposures (asbestos, arsenic, chromium, cadmium, formaldehyde, chloromethyl ether).

Clinical Presentation About 6% of patients with lung cancer are asymptomatic; most, being smokers, have a habitual cough, but this will change as the cancer starts to produce effects.

1. Local. Symptoms from the primary tumor depend on its location. Central tumors produce a cough, hemoptysis, wheezing, stridor, dyspnea, pain, and pneumonia. Peripheral lesions cause a cough, chest wall pain, shoulder and arm pain, pleural effusion, dyspnea, and Horner's syndrome.

2. Regional. Extension of the primary tumor to the lymph nodes, nerves, esophagus, superior vena cava, pericardium, and ribs may cause pain or other symptoms such as dysphagia, phrenic nerve palsy, superior vena cava syndrome, voice hoarseness, pericardial rub, distended neck veins, and tachycardia.

3. *Systemic.*   Metastases may cause pathological fractures, jaundice, abdominal pain and masses, neurological deficits, intellectual deterioration, weight loss, anorexia, weakness, and malaise.

Lung cancer paraneoplastic syndrome is associated with many syndromes that affect the cardiovascular, neurological, renal, gastrointestinal, hematologic, metabolic, skeletal, and dermatologic systems. Signs and symptoms may include fever, dementia, increased strength with repeated contractions (myasthenic syndrome), erythrocytosis, hypercalcemia, arthropathy, autonomic and peripheral neuropathies, and anorexia.

Examination

❏ History: Look for changes in cough, hemoptysis, smoking history, alterations in mental status, weight loss, and anorexia.
❏ Observation: Gauntness, skin coloration (anemia, jaundice, grayness, and dermatitis), reduced energy levels, mental processing, miosis, ptosis, anhydrosis, hemifacial flushing, voice hoarseness, and finger clubbing are all possible signs of lung cancer.

Pancoast's Syndrome

Superior sulcus tumors and breast cancers frequently invade the upper chest wall and brachial plexus, giving rise to Pancoast's syndrome. The cancer will usually invade the upper two ribs, leading to scapular, shoulder, and arm pain together with the neurological symptoms arising from the brachial plexus effects. These include radicular and somatic pain and parasthesia in the C7, C8, and T1 distributions. The stellate ganglion is often affected, causing Horner's syndrome (ipsilateral miosis, anhydrosis, ptosis, and facial flushing). X-rays and sputum analysis will usually generate the diagnosis, although often the anteroposterior x-ray will not show the lesion and special oblique views have to be taken.

If the ribs have been affected, passive neck side flexion away from the painful side may be limited and painful, with a spasm end feel, and isometric side flexion toward the side is painfully weak. There is sensation loss in the lower brachial plexus distribution, usually ulnar, along with intrinsic hand weakness and wrist flexor and finger flexor paresis. The presence of Horner's syndrome is a complete contraindication to any treatment until this has been diagnosed.

Breast Cancer

This is the most common cancer, accounting for 30% of all malignancies and 18% of all cancer-related deaths. The lifetime risk of cancer in women is about 10% and increasing, with the rate in women being 102/100,000 in females and 0.7/100,000 in males, with 27 and 0.3 deaths respectively.

Risk Factors

❏ Age: Incidence increases with age, going from 1/100,000 before 25 years to 400/100,000 at 80. The median age at diagnosis is 57.

❏ Sex: Females are more at risk than males by 146:1.

❏ Race: Risk is 1.2 times higher in white females than black.

❏ Genetics: The risk is uncertain in first-degree relatives, but 1.5 times higher in second-degree relatives.

❏ Previous Pathology: There is no increase in risk with fibrocystic changes. Following unilateral cancer, there is a 4 to 5 times increased risk of developing cancer in the contralateral breast.

❏ Endocrinal: Early menarche (before 12 years) increases the lifetime risk of cancer. Prolonged estrogen stimulation for postmenopausal problems increases the risk. There is no demonstrated relationship between oral contraceptives and breast cancer. There is an increased risk with late menopause (after 54) and a lower risk with early menopause. Early first parity (before age 18) lowers the risk, first parity after age 30 increases it, and not having children increases it further.

Clinical Presentation The primary tumor presentation will almost certainly not be a presentation problem for the therapist because this is usually a painless palpable breast mass. However, it is possible that the patient has missed its development and presents with symptoms of extension of the tumor into the brachial plexus or upper ribs (Pancoast's syndrome) or bone or neurological metastases have developed and brought the patient to the therapist.

Notes

1. Cameron RB (ed): *Practical Oncology.* Norwalk, CT, Appleton & Lange, 1994.

2. Holleb AI et al: *Clinical Oncology.* Atlanta, American Cancer Society, 1991.

3. Cameron RB (eds): Introduction to the cancer patient, in RB Cameron (ed), *Practical Oncology.* Norwalk, CT, Appleton & Lange, 1994.

4. Pfeifer JD, Wick MR: The pathological evaluation of neoplastic disease, in AI Holleb et al (eds), *Textbook of Clinical Oncology,* Atlanta, American Cancer Society, 1991.

5. Foly KM: Diagnosis and treatment of cancer pain, in AI Holleb et al (eds), *Clinical Oncology,* Atlanta, American Cancer Society, 1991.

6. Weissman DE: Principles of pain management, in RB Cameron (ed), *Practical Oncology,* Norwalk, CT, Appleton & Lange, 1994.

7. Cyriax J: *Textbook of Orthopedic Medicine,* vol 1. London, Balliere Tindall & Cassell, 1982.

8. Horowitz SM: Wrist pain in a 32-year-old man. Clin Orthop Rel Res 307:280, 1994.

9. Lopez-Barea F: Tumors of the atlas: 3 incidental cases of osteochondroma, benign osteoblastoma and atypical Ewing's sarcoma. Clin Orthop Rel Res 307:182, 1994.

10. Grod JP, Crowther ER: Metastatic bone disease secondary to breast cancer: an all too common cause of low back pain. JCCA 38:139, 1994.

11. Stern PJ et al: Cervical spine osteoblastoma presenting as mechanical neck pain: a case report. JCCA 38:146, 1994.

12. Roth P: Neurologic problems and emergencies, in RB Cameron (ed), *Practical Oncology,* pp 57–59. Norwalk, CT, Appleton & Lange, 1994.

CHAPTER 8

Summary of Chapters 1 Through 7

The differential diagnostic examination is a vital precursor to any biomechanical examination; it must be carried out to ensure that the physician has referred appropriate pathology or, in the case of direct contact, that the patient has walked into the appropriate setting. In addition, the examination is necessary to pinpoint the pathology. Diagnoses such as shoulder pain, low back pain, internal derangement, and rotator cuff syndrome are of no value in determining what treatment is required. The routine examination of the patient must include an examination that will produce a differential diagnosis or indicate the need for a biomechanical examination when a differential diagnosis is not attainable from the information generated from the examination.

The examination outlined in this chapter is that advocated by James Cyriax, M.D., and is based on selective tissue tension testing. The routine differential diagnostic examination involves the stressing of a specific tissue while that tissue's function is as isolated as possible from the other tissues of the musculoskeletal system. For the purposes of this examination, the tissues were classified as *inert, contractile, neurological,* and *vascular,* each of which was tested according to the principles of selective tissue tension testing. Special tests and peripheral screening tests are employed when there are specific indications for them. The following tests are routinely carried out in the differential diagnostic examination:

- ❏ History
- ❏ Observation

❑ Musculoarticular (active, passive resisted, stress)
❑ Dural
❑ Neurological (myotome, dermatome, reflexes)
❑ Special

Comparison of Systemic and Musculoskeletal Pain

Systemic	Musculoskeletal

• Disturbs sleep
• Deep aching or throbbing
• Reduced by pressure
• Constant or waves of pain and spasm
• Is not aggravated by mechanical stress
• Associated with
   jaundice
   migratory arthralgias
   skin rash
   fatigue
   weight loss
   low-grade fever
   generalized weakness
   cyclic and progressive
     symptoms
   history of infection
	• Generally lessens at night
	• Sharp or superficial ache
	• Usually decreases with cessation of activity
	• Usually continuous or intermittent
	• Is aggravated by mechanical stress
	• Usually associated with nothing specific

The diagnosis is arrived at only after all of the routine and indicated special tests have been carried out and all the information has been processed. Generally, a number of provisional diagnoses are generated (the more experienced you are, the fewer there are) and the most probable is selected for treatment. If this does not turn out to be the correct one (the treatment does not work), the next most likely is treated, and so on. Usually, however, the differential diagnosis examination is negative, in that it does not generate a diagnosis. In this case, more information is required. The best method of acquiring this is with the biomechanical examination, which will generate a joint pathomechanical diagnosis. If the therapist is not familiar with a biomechanical examination, treatment will have to be based on the best information from the differential examination. This treatment will usually be an exercise program designed to increase range of motion. To do this, secondary examination techniques such as repeated movements can be utilized to assess the potential effects of an exercise program over a short period.

The following table looks at some potential implications of certain characteristics gained from the subjective examination and the observation of the patient in different types of conditions and patients.

Characteristic	Serious Pathology	Chronic Pain Syndrome	Secondary Gain
Appearance	Tired and often ill looking	May look tired but not ill	Normal
Pain areas	Local and/or radiating	Multiple associated areas	Local, sometimes with extensive radiation
Pain behavior	Constant and may not be affected by mechanical stress	Exacerbations on anything but particularly emotional stress	Exacerbated by work activities or postures
Pain description	Usually reasonable, although patient may be depressed	Nonspecific, and concentrates on patient's suffering	Matter of fact and unconcerned
Numbness	None or objective	Widespread, nonobjective, and hyperesthetic	None, or if claimed, nonobjective
Tenderness	None or over bone	Widespread	Local and inconsistent if patient is distracted
Attitude	Worried, angry, or depressed	Egocentric, misunderstood, and either hostile or apathetic	Mainly concerned that you believe him or her
Previous treatment results	No or very short-term response, patient concerned with the lack of results	Often very proud of the lack of results	Unconcerned with the lack of results more interested in making sure that everything is documented
You are	Worried	Despondent	Annoyed

The following tabulates general signs from the objective examination that are potentially serious, particularly when found in combinations:

Clinical Sign	Potential Serious Cause	Probable Benign Pathology
Full range of motion with normal end feels in patients with significant pain	Visceral conditions Bone cancer	Therapist error Amplification or fabrication
No range of motion	Possible fracture	Anxiety
Multidirectional movements with spasm end feels	Possible fractures	None
Multidirectional painful weakness	Fracture Bone cancer	Hyperacute arthritis
Multisegmental paresis and/or hypoesthesia	Neurological cancer Cauda equina syndrome Neurological disease	Central stenosis Multiple-level lateral stenosis
Anesthesia	Central nervous system pathology Neuroma	Peripheral neuropathy
Paralysis	Central nervous system pathology Neuroma	Peripheral neuropathy
Empty end feel	Serious pathologies that affect tissues that cannot cause spasm	Subdeltoid bursitis
Progressive pain	Cancer Infection	Inflammation
Signs are worse than the symptoms	Neurological disease	None
Night pain	Cancer Infections	Acute inflammation
Bony point tenderness	Bone cancer Bone infection	Referred tenderness
Expanding pain	Bone or neurological cancer Infections	Increasing disk herniation

If there is any cause for concern about the patient's general health, the following can be sought either from the history or from the objective examination:

History
- ❏ Fever
- ❏ Unexplained weight loss
- ❏ Malaise
- ❏ Sweating, especially at night

❏ Changes in coughing habits or product
❏ Fatigue
❏ Changes in urination habits (hesitancy, retention, incontinence)
❏ Changes in the urine (blood, pus)
❏ Sleep disturbances
❏ Drop attacks
❏ Episodic syncope
❏ Repeated dropping of objects or stumbling
❏ Other joint problems
❏ Pathological fractures
❏ Diabetes
❏ Osteoporosis
❏ Recurrent infections

Observation

❏ Jaundice
❏ Grayness
❏ Cyanosis
❏ Edema
❏ Horner's signs
❏ Nystagmus
❏ Dysarthria
❏ Dysphasia
❏ Facial drooping
❏ Ptosis
❏ Aniscoria
❏ Ataxia

Pulse Rate and Rhythm

❏ Dysrhythmia
❏ Tachycardia
❏ Bradycardia

Respiration Rate and Depth

❏ Rapid
❏ Shallow
❏ Labored

Blood Pressure

❏ Hypotension
❏ Hypertension

Abdomen

❏ Ascites
❏ Masses
❏ Tenderness
❏ Aortic pulsatile mass

Differential Diagnostic Examination

The following lists the very significant findings of the general differential diagnostic examination together with an indication of why they are significant. The following indications are used.

!   Be careful with this patient and watch his or her progress carefully. If therapy worsens matters or does not help, quickly refer the patient back to the physician.

*   The patient potentially has a problem that is outside our scope of practice either as the presenting complaint or coincidental with it, or the musculoskeletal problem will likely require prolonged treatment or specialist intervention. It is as well to discuss this patient with the physician so that arrangements can be made for specialist referral or time of work, medication, and so on. It is not necessary to discontinue treatment if the problem is of musculoskeletal origin.

**   This has all the makings of a very nasty condition and should be examined with extreme caution if found in the history. It should almost certainly be referred to the physician for further testing.

History

- ❑ Trauma !
- ❑ No previous history of type !
- ❑ Worsened with treatment !
- ❑ No difference with treatment !
- ❑ Cancer **

Symptoms

PAIN

- ❑ Radicular (lancinating) !
- ❑ Causalgia !
- ❑ Constant, worsened by activity or position !
- ❑ Constant, not worsened by activity or position **
- ❑ Exacerbated by eating or diet **
- ❑ Strongly exacerbated by emotional stress **
- ❑ Claudicational !
- ❑ Worsening !
- ❑ Nocturnal **
- ❑ Deep and diffuse *
- ❑ Reproducible by physical posture or activity
- ❑ Not reproducible by physical posture or activity **
- ❑ Immediate *

❏ Very extensive !
❏ Nonsegmental
❏ Unilateral and segmental
❏ Bilateral and segmental !
❏ Bilateral and multi- or nonsegmental *
❏ Hemilateral !
❏ Saddle area *
❏ Forbidden area (skin across the back at L1 or L2 level) *
❏ L1 or 2 dermatome *
❏ Bilateral face **
❏ Hemifacial if not TMJ (Temperomandibuler Joint) disorder *
❏ Hemifacial and contralateral body-limb **

ANESTHESIA AND PARESTHESIA

❏ Anesthesia ** (unless peripheral neuropathy diagnosed)
❏ Unilateral and segmental paresthesia !
❏ Bilateral segmental paresthesia !
❏ Bilateral multisegmental **
❏ Quadrilateral **
❏ Bisegmental upper limb paresthesia !*
❏ Trisegmental lower limb paresthesia !*
❏ Saddle-area paresthesia **
❏ Hemifacial **
❏ Full face **

OTHER COMPLAINTS

❏ Bladder, bowel, or genital dysfunction **
❏ Dysmenorrhea **
❏ Vertigo *
❏ Dizziness !
🖥 Central neurological (cardinal) !**

OBSERVATION

🖥 Central neurological signs (cardinal signs) **
❏ Patchy or hemifacial sweating **
❏ Hemilateral sweating **
❏ Unilateral segmental atrophy !
❏ Bilateral segmental atrophy *
❏ Acutely painful angular deformity **
❏ Severe bruising *
❏ Nontraumatic swelling over bone **
❏ Nontraumatic effusion !
❏ Reddening **

ACTIVE RANGE OF MOVEMENT

❏ Severely restricted or no movement **
❏ Nontraumatic capsular pattern !

❏ No restriction, and no pain reproduced at end range **
❏ Reproduces lancinating pain !
❏ Reproduces paresthesia !
❏ Reproduces CNS signs or symptoms **

PASSIVE MOVEMENT

❏ Empty end feel ** (acute subdeltoid busitis is the exception)
❏ Multidirectional spasm **
❏ Large increase over active range !
❏ Cog-wheeling movement *
❏ Painful crepitus *

ISOMETRIC RESISTED TEST (CONTRACTILE)

❏ Painful weakness !

STRESS TEST

❏ Craniovertebral instability **
❏ Other ligamentous instability *

MYOTOME (KEY MUSCLES)

❏ More than one-level weakness in the upper limb *
❏ More than three-level weakness in the lower limb *
❏ Bilateral weakness *
❏ Quadrilateral weakness **
❏ Paralysis ** (unless a peripheral neuropathy is diagnosed)

DERMATOME

❏ More than one-level hypoesthesia in the upper limb *
❏ More than three-level hypoesthesia in the lower limb *
❏ Bilateral hypoesthesia *
❏ Quadrilateral hypoesthesia **
❏ Facial **
❏ Anesthesia ** (unless a peripheral neuropathy is diagnosed)

REFLEXES

❏ Deep tendon hyporeflexia !
❏ Deep tendon hyperreflexia **
❏ Clonus **
❏ Babinski response **
❏ Hoffman's reflex strongly positive **
❏ Dynamic Hoffman's reflex **

DURAL

❏ Severely limited !
❏ Produces lancinating pain !
❏ Produces paresthesia !

❑ Bilateral !
❑ Crossed !

SPECIAL TESTS

❑ Fracture tests **
❑ Vertebral artery **
❑ Cranial nerve test in neutral head position *
❑ Cranial nerve tests in altered head positions **
❑ Long tract tests **

Many of these items need to be considered in context rather than as absolutes. Cranial nerve and long tract congenital anomalies do exist as isolated nonsignificant entities, but if they are associated with symptoms or other signs, do not assume this. It is better to be overcautious than cavalier; the worst that happens if you are wrong is that the patient has further tests.

Viscerogenic Causes of Spinal Pain

Cervical	Thoracic	Lumbar	Sacroiliac
Tracheobronchial irritation	Pleuropulmonary disorders	Metastatic lesions	Prostatitis/cancer
Cervical bone tumors	Peptic ulcer	Renal disorders	Gynecologic disorders
Cervical cord tumors	Pancreatitis or cancer	Prostatitis/cancer	Lower bowel disorders
Pancoast's tumors	Cholycystitis	Testicular cancer	Endocarditis
Vertebral osteomyelitis	Renal disorders	Abdominal aortic aneurysm	Spondyloarthropathies
			• ankylosing spondylitis
			• Reiter's syndrome
			• psoriatic arthritis
			• Crohn's disease
	Mediastinal tumors	Endocarditis	Paget's disease
		Aortic aneurysm	Sign of the buttock causes
		Endocarditis	
		Acute pancreatitis	
		Small intestine obstruction	
		Crohn's disease	
		Gynecologic disorders	
		Tuberculosis	

Appropriate Findings and General Treatment Guidelines

Conditions	Findings	Treatment Protocol
Disc Lesions		
Small protrusion	Ipsilateral extension quadrant-limited with springy end feel	Extension or unilateral extension
Others (large protrusion, prolapse, extrusion)	All movements severely reduced with severe pain	Neutral to extension (gentle manual traction)
Segmental Subluxation		
Anteroposterior	Flexion and extension very restricted and painful; rotation minimally affected	Extension (manual traction and traction manipulation in extension)
Transverse	One rotation maximally affected, flexion and extension minimally so; will show mainly on the biomechanical examination with transverse mobility test	Neutral (manual traction and traction manipulation)
Facet Lesions		
Arthritis	Capsular pattern (ipsilateral extension extension quadrant much less than contralateral flexion quadrant) with spasm end feel on extension quadrant	RICE (rest, ice, compression and elevation) until the spasm is absent then pain modalities including grade 1 and 2 mobilizations
Arthrosis	Capsular pattern (ipsilateral extension quadrant much less than contralateral flexion quadrant) with hard capsular end feel on extension quadrant and less so on flexion quadrant	Flexion and extension mobilizations
Fibrosis	Ipsilateral extension quadrant decrease = contralateral flexion quadrant with very hard capsular end feel on both quadrants	Flexion and extension mobilizations
Subluxation	Flexion *or* extension quadrant-limited with pathomechanical end feel	Flexion or extension mobilizations or manipulation

The Biomechanical Evaluation

Although this book concerns differential diagnosis rather than biomechanical evaluation, the latter will be mentioned in some of the case studies to follow. I have therefore included the short section that follows to review the principles of biomechanical evaluation and diagnosis as I know it.

Although manipulative therapy is practiced by many health care professions including physical therapy, osteopathy, chiropractic, and medicine, biomechanically based examination and treatment has been adopted almost exclusively by physical therapy. It is based on anatomy and the extrapolated or proven biomechanics that arise from that anatomy. The generated diagnosis is nonmedical, specific, and distinctly biomechanical in flavor.

We are having trouble proving that the selective tissue tension examination does or does not work, and the biomechanical examination is proving extremely recalcitrant in this regard, but from a practical perspective it appears to work, and in the absence of proof to the contrary, it is the examination that the physical therapy diagnosis will be based on in this book.

Speculations concerning biomechanics, pathomechanics, indicated treatments, and so on are simply discussions and should be judged on their merits and not taken as definitive. I offer no apology for this, for if such speculations are not forthcoming from clinicians, researchers will have very little to do in the important arena of enhanced patient care. Most of the research that has come about in manual therapy concerns its practicality as a treatment. Effectiveness, efficiency, validity, and reliability have all been studied, more often than not demonstrating that manual therapy does work as well or better than other modalities. In this regard, it is among the most researched areas in physical therapy, but, with one or two notable exceptions,[1,2] there is very little research into the basic underpinning of manual therapy, especially regarding the validity of examination procedures. In the absence of rigorous scientific proof, construct validity and clinical experience with the procedures must replace hard research. It is to be hoped that further union between the researcher and the clinician will remedy the situation, but until significant amounts of clinically relevant research are forthcoming, the clinician can only work with what is available.

John McM. Mennell defined *joint dysfunction* as "a loss of joint-play movement" and *joint-play movement* as a "movement that cannot be produced by the action of voluntary muscles."[3] Alan Stoddard, a British osteopath and medical practitioner, extended the idea of joint dysfunction to include hypermobility and how prolonged hypomobility could lead to hypermobility.[4] Stoddard made the following statement in the first edition of his book in 1959, which is very appropriate in the current climate of turf protection (albeit under other guises):

> The art of manipulation is not the sole prerogative of the osteopath. Rather it is the prerogative of the patient. It is desirable, therefore, to disseminate as widely as possible the available knowledge of this work so that the maximum numbers of suffering humanity may derive benefit.

Maigne,[5] discussing vertebral manipulation stated that

> Their (vertebral manipulation techniques) reputation is often bad. This is due partly to their misuse by laymen who have tried to use manual techniques as a miracle cure for various disorders, and partly to doubtful pathogenic interpretations.

He also said,

> With a good knowledge of indications and contraindications, a selection of effective and harmless maneuvers, and with codification of their use, manipulations must have their place in our therapeutic arsenal.

The late David Lamb,[6] who was always concerned with the role of manual therapy as part of the overall rehabilitation of the patient rather than as the sole or even primary treatment said,

> Physiotherapists have always been concerned with total rehabilitation following orthopedic, neurological, circulatory and respiratory disorders to itemize a few. It is a natural extension of this training that manual therapists should be concerned with the restoration of total bodily function using comprehensive analysis of somatic dysfunction, selection of appropriate technique, and advice on management and prophylaxis, thus helping to attain total body harmony and wellness.

I have spent some space introducing the subject of manual therapy because it is becoming a contentious issue both within the profession and between professions. Many in our own profession, who plainly do not fully understand the role of manual therapy, see it as a passive treatment. They should, instead, see it for what it is, an adjunctive treatment to the total rehabilitation of the patient that is effective[7] and safe (it is a good deal safer to take a series of manipulative treatments for neck pain than it is to take aspirin for the same problem over the same time period[8]). Outside of our profession, chiropractic is trying to limit our use of manual therapy, and in some instances they are trying to prevent us from effectively treating the spine at all (manually and nonmanually). Manual therapy will greatly facilitate your treatment of many if not most of your nonsurgical orthopedic patients, and the sooner you learn to incorporate this subdiscipline into your practice, the sooner you will be more effectively treating your patients.

Biomechanical Terminology Definitions

For the most part, these definitions have evolved from a body of work by MacConaill and Basmajain.[9-11]

❏ *Arthrokinematics.*   The motion that occurs at the joint surface during and as part of the physiological motion. Also called *glides* or *slides,* for *swing* and *spin* when no linear displacement occurs.

❏ *Arthrokinesiology.*   The study of movements at joints.

❏ *Biomechanical examination.*   The specific and nonspecific examination of an articular complex's motion state that reaches a motion dysfunction diagnosis.

❏ *Close pack position.*   The close pack position is the position of maximum inert stability and is characterized by
a. maximum tautness of the joint capsule and major ligaments
b. maximum articular surface congruency
c. least intra-articular volume
d. least transarticular pressure
e. least availability of traction or angulation or glide

❏ *Degrees of freedom.*   The number of independent axes around which a bone can move. There is a maximum of three degrees of freedom (one for each dimension), and for the most part, the number of degrees of freedom depends on the joint surface at which the movement is occurring. The unmodified ovoid surface potentially has three degrees of freedom; the modified ovoid potentially has two degrees of freedom; the unmodified sellar potentially has two degrees of freedom; and the modified sellar potentially has one degree of freedom.

❏ *Mechanical axis.*   An imaginary line extended perpendicular to the average plane of the joint that replaces the bone when modeling osteokinematics.

❏ *Passive arthrokinematic (accessory) intervertebral movement.*   The passive assessment or treatment of an intervertebral joint through its glides.

❏ *Passive arthrokinematic movement.*   The passive assessment or treatment of any joint through its glides, generally used in connection with the peripheral joints.

❏ *Passive intervertebral movement (PIVM).*   A nonspecific term for any intervertebral movement whether physiological, arthrokinematic, or osteokinematic.

❏ *Passive physiological intervertebral movement (PPIVM).*   The assessment or treatment technique whereby one vertebra is moved in physiological ranges on another.

❏ *Passive physiological movement (PPM).*   The assessment or treatment technique whereby one bone is moved in physiological ranges on another (flexion, extension, side flexion, rotation, abduction, adduction). It is used when testing or treating a peripheral joint as distinct from PPIVM.

❏ *Osteokinematics.*   The movement of the bone around its mechanical axis.

❏ *Ovoid Surface.*   A surface that is entirely convex or concave. Unmodified ovoids have equal curvature in all directions; modified have not.

❏ *Sellar Surface.*   A surface that is concavoconvex. An unmodified sellar has its convexity perpendicular to its concavity, a modified convex surface is not perpendicular to its concave.

The Integration of the Examinations of the Musculoskeletal System

The examination of the musculoskeletal system falls into two main parts, the initial examination for medical conditions, which is the differential or scanning examination, and the biomechanical examination. At the end of the differential diagnostic examination, either a medical diagnosis— disk lesion (protrusion, prolapse, or extrusion), acute arthritis, specific tendonitis or muscle belly tear, spondylolithesis, or stenosis—can be made or the examination is considered negative. A negative examination does not imply that there were no findings but rather that the results of examination were insufficient to generate a diagnosis upon which specific treatment could be based. In this case, further examination is required. The inability to effectively treat following the scanning examination requires that a biomechanical examination be carried out prior to any treatment being initiated.

The biomechanical examination will provide information concerning the motion state of the joint. It consists of optional screening tests that help focus on the problem area and specific stability and mobility tests that determine whether the spinal segment or peripheral joint is hypomobile, hypermobile, stable, or unstable (that is, the motion state of the segment or joint). These tests will include passive accessory motion, articular stability, and conjunct rotation assessments.

Screening tests are quick, noncomprehensive tests that allow the therapist to include a joint or group of joints as possibly contributing to the patient's symptoms. Among the screening tests are Faber's test, squatting, and active, passive, and resisted movement testing of each joint.

Biomechanical screen tests include various kinetic tests, manubrial testing, position testing, and quadrant tests. The purpose of screen testing is to rapidly evaluate the probability that a joint or group of joints are dysfunctional and whether they require more detailed biomechanical testing. Biomechanical screening tests are especially useful when the remote cause of a dysfunction is being investigated because it allows the numerous areas that have to be examined to be *provisionally* excluded from a more definitive examination. However, it must be constantly remembered that screening tests are not all-inclusive and that false negatives are common, so these tests must be subordinate to other considerations in the examination of the patient.

Motion Dysfunction States

For the purposes of this text, motion dysfunction is the basis of biomechanical assessment and treatment. Is the joint or segment too stiff or too loose, and if it is too stiff, what is the limiting factor? In determining the motion status of the joint or segment, the patient's symptoms are not considered because they can confuse the issue. That is not to say that the symptoms are unimportant, because they obviously are when it comes to determining relevance of findings and effect of treatment, but for the diagnosis of the dysfunction at a given joint or segment, they do not help.

Movement dysfunctions fall into one of two major categories: either there is too little movement or too much. From these two main divisions, subdivisions of dysfunctions can be considered.

Reduced Movement

There are three main types of hypomobility if we exclude ankylosis (which is not treatable by us):

1. Myofascial

2. Pericapsular

3. Pathomechanical or subluxation

Myofascial Hypomobility This is caused by shortening of muscle and fascia.

Causes
- ❏ Hypertonicity
- ❏ Post-traumatic scarring or adhesions
- ❏ Adaptive shortening

Effects
- ❏ Reduces the passive physiological movement but not the passive arthrokinematic (accessory) movement, the glide
- ❏ Not a capsular pattern restriction
- ❏ Demonstrates the constant-length phenomenon
- ❏ The end feel may be capsular if scarred, a resistant feeling, or elastic

Pericapsular Hypomobility This is caused by shortening of the joint capsule or ligaments.

Causes
- ❏ Scars or adhesions
- ❏ Adaptation to a chronically shortened position
- ❏ Arthritis
- ❏ Arthrosis
- ❏ Fibrosis

Effects
- ❏ Reduces the physiological and the arthrokinematic movements
- ❏ Frequently causes a capsular pattern of restriction
- ❏ Does not demonstrate the constant-length phenomenon
- ❏ The end feel is premature and hard capsular or spasm if inflamed.

Pathomechanical or Subluxation Hypomobility A biomechanical problem with the joint jamming at one end of the range of movement and blocking motion away from that end of the range.

Causes
- ❏ Sudden macrotrauma

❏ Repeated or prolonged microtrauma
❏ Microtrauma imposed on an instability

Effects

Either limitation of gross motion or conjunct rotation such that

❏ The physiological motion away from the subluxation is limited.
❏ The arthrokinematic motion away from the subluxation is limited.
❏ The physiological motion toward the subluxation is full range or at least has a normal end feel and appears full range.
❏ The arthrokinematic motion toward the subluxation is full range.
❏ The end feel away from the subluxation is abnormal and abrupt, almost bony.
❏ The end feel toward the subluxation is normal.

Excessive Movement

1. Hypermobility

2. Instability

Hypermobility The terms *hypermobility* and *instability* are frequently used synonymously, or the term *hypermobility* is used to describe normal hyperflexibility. Neither use is helpful clinically. For purposes of the discussion of clinical biomechanics within this text, *hypermobility* will be defined as "that condition when the physiological range of motion is increased beyond normal but there is no new movement present that should not be present." The stress/stability tests are negative; consequently, this condition is found with mobility tests not stability tests.

Causes

❏ Cumulative stress (creep) caused by neighboring hypomobility
❏ Low-level but prolonged or repeated stress through overuse or remote dysfunction
❏ Sudden macrotrauma that does produce instability (rare)
❏ Neurological palsy with hypotonia and reduced muscle control
❏ Neuromuscular incoordination caused by neurological or neurophysiological dysfunction

Effects

❏ Increase in gross passive physiological movement if tissues not irritable
❏ Increase in arthrokinematic range if tissues not irritable
❏ End feel with (a) and (b) soft and late capsular
❏ Normal gross passive physiological movement if tissues irritable

❑ Normal gross arthrokinematic movement if tissues irritable
❑ End feel late spasm if tissues irritable

Instability There are many definitions of *instability*. Again, many do not help the clinician too much. The definition that will be used in this book is that "instability exists where there is a movement that should not exist or is not normally perceptible to the examiner on testing." This fits in with our understanding of stress/stability tests.

There are two types of instability, ligamentous and articular/segmental. Ligamentous instability occurs as a result of deficiency in the ligament, is uni- or occasionally bidirectional (depending on the width of the ligament), and will soften the normal end feel stress test and allow movement during the test. Articular instability results from deficiencies in the labrum or articular surface of the joint. If the surrounding pericapsular tissues are normal, the end feel is normal, but there is movement in directions where there should be no movement. If the labrum alone is torn, it results in unidirectional instability, if there is a generalized thinning of the articular cartilage, there is omnidirectional nonphysiological movement.

Causes

❑ Sudden macrotrauma (ligamentous)
❑ Hypermobility allowed to progress (ligamentous)
❑ Degeneration of interposing hyaline or fibrocartilage (articular)
❑ Labral and meniscal tears
❑ Segmental degeneration
❑ Congenital and developmental

Effects

❑ Presence of nonphysiological movement (i.e., a movement exists that should not)
❑ End feel soft capsular if ligamentous instability
❑ End feel normal if articular instability
❑ Hypermobility if spinal but not necessarily so if peripheral
❑ Recurrent subluxations

Biomechanical Examination

The purpose of the biomechanical assessment is to

1. determine which peripheral/spinal joint is dysfunctional
2. determine the presence, direction, and type of movement

dysfunction (hypomobility, hypermobility, or instability), and from this,

3. determine an appropriate treatment.

Hyper- and Hypomobility

To determine mobility, passive physiological movement tests (PPMs) are usually utilized first. These will give an idea of range of motion and, with some stabilization, the end feels. End feel is particularly important in joints with very small ranges of motion such as occurs at the spinal segments because evaluating range becomes extraordinarily difficult when there are only three or four degrees of range available even in the absence of dysfunction. Once the physiological range has been assessed, it can be classified as normal, reduced, or excessive. If reduced, passive arthrokinematic (accessory) motion (PAM) testing is carried whenever practical to determine if the reduction of motion is caused by articular or extra-articular lesions. With a few exceptions, muscle cannot restrict arthrokinematic (gliding) motion at a joint, especially if the glides are tested in the anti–close pack (rest) position of the joint.

Positive findings for hypomobility are reduced range of motion in a capsular or noncapsular pattern, depending on the cause, and a change in end feel, again depending on the cause (discussed later). For hypermobility, one of two results will be obtained, depending on whether the attenuated articular restraints are irritable or not. If they are not irritable, the physiological range of motion will be increased and the end feel will be a softer than expected capsular one. If they are irritable, the range will be approximately normal, but with a spasm end feel because the reflex muscle contraction prevents motion into the abnormal and painful range.

Instability

Articular instability is presumed to occur with cartilage (hyaline or fibro) degeneration or damage and subsequent deficit. In the spine, it seems likely that ligamentous (disk) instability must occur simultaneously with articular instability (zygapophyseal and uncovertebral joints) for the instability to be clinically detectable.

If the passive physiological movement tests of the spinal joints have normal range and end feel, the segment can usually be considered normal, because instability will almost invariably produce a hypermobility. Articular instability is presumed to occur with cartilage (hyaline or fibro) degeneration and thinning. In the spine, it seems likely that ligamentous (disk) instability must occur simultaneously with articular instability (zygapophyseal and uncovertebral joints) for the instability to be clinically detectable.

This articular deficit leads to reduced congruency of the articular surfaces, allowing slipping between them. In addition, the degeneration permits the bone ends to move closer to each other thereby slackening off the capsule and ligaments. To test this type of instability in the spine, we will make the segment try to do movements that would normally not be detectable. These tests will include transverse, anterior, and posterior translations and pure (axial) rotation. Although these movements do exist to some small extent, they should not be detectable as actual shifts in the bone.

The assessment of any spinal region must be of sufficient detail to determine the presence and cause of hypomobility and instability. However, the examination process should flow so that a positive or negative test leads naturally to a second test. For example, reduced physiological motion should lead to arthrokinematic testing to determine whether the hypomobility is myofascial or articular. Excessively mobile physiological tests should lead to stress testing to determine the stability of the segment.

A general algorithm that can be used in principle in every area is as follows:

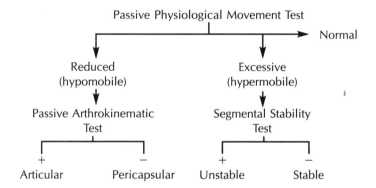

Notes

1. Jull G et al: The accuracy of manual diagnosis for cervical zygapophyseal joint pain syndromes. Med J Aust 148:233, 1988.

2. Gonnella C et al: Reliability in evaluating passive intervertebral motion. Phys Ther 62:436, 1982.

3. Mennell JM: *Joint Pain: Diagnosis and Treatment Using Manipulative Techniques,* pp 2–5. Boston, Little Brown and Company, 1964.

4. Stoddard A: *Manual of Osteopathic Technique.* 2d ed., pp 13–24. London, Hutchison, 1977.

5. Maigne R: Manipulation of the spine, in JB Rogoff (ed), *Manipulation, Traction and Massage,* 2d ed., pp 59–63. Baltimore, Williams and Wilkins, 1980.

6. Lamb DW: A review of manual therapy for spinal pain, in JD Boyling, N Palastanga (eds), *Grieve's Modern Manual of Therapy,* 2d ed. Edinburgh, Churchill Livingstone, 1994.

7. Koes BW et al: The effectiveness of manual therapy, physiotherapy and treatment by the general practitioner for non-specific back and neck complaints: a randomized clinical trial. Spine 17:28, 1992.

8. Dabbs V et al: A review of the literature and comparisons to the use of NSAIDs for cervical pain. J Manipulative Physiol Ther 18:530, 1995.

9. MacConaill MA, Basmajian JV: *Muscles and Movements: A Basis for Human Kinesiology.* Baltimore, Williams and Wilkins, 1969.

10. MacConaill MA: Spurt and shunt muscles. J Anat 126:619, 1978.

11. MacConaill MA: A generalized mechanics of articular swings. 1. From Earth to outer space. J Anat 127:577, 1978.

CHAPTER 10

The Cervical Spine

In the region-specific examinations, the peculiarities of anatomy and pathology of each area are taken into consideration in testing and in the interpretation of data. The examination is sequenced so as to make it as efficient as possible. This generally means having the patient change position as little as possible, that is, doing as many tests as possible in one position. In the acute patient's examination, this method also results in as little aggravation as possible. In this chapter, only those examination findings specific to the area being examined will be discussed.

Cervical Spine

It is extremely important when examining a patient whose neck you are potentially going to treat that you rule out, at least as much as possible, the presence of craniovertebral instability and vertebrobasilar compromise. This is particularly important but not exclusive to post-traumatic patients. The examination of the neck will be discussed in two parts, the nontraumatic and the post-traumatic neck patient.

History

There is of course considerable overlap in the examination of the traumatic and nontraumatic neck; some of the difference is in the detail of the examination and some in the sequencing. The differences will be made clear as they become significant.

The cervical spine presents some unique considerations as far as safety and differential diagnosis are concerned. Among the more serious nontraumatic conditions that must be recognized are

❑ Vertebral artery anomalies and nontraumatic pathologies
❑ Compression of the spinal cord
❑ Craniovertebral instabilities from disease processes
❑ Coexisting neurological disease or central nervous system neoplasms

Cardinal signs and symptoms include

❑ Facial paresthesia/anesthesia/causalgia
❑ Perioral paresthesia/anesthesia/causalgia
❑ Bilateral paresthesia/anesthesia/causalgia
❑ Quadrilateral paresthesia/anesthesia/causalgia
❑ Hemilateral paresthesia/anesthesia/causalgia
❑ Periodic consciousness loss (syncope)
❑ Post-traumatic pulsatile tinnitus
❑ Sudden profound deafness
❑ Non-acute visual field deficits
❑ Dysphasia
❑ Dysarthria
❑ Dysphonia
❑ Horner's signs (ptosis, endophthalmos, anhidrosis, miosis, facial flushing)
❑ Ataxia
❑ Babinski's response
❑ Clonus
❑ Hyperreflexia
❑ Drop attacks
❑ Aniscoria (symmetrical pupils)
❑ Abnormal pupil light reflexes
❑ Nystagmus (especially downbeat)
❑ Facial droop and lower facial muscle weakness
❑ Sensorineural hypoacusia
❑ Trapezius/sternomastoid atrophy and weakness
❑ Tongue atrophy and weakness
❑ Painless dysphagia
❑ Paralysis in a nonperipheral nerve distribution

The history must include questions that will elicit any symptoms that might be suggestive of any central nervous system conditions. These symptoms relate to compromise of the function of the spinal cord long tracts, brainstem, thalamus, cerebellum, or cerebrum, and include the so-called cardinal signs and symptoms. If any of the symptoms are un-equivocal, especially if they are combined with other such symptoms, the patient should be referred back to the physician immediately. Symptoms that are pathognomonic of either spinal cord compromise or vertebral artery insufficiency should preclude further movement examination, because there is the very real risk of making a bad situation a lot worse. The patient's neck should be stabilized with a hard collar and the patient should be transported to the Emergency Room.

Rheumatoid arthritis, ankylosing spondylitis, Down's syndrome, Reiter's disease, or recurrent upper respiratory tract infections in children (potential Grisel's syndrome) in the history are all cautions, especially when treating the neck, because they may result in destabilization of the craniovertebral joints. About 30% of rheumatoid arthritic patients have neck pain, and about 30% have anterior or vertical instability of the atlantoaxial segment.[1] The numbers are high enough to suggest that treatment of the craniovertebral joints in a rheumatoid patient is, at the least, very risky. Certainly any of these conditions demands that exhaustive clinical testing of stability of these segments be undertaken, and perhaps all of these patients should have flexion/extension x-rays taken prior to beginning treatment.

Is there a history of trauma? If so, when was the trauma and what was the mechanism? The most common cause of trauma to the neck is the hyperextension injury in rear-end collisions, and there is overwhelming evidence implicating hyperextension forces as the most damaging when the patient is not suffering from life-threatening injuries.[2-9] Of course, there are other forms of cervical trauma and the following discussion on the examination of the whiplash patient equally applies to them. Trauma may destabilize the craniovertebral joints, cause severe zygapophyseal joint damage, fracture cervical vertebras, tear and/or herniate intervertebral disks, tear the pharynx or esophagus, damage the vertebral artery, or produce central neurological lesions.[10-14]

The injury is further worsened if the head is rotated or extended at the time of impact and if the patient is unaware of the impending impact.[9] Were there neurological symptoms such as lancinating pain, paresthesia, or anesthesia? The presence of neurological symptoms usually indicates more severe damage to the skeletal system, which of course is further from the axis of rotation and therefore subjected to larger torque forces.[9,15-17] Generally, the more intense the pain, the higher the level of damage.

Did the pain or the neurological symptoms start immediately, suddenly, and severely, or were they delayed or of gradual onset? An immediate onset of severe pain suggests quite profound structural damage to muscles, ligaments, or bone rather than simple inflammation, which has a more delayed and gradual onset.

The following lists the more important and research established indications of more severe pathology from whiplash injury.[9,15-17]

- ❏ Hyperextension injury
- ❏ Craniofacial impact
- ❏ Severe range of motion loss
- ❏ Rotated or inclined head position
- ❏ Initial high multisymptom score
- ❏ Preaccident headache (demonstrates poor prognosis rather than tissue damage)
- ❏ Neurological symptoms (lancinating pain, paresthesia, numbness)
- ❏ High headache intensity
- ❏ Immediate, severe neck pain
- ❏ Intensity of neck pain
- ❏ Unpreparedness
- ❏ Stationary car

Scotoma is defined as a loss of function within the visual field. It is commonly central in nature and may be blank or deformed. The patient complains of difficulty in reading or watching television and often states that he or she must read or look from the side of the eye. This is not caused by conditions that bring the patient into the orthopedic therapist but may consist coincidentally and can be caused by retinopathies, optic neuropathy, pituitary tumors, carotid aneurysms, and papilloedema. The loss of a small visual part of the field in one eye may be the result of uncorrected or partially corrected childhood strabismus (squint). Suppression of a small area of vision can occur as a result.[18]

Hemianopia or *quadranopia* is visual loss in half or a quarter of the visual field. The condition is bilateral because the lesion lies at or posterior to the optic chiasm. There may be hallucinations within the field such as flashing lights (scintillations), in which case the patient is very aware of the condition. If these are not present, and the central visual areas are unaffected, the patient may not know that half the vision is lost in both eyes because the blind area moves with the head. Vertebrobasilar compromise that affects the visual cortex via the calcerine arteries may cause homonymous hemianopia or quadranopia, depending on how extensive the affected area is.[19,20] In homonymous hemianopia, the visual loss is bilaterally right or bilaterally left and results from a lesion behind the optic chiasm. In addition to vertebrobasilar compromise, cerebral stroke and tumors affecting the pathways behind the chiasm can cause this type of visual field loss. In heteronymous field loss, the loss is left and right and is caused by a lesion at the chiasm, which may be a pituitary gland tumor or a craniopharyngioma, an aneurysm of the circle of Willis, a meningioma or metastatic carcinoma, or another, much rarer condition. The presence of hemianopia or quadranopia, whether homonymous or heteronymous, requires further medical investigation.

Blurred vision is one of the more common symptoms of vertebrobasilar compromise[21] but also occurs with other conditions. Blurred vision may be a visual acuity problem or diplopia (double vision). It is sometimes difficult for the patient to tell whether his or her vision is simply blurred or is doubled. Ask about recent eye examinations, but do not take any answer as definitive.

Diplopia may be caused by corneal or lens diseases, but in the population we see, the concern must be with ocular paralysis. A third, fourth, or sixth cranial nerve palsy or a supranuclear lesion can produce this symptom. If, for example, one eye cannot converge because of medial rectus paralysis or paresis, near vision will be affected, because this requires convergence to fuse the images from each eye. If one eye cannot converge, two images will be generated. This will be correctable by having the patient move his or her head around until the nonconverging eye is carried over the image and the normal eye overconverges and fuses the image. Alternatively, the visual target can be moved until it comes into the field of the nonconverging eye. Causes of diplopia include basal skull tumors, meningiomas, head injuries, neuromas, vertebrobasilar compromise, aneurysms, chronic meningitis (tuberculosis, syphilitic), herpes zoster (shingles), and undetermined causes.[20,22]

Facial paresthesia or numbness may be a serious symptom. The trigeminal nucleus runs from the midbrain to at least the third cervical level, with the chief sensory nucleus situated in the midbrain and vascularized by the basilar artery. Carotid artery dissections and vertebrobasilar ischemia have been shown to cause these symptoms, usually in the maxillary and/or mandibular distributions of the trigeminal nerve.[20,22] It is not wise to assume that paresthesia in this area is caused by segmental facilitation or is an aberrant part of the tongue-neck syndrome until the possibility that it is caused by more serious pathology is eliminated. The symptom is particularly significant if it is associated with ipsilateral sensation loss or decrease in the face. Perioral anesthesia, as was discussed in Chapter 2, is a very significant sign and symptom.

Taste disturbances in the form of bitter or metallic tastes or reduced or absent taste (hypogeusia or ageusia) may occur with trigeminal, facial, glossopharyngeal, or vagal nerve lesions and demands a cranial nerve examination, especially when combined with other symptoms that could emanate from pathology of these structures. Because taste is so dependent on the sense of smell, taste loss may also be caused by hyposmia or anosmia.[20]

Hyperacusia, commonly in the form of increased sensitivity to loud sounds (70 to 90 decibels above threshold), may be caused by paralysis or paresis of the stapedius or tensor tympani muscles. The facial nerve and the tensor tympani innervate the stapedius by the trigeminal nerve; both muscles take part in the auditory attenuation reflex. This occurs when a loud or very high pitched sound stimulates the cochlea. The stapedius and tensor tympani muscles contract, reducing the connectivity of the auditory ossicles from each other and the tympanum and also allowing the tympanic membrane to relax, thus cutting down the intensity of the sound reaching the cochlea. This can be tested, provided that there is no difference between the ears in hearing levels at low decibel levels, by plugging a stethoscope into the patient.[18,23]

Hypoacusia (reduced hearing) can be mechanical in origin (conduction), when the sound waves do not reach the cochlea because of mechanical impairments such as wax buildup, auditory ossicle fracture or dislocation, tympanic membrane rupture, eustachian tube obstruction, and so on. It is generally a low-frequency hearing loss. Alternatively, and more seriously, it can be caused by ischemia or damage to the cochlea or to the neural projections from the cochlea. This is termed *sensorineural hypoacusia* and is usually a high-frequency loss. Unless the hearing loss is sudden and/or profound, the patient may not realize that his or her hearing is impaired. Perhaps better questions are, Do you have problems hearing conversations in noisy rooms? Are you still holding the telephone to the same ear? This can occur with sensorineural hypoacusia, and deafness may be the only symptom. Because the cochlear nuclei are connected to both parietal areas of the cortex, it generally takes severe neurological damage to interfere with hearing in cases with lesions distal to the eighth nerve. In fact, usually the damage is so severe that testing is impossible because of the other neurological impairments.[23] However, reduced hearing has been reported in some cases of vertebrobasilar ischemia.[24,25]

Tinnitus[20,22] may be defined as "sounds that do not have an external source" and is classified into two main categories, objective and subjective. In objective tinnitus, the examiner can also hear the sounds, which include crepitus from middle ear muscles, vascular bruit, auditory ossicle crepitus and clicks, eustachian tube opening and closing, and palatal and hyoid movements. Of these, vascular tinnitus is potentially the most serious. It is pulsatile in nature and may indicate bruit from the large blood vessels in the neck or from an intracranial arteriovenous fistula. Other causes include raised intracranial pressure, intracranial tumors, and carotid occlusion. Pulsatile tinnitus may be heard through a stethoscope over the mastoid and may be eliminated by gently compressing the jugular vein.

In 100 consecutive cases of pulsatile tinnitus, carotid disease, glomus tumors, and hypertension were found to be the most common causes.[26] A recent onset of pulsatile tinnitus of itself is reason to send the patient to the physician. If pulsatile tinnitus occurs after head or neck trauma, the patient requires further medical investigation because this could be indicative of intracranial bleeding, traumatic hydrocephalus, or destabilized arteriovenous fistulas.

Subjective tinnitus can only be heard by the patient. Approximately 90% of the general population have physiological tinnitus, but under usual circumstances it is suppressed by ambient room noise. It can only be heard when the decibel level is below 17 decibels; because the average noise level in a living room is about 34 decibels, most people do not hear their own tinnitus. Subjective tinnitus can be low in frequency, when it sounds like roaring or rustling. The ocean noise that is heard on holding a sea shell to your ear is low-frequency tinnitus and results from the shell blocking external sounds; it is not actually the ocean (sorry to burst any bubbles). High-frequency subjective tinnitus is described as *whistling, ringing, chirping,* and even *musical.* The frequency of the tinnitus is usually related to the frequency of the hearing loss because the hearing loss reduces external noises and allows the tinnitus to be heard. High-frequency tinnitus is usually associated with sensorineural deafness and Low-frequency tinnitus with conduction deafness. The notable exception to this is the tinnitus accompanying Meniere's disease, which, although it causes a sensorineural hypoacusia, is more commonly related to low-frequency tinnitus. The presence of tinnitus in the history is indicative of hearing loss, which may itself be indicative of vertebral basilar compromise.[27]

Dizziness is an important finding in the history. Most dizziness has a benign cause, but rarely the cause will be serious. *Dizziness* may be defined as "a sense of imbalance." It is one of the most common complaints made to family practitioners, being fourth most common in women and seventh most common in men, and is in general age dependent, being more common in the elderly than in the young.[28] However, traumatic dizziness, including that caused by vertebral artery injury, tends to occur in the younger population. The average age for vertebral artery injury is about 37 years.[29,30] However, Terrett[30] made the point that this was because this was the peak age at which people required manual care for neck pain.

Dizziness may be caused by disturbances in the vestibular system or its vascularization, or by more mundane causes such as fever, hunger, shock, and emotion. The vestibular system is usually thought of as the vestibular apparatus in the inner ear, the eighth cranial nerve, the vestibular nuclei, and their neurological projections. However, from a more functional perspective, the total system also includes mechanoreceptors from all over the body, but particularly from the cervical spine and the eyes and their extraocular muscles. In addition to the structures that form the vestibular system, we should not forget the vertebrobasilar system, which supplies most of it.

There are numerous causes of dizziness, including[31]

❏ Central nervous system trauma (petechial hemorrhaging, TBI (Traumatic Brain Injury), concussion)
❏ Central nervous system disease (multiple sclerosis, cerebellar diseases)

❑ Vertebrobasilar compromise (trauma or degeneration)
❑ Central nervous system neoplastic disease (eighth cranial nerve neuromas, cerebellopontine tumors)
❑ Vestibular neuronitis (Ramsay Hunt syndrome, viral infections)
❑ Acute or chronic otitis media (bacterial or viral infections)
❑ Labyrinthine disease (Meniere's disease)
❑ Labyrinthine concussion (cupulolithiasis, canalolithiasis, perilymph fistulas)
❑ Medication (relaxants, NSAIDs, steroids, streptomycin, aspirin, diuretics)
❑ Toxins (alcohol, tobacco, carbon monoxide)
❑ Migraine
❑ Metabolic and hematologic disease (anemia, diabetes)
❑ Cardiovascular disease (dysrhythmias, congestive failure)
❑ Cervical dysfunction (inflammation, instability, hypomobility)
❑ Temporomandibular joint dysfunction
❑ Psychiatric

One study found that 100% of vertebrobasilar compromised patients complained of dizziness[21]; another found that only about two thirds experienced dizziness.[30] This of course does not mean that all patients complaining of dizziness have vertebrobasilar ischemia. There are many other causes, most of which are benign. The term *dizziness* is very nonspecific and must be better defined by the patient before any assessment of its severity or cause can be made. The most common method of classification is into those cases of dizziness that are caused by (1) a central lesion, vestibular nuclei and their projections, and (2) peripheral dizziness, caused by damage to the peripheral apparatus. This system is fine once the diagnosis has been made, but it does not really help to make the diagnosis, or at least not easily. A better system classifies the patient's symptomatology as follows[32]:

Type 1	Vertigo/oscillopsia
Type 2	Presyncope
Type 3	Dysequilibrium

Type 1 dizziness is *vertigo* or *oscillopsia.* Many use the term *vertigo* to imply any illusory movement, but only the illusion of rotatory motion is true vertigo.[33-35] This rotation can be in any plane but is commonly around a vertical axis. Rotation around a sagittal axis is much less common and can have serious implications, because it is more likely to be the result of cerebellopontine tumors than is the more common vertigo. If the environment spins, the condition is termed *objective vertigo,* and if the patient spins, *subjective vertigo.* It used to be thought that there was some clinically significant difference between the two, but now most clinicians involved in the condition think otherwise. Oscillopsia (visual oscillations) is the illusion of linear motion, a bobbing up and down, side to side, or forward and backward. It is usually caused by vestibular dysfunction, but may be caused by paresis with subsequent nystagmus of one or more extraocular muscles. All forms of vertigo are caused by problems in the vestibular system.

Most commonly the cause of vertigo or oscillopsia lies in the vestibular labyrinth, the eighth cranial nerve, the cerebellum, the vestibular nuclei, or their neurological projections. These structures can be compromised by

- ❏ Labyrinthine damage or inflammation
- ❏ Meniere's disease
- ❏ Brainstem concussion and contusion
- ❏ Eighth cranial nerve neuroma
- ❏ Brainstem tumors
- ❏ Medications
- ❏ Sudden onset of ophthalmoplegia
- ❏ Cerebellar disease
- ❏ Migraine
- ❏ Cervical joint dysfunction

The presence of vertigo is usually benign and usually caused by labyrinthine disorders but may be caused by more serious pathologies such as cerebellopontine tumors, Arnold Chiari malformations, and vertebrobasilar insufficiency. However, even when the vertigo is considered by the therapist to be benign, the patient must be discussed with the physician. This disorder needs to be treated as quickly as possible because not only is it very uncomfortable for the patient, it often makes function dangerous and will interfere with the recovery of the patient's neck.

Type 2 or *presyncope dizziness* is light-headedness, nausea, fainting, giddiness, wooziness, and so on, and is the most common type of dizziness. It may or may not be caused by vestibular system dysfunction, as was discussed earlier. In the study that looked at symptom frequency in vertebrobasilar ischemia, dizziness was quoted as being present in all patients but vertigo was complained of in only 40%. The causes for this type of dizziness are more numerous, so assessment can be more difficult. Among the causes are

- ❏ Central nervous system trauma
- ❏ Central nervous system disease (multiple sclerosis, Parkinson's disease, syringobulbia, syphilis)
- ❏ Vertebrobasilar ischemia
- ❏ Neoplastic disease (neuroma, cerebellopontine tumors)

- ❏ Acute and chronic otitis media
- ❏ Vestibular disorders
- ❏ Medication
- ❏ Surgery
- ❏ Toxins (alcohol, carbon monoxide, tobacco)
- ❏ Migraine
- ❏ Metabolic disease (diabetes, hypoglycemia, hyperventilation)
- ❏ Cardiovascular disease (cardiac or valvular dysrythmia, postural hypotension)
- ❏ Cervical joint dysfunction
- ❏ Temporomandibular joint dysfunction
- ❏ Fever
- ❏ Psychiatric
- ❏ Allergic Reactions

Disequilibrium, type 3 dizziness, is actually being off balance and is commonly confined to the older patient. The patient must reach out to save him or herself from falling or alternatively does fall. Older individuals may lose their balance when extending their neck because of impairment of their peripheral sensory afferents in the neck and decreased protective postural mechanisms. If one or both vestibular labyrinths are dysfunctional, the elderly patient may be permanently unbalanced, whereas the younger is able to compensate for the loss of vestibular function. Degenerative disease of the cerebellum may also cause disequilibrium, and again the potential for accommodation using other systems is less in the older person than the younger. If type 3 dizziness is seen in isolation—that is, no other type of dizziness is related—it is extremely unlikely for the cause to be vertebrobasilar compromise.

Vertebrobasilar ischemia can cause all three types of dizziness. It presumably creates the dizziness by ischemia of one or more of the vestibular nuclei and nerve, the cerebellum, and the vagus nucleus. Many of these conditions will be apparent on taking the patient's history.

Postural (orthostatic) hypotension makes itself known when the patient suddenly sits or stands up but not when sitting or lying down. Temporomandibular joint dizziness is more of a mild lightheadedness and is associated with temporomandibular joint pain.

With medication-induced dizziness, the dizziness will be worse just after ingestion and will ease with time until the next dose. Among the medications that are capable of producing dizziness as an adverse effect are[36,37]:

- ❏ Steroidal and nonsteroidal anti-inflammatories
- ❏ Muscle relaxants
- ❏ Analgesics
- ❏ Sedatives
- ❏ Antihistamines

- [ ] Vasodilators
- [ ] Antianginals
- [ ] Antidepressants
- [ ] Hyper- and hypoglycemic medications
- [ ] Oral contraceptives
- [ ] Antibiotics (especially the aminoglycosids)
- [ ] Antiallergenics
- [ ] Loop diuretics

Undiagnosed neurological disease states will provide an interesting though probably insolvable problem for the OMT (Orthopedic Manual Therapist). However, other signs that should be apparent on a detailed neurological examination will point the way and cause the therapist to refer to the physician. Some cardiopulmonary diseases will be obvious, such as congestive failure, that cause dizziness, and the dizziness will be associated with dyspnea. However, others, such as undiagnosed cardiac dysrhythmia, will not be obvious and will be referred to the physician as dizziness of unknown origin when other causes cannot be ascertained. Psychiatric dizziness may be obvious after talking to the patient for more than a few minutes.

Post-traumatic dizziness is probably more indicative of serious causes that affect the orthopedic therapist's treatment than is nontraumatic dizziness. According to one study,[38] approximately 20% of all neck injury patients have damage to one vertebral artery. In this series, 25% of hyperflexion injuries and 10% of hyperextension injuries had injured the artery, but only one-fifth of the patients with an injured artery demonstrated any symptom that could have been ascribed to the artery. That symptom was blurred vision.

Among the traumatic pathologies that may cause dizziness are[31]

- [ ] Vertebral artery injury
- [ ] Intracranial bleeds
- [ ] Cerebral concussion
- [ ] Brainstem concussion
- [ ] Labyrinthine concussion
- [ ] Cervical joint injury

Most post-traumatic dizziness seen by the orthopedic therapist will be caused by cervical joint dysfunction, but it is of course important to exclude the more serious causes before assuming the least serious.

The onset of the dizziness in relation to the onset or exacerbation of neck pain, or in the case of trauma in relation to the trauma, may help differentiate the cause. If there is no relationship between the dizziness and the neck pain, it is probable that the one is independent of the other. If the dizziness follows cervical trauma, was it immediate or delayed? Severe cervical pain following a neck injury is usually felt hours or even days after the injury, so if the dizziness has been caused by the cervical joint injury, its onset should be approximately simultaneous with the onset of the more severe cervical pain.

Dizziness coming on immediately after the trauma and associated with delayed pain could be caused by vertebral artery injury or compression, labyrinthine concussion, or cerebral concussion. Vertebral artery injury has been known to cause immediate dizziness that lasted a few minutes and then disappeared. Presumably there was a short-term vasospasm response to the insult. Ask about other symptoms of brainstem ischemia that may have occurred at the same time, and if these were present, assume that the cause was vertebral artery injury and ask the physician for further tests. If a history of these symptoms is absent and there is amnesia, the dizziness is probably related to concussion; however, objective tests must be done to exclude other causes. Labyrinthine concussion may be of immediate onset or delayed. If the traumatic forces have displaced the otoconia, it may take some time for them to reach an anatomic position of sensitivity (usually the posterior canal), and the patient may not put his or her head into a sensitizing position for some time. Traumatic hydrops (inflammation) may also take time to arise and produce symptoms. Other results of labyrinthine concussion such as perilymph fistulas and tympanic membrane rupture may be more immediate. Labyrinthine concussion is often associated with an ear noise such as popping or cracking at the time of the injury, and pain may be felt in the ear.

Delayed dizziness may be caused by the effects of labyrinthine concussion as already described, by cervical joint inflammation or instability, or by delayed vertebrobasilar compromise. The last cause may result from the patient increasing his or her range of motion and compressing the vertebral artery. There may be increasing dissection of the artery with increased bleeding, a pseudoaneurysm may have ruptured, or the treatment may have damaged or otherwise compromised the previously nontraumatized artery.

Disequilibrium may include ataxia, stumbling, falling, and drop attacks. The patient's method of relaying this information may not be straightforward. One patient complained that he felt as if he had a magnet in his pocket that caused him to be attracted to furniture or a wall on the left side of his body. He was describing lateral ataxia, and he was having transient ischemic attacks. *Drop attacks* are sudden collapses without losing consciousness. The victim is usually an elderly female, and she generally falls forward. Often, the immediate precipitating factor is extending the head. Recovery is immediate, and apart from any scrapes incurred from the fall, there are no other symptoms. Causes have been ascribed to neoplastic and other diseases of the cerebellum, cysts of the third ventricle, and vestibular hypofunction, particularly Meniere's disease. Although drop attacks are one of the four big Ds of vertebrobasilar ischemia (drop attacks, diplopia, dizziness, and dysarthria)[39] most neurologists do not consider this condition to be a major cause of drop attacks. One study put the rate of drop attacks with vertebrobasilar insufficiency at between 10% and 15%.[40] Although most drop attacks are relatively benign in nature, the cause of the attack must be ascertained, or at least serious causes must be excluded, before any mechanical treatment to the neck is undertaken. Consequently, patients relating drop attacks in their history must be referred back to the physician for an adequate workup that will exclude the more serious causes.

Paresthesia other than that distributed segmentally may indicate serious problems. Hemilateral paresthesia occurs with brainstem lesions, especially Wallenberg's or lateral medullary syndrome. Bilateral upper limb paresthesia has been found to be present in vertebrobasilar compromise[21] and may present with cervical myelopathy. Bilateral lower limb paresthesia has also been shown to occur in cervical myelopathy, but it may also be caused by thoracic spinal cord compression or ischemia and cauda equina syndrome. Quadrilateral paresthesia is almost certainly caused by spinal cord compression, disease, or ischemia. Facial paresthesia and perioral paresthesia have already been discussed in Chapter 1 and are certainly possible symptoms of vertebrobasilar compromise.

Dysphagia is of one of the most common symptoms of lateral medullary (Wallenberg's) syndrome, and complaints of swallowing difficulty must be taken seriously.[41] Hyperextension injuries have the potential to damage the hyoid muscles and even tear the pharynx and/or esophagus, leaving a retropharyngeal or retroesophageal hematoma.[3] In the early phase of these conditions, pain will be associated with the swallowing difficulty. It is the dysphagia that is not and has not been associated with pain that is important to the orthopedic therapist. The glossopharyngeal and vagus nerves mainly control swallowing, but the tongue must be able to function to form a bolus of the food. Consequently the therapist must look for evidence of paresis of the ninth, tenth, and twelfth cranial nerves in particular when this complaint is made. Dysphagia has been reported by some therapists when dealing with temporomandibular joint dysfunction but this diagnosis must only arrived at reluctantly after more serious causes have been eliminated.

An undiagnosed change in speech, *dysarthria,* is important because it might herald serious lesions in the medulla. Compromise of the medulla by tumor or ischemia may produce slow, slurred speech. There is no loss of cognition and the patient usually recognizes the problem.

Painless *dysphonia* is generally caused by a vocal cord paresis. The voice is hoarse and rasping. The control of the vocal musculature is from the vagal nucleus and this is part of the lateral medullary syndrome. Painful voice loss occurs post-traumatically with damage to the larynx and nontraumatically with laryngitis. Painless dysphonia requires laryngoscopic examination because it is a common symptom of Wallenberg's syndrome.[41]

Headaches

Headaches can be grouped into two main divisions, benign and nonbenign. Of the benign headaches approximately 20% are of vascular origin, with the remainder being variously attributed to tension, psychogenic overlay, fatigue, depression, and cervical spine dysfunction.[42]

Anatomy of a Headache[43]

On first consideration, it is difficult to understand how upper cervical dysfunction can generate supraoccipital headaches on a consistent basis. The general misunderstanding is that there is no cervical sensory reference to the head area because the C1 dorsal ramus has no sensory component. This has led to the erroneous belief that only the trigeminal nerve has sensory input to the vertex and frontal regions. In fact, there is considerable sensory input into the C1 root, but not from a cutaneous source.

Sensorially, the C1 dorsal ramus supplies the suboccipital muscles, the ventral ramus supplies the atlanto-occipital joint, and its sinuvertebral nerve together with those of C2 and C3 supplies the median atlantoaxial joint and the dura of the posterior cranial fossa. The ventral ramus of C1 joins with the hypoglossal nerve to form recurrent meningeal branches that supply the dura near the occipital condyles. Together with C2 and C3, the ventral ramus also innervates the longus capitus, longus cervicis, rectus capiti anterior, and lateralis.

The second cervical dorsal ramus supplies the occipital skin, semispinalis capitus, longissimus capitus, and splenius capitus. It directly innervates the lateral atlantoaxial joint and, via its sinuvertebral connections, the median atlantoaxial joint and the dura of the posterior cranial fossa. From its input into the cervical plexus, the ventral ramus supplies the prevertebral muscles, the sternomastoid, and trapezius. The ventral ramus of C2 connects with the hypoglossal and vagal nerves via the cervical plexus to form meningeal branches that also supply the posterior cranial fossa.

The C3 dorsal ramus forms the third occipital nerve and the deep medial branch. The third occipital nerve supplies the semispinalis capitus and the skin of the suboccipital area. The deep medial branch supplies the upper multifidi. The C3 dorsal ramus via its occipital nerve supplies the C2-3 zygapophyseal joint. The ventral ramus of C3 as a component of the cervical plexus innervates the prevertebral muscles, the sternomastoid, and the trapezius.

Vasomotor function to the extra and intracranial parts of the vertebral artery is served by the vertebral nerve formed from C1-C3 ventral plexi. Cell bodies in the C1 and C3 dorsal root ganglia sensorially supply the intracranial (fourth) portion of the vertebral artery.

To summarize, the dorsal and ventral rami of C1-C3 innervate the anterior and posterior suboccipital muscles, the dura of the posterior cranial fossa, the atlanto-occipital and atlantoaxial joints (lateral and median), the C2-3 zygapophyseal joints, all of their ligaments, the sternomastoid, the trapezius, the prevertebral and upper posterior cervical muscles, and the vertebral artery. Consequently, pain can arise from any of these structures and can be referred to any of the segmentally associated tissues. In addition, if vasomotor function can be affected by nociceptive sensory input into these segments, the possibility of pain from vertebral artery ischemia is present.

When the anatomy of the trigeminal nerve is considered, further indirect pain and other symptoms can be seen to be caused by nociceptive input and radiation via the trigeminocervical nucleus. The spinal nucleus of the trigeminal nerve extends through the medulla to at least the upper three levels of the cervical cord, which implies that sensation, cutaneous or otherwise, from the upper cervical spine is intimately connected with sensation from the occiput, vertex, frontal area, and face via the trigeminocervical nucleus. This relationship and potential for referral has been demonstrated experimentally.

Distribution

The following distribution of headaches is strongly based on Jull's study of 203 cervical patients treated in an Australian physical therapy clinic.[44] Ninety-six of the 203 complained of headaches. This distribution was almost identical to that in another study with a larger sample.[45] However, the subjects were of a clinical population and so more typical of patients presenting to the orthopedic therapists. Thus, this has more significance for the clinical therapist than do the general population statistics.

Approximately 47% of cervical patients have headaches as part or all of their symptomatology. Females in all age groups except those over 60 years, for whom incidence was equal, suffered headaches with more prevalence than males. On average, for all age groups, women suffered from headaches about three times more often than men. The age group with the highest incidence was 20 to 40 years, when approximately 42% of the headaches occurred. The age group 40 to 60 years accounted for about 24% of the reported headaches.

Vertebral Level of Origin

Based on reproduction of symptoms from posteroanterior and anteroposterior pressures over the spinous process or over the zygapophyseal articulation, headaches could approximately be reproduced at

- ❑ C0-1 (60%)
- ❑ C1-2 (40%)

❏ C2-3 (55%)
❏ C3-4 (20%)
❏ C4-5 (10%)
❏ C5-6 (5%)
❏ C6-7 (8%)
❏ C7-T1 (2%)

Headaches from the upper three levels (C0-1, C1-2, and C2-3) were nearly three and a half times more frequently reproduced by posteroanterior pressures over the joint than they were at the lower levels. The lower levels were about three and a half times more likely to reproduce nonheadache symptoms with posteroanterior pressures over the joint or spinous processes.

Region of Symptoms

Half of all headaches were reported to include the occipital or suboccipital areas, and 38% of headache patients experienced accompanying cervical pain. In only 12% of headache patients was cervical pain not reported. The absence of cervical pain does not exclude the spine as being the source of the headache, but its absence is unusual.

Pain Type

Aching was the most commonly reported pain and is reported in about 75% of patients. Some patients described a tightness around the head as with a tight band, others reported stabbing and shooting pains. Throbbing was described by 7% of patients. Tightness or heaviness has been related to tension, stabbing pain in the eye has been associated with cervical spine disorders, and intense throbbing has been related to vasculogenic headaches.

Severity

Based on normal activity ability or disability and the patient's reliance on analgesics, 20% of patients rated their headaches as severe, 73% as moderate, and 7% as mild.

Frequency and Duration of Headaches

❏ 61% of patients reported daily headaches.
❏ 28% reported headaches at least 2 or 3 times a week.
❏ 10% had headaches irregularly.
❏ 66% stated that the headaches lasted a few hours.
❏ 33% suffered headaches all day.
❏ 58% of patients reported waking with the headache.

Associated Symptoms

About 45% of cervical headache patients complained of associated symptoms, the most common of which were

- ❑ Nausea
- ❑ Visual disturbances (such as flashing lights, photophobia, and blurring)
- ❑ Dizziness

Nonnociceptive symptoms such as visual, balance, and vascular disturbances have been ascribed to the cervical spine by various authors. Various mechanisms for the causes of these symptoms have been proposed, including subluxation of the lateral atlantoaxial joint, which compresses the second cervical ventral ramus and causes neck-tongue syndrome via the ramus's connection with the hypoglossal nerve. Experimental evidence suggests a link between nociceptive stimulation of the periarticular tissues of C0-1 and C1-2 and giddiness, nausea, and tinnitus. The proposed connection is via the upper cervical nerves and the vagal, accessory, and hypoglossal nerves and the superior cervical ganglion. Vertebrobasilar ischemia caused by mechanical obstruction from disk prolapse, instability, or osteophytosis, or from sympathetic irritation has been proposed to account from many of the nonnociceptive symptoms associated with headache.

Causal/Contributive/Precipitating Factors

Postures, movements, or activities that put strain on the neck have been associated with headaches. In one study, 51% of patients associated their headaches with particular sustained neck flexion during reading, studying or typing, and driving a car, 65% of headache patients reported a chronic course running between 2 and 20 years, and only 7% reported pain of less than 1 week's duration.

Trauma was reported in 44% of 6000 headache patients in one study[46] and in 40% of 96 in another, with 16% of the 96 having been involved in a motor vehicle accident. The role of trauma may be understated because the trauma often occurs some considerable time before the onset of the headache and so may be forgotten. Tension may well initiate a headache in a patient predisposed by some previous and forgotten traumatic incident.

Degenerative joint disease has also been inculpated as a cause of headaches, with some authors denying a significant role played by trauma in the genesis of the headache.[47] As with trauma, the degeneration may not in and of itself generate the headache, but if stress or some microtrauma is superimposed, the patient may become symptomatic. This would explain those patients who have quite advanced degeneration but whose headache has only recently occurred.

The following characteristics may provide for differentiation of cervicogenic headaches and those from other benign causes.

- ❏ Females more commonly affected than males
- ❏ Occipital and suboccipital pain with radiation to the frontal and retro-orbital regions
- ❏ Aching pain most common, with occasional shooting or stabbing
- ❏ Vascular or sympathetic symptoms common
- ❏ Onset usually associated with sustained neck flexion, tension, or neck pain and motion
- ❏ Patients often waking with the pain
- ❏ Frequently chronic
- ❏ Trauma related about as often as not
- ❏ Standard radiographs usually considered normal
- ❏ Articular dysfunction usually demonstrated by craniovertebral biomechanical joint examination

From a safety aspect, noncervical headaches must be recognized. Often the distribution is different and often the headache is not associated with neck pain. The quality of the pain may also be different. Deep, diffuse headaches that are dull in nature can be caused by increases in intracranial pressure from bleeding or neoplasm.[48] If there is increasing pressure, there will be other signs and symptoms during the process. Ask about concentration difficulties, drowsiness, reading problems, and so on. If these or other symptoms exist, the patient should be referred back to the physician. It is also worth noting that there is frequently an inverse relationship between the severity of the headache and the seriousness of the pathology causing that headache.[49-51]

Migraine[20,52,53] is another type of headache that must be considered by the therapist, because it must be managed medically. Classical migraine (migraine with aura) can take many forms but tends to be unilateral, throbbing, and severe. In classical migraine, cranial nerve and/or long tract symptoms precede the headache. These symptoms may include scintillating hemianopia or quadranopia, blurred vision, tinnitus, hypoacusia, facial or limb paresthesia, taste or smell disturbances, vertigo, nausea, aphasia, dysphasia, and more. The most common are visual symptoms. Classical migraine criteria according to the International Headache Society are[48]

1. At least two attacks that fulfill
2. At least three of the following characteristics
  - ❏ One or more fully reversible aura symptoms, indicating cerebral cortical and/or brainstem dysfunction

❏ At least one aura symptom develops gradually over more than 4 minutes or two or three symptoms occur in succession

❏ The aura symptom lasts less than 60 minutes (if more than one aura symptom is present, accepted duration is proportionally increased)

❏ Headache follows aura with a free interval of less than 60 minutes (it may also begin before or simultaneously with the aura)

3. History and examination do not suggest an organic or metabolic disorder, the latter is ruled out by appropriate investigations, or the migraine attacks do not occur for the first time in close temporal relation to an organic or metabolic disorder.

Alternatively, the Albert Einstein College of Medicine in New York gives the following:

Recurrent idiopathic headache associated with at least two or the following:

1. Nausea with or without vomiting

2. Unilateral pain

3. Throbbing quality

4. Photophobia or phonophobia

5. Pain is increased by menses and there is a positive family history (this last can be removed without altering the specificity of the criteria).

It is apparent from these symptoms that the patient could just as easily be suffering a transient ischemic attack as a migraine. If this is the first attack to be provisionally diagnosed as such, the diagnosis is very tentative and can only be made after the patient has survived a series of attacks without stroking.

In migraine equivalent, there are prodromal symptoms (as listed earlier) but no subsequent headache. Migraine variant or common migraine is essentially the opposite, with the patient suffering the headache but not the prodromal symptoms.

When there are definite signs and/or symptoms of neurovascular involvement, migraine and migraine equivalent demands that the therapist be very cautious about accepting this diagnosis unless it has received a good deal of consideration by the physician. Certainly, do not undertake to treat this patient if he or she has not survived at least three episodes and the physician is fully aware of the problem.

Headache is a common symptom in patients suffering from cervical spine dysfunction. Most commonly, the source of the symptoms lies in the upper three cervical levels and includes some degree of hypomobility in one or more joints of these levels (discussed earlier). In many cases, the headache is accompanied by other symptoms, which on the surface can appear somewhat bizarre. These include visual disturbances, disequilibrium, tongue symptoms, and so on. Most of these can be explained away by applied anatomy, but the cause that is most sinister is vertebrobasilar ischemia. It is important for the therapist to preclude this as a cause before becoming embroiled in other differential diagnostic problems.

Summary

In summary, for you to diagnose the patient's headache as cervical in origin, the majority of the following should be present:

1. It should follow the typical cervical distribution:
   Suboccipital → occipital → occipitofrontal → frontal → orbital
      or
   Suboccipital → occipital → occipitotemporal → frontal → orbital
2. It should be associated with neck pain.
3. It should be associated with neck postures or movements.

It should not be

1. Diffuse
2. Deep
3. Isolated to the eyes
4. Extreme
5. Associated with neurological symptoms
6. Associated with intellectual impairment such as drowsiness, inability to concentrate, or inability to retain information

If any of these are present, make sure that the physician is aware of them and that you have an adequate explanation for their presence.

Meningitis[20]

A potentially serious and confusing cause of headaches is meningitis. Viral meningitis is much less dramatic than bacterial and is more likely to reach the therapist. Symptoms include

❏ Mild to moderate fever (38 to 40°C)
❏ Headache
❏ Neck stiffness
❏ Reduced neck and trunk flexion
❏ Photophobia
❏ Painful eye movements

Less common signs and symptoms are

❏ Reduced straight leg raise
❏ Sore throat

❑ Nausea
❑ Diplopia
❑ Strabismus
❑ Transient Babinski's response
❑ Back and neck pain
❑ Limb paresthesia
❑ Drowsiness or confusion

Objective Examination

The following examination is the routine examination of the nonacute and nontraumatic neck patient. The special tests and cranial nerve tests will be discussed after the routine examination.

Standing and Walking (Observation)

❑ Gross deformities such as torticollis
❑ Spine surgery or thyroidectomy scars
❑ Sternomastoid or trapezius atrophy (possible eleventh cranial nerve neuroma)
❑ Deltoid, supraspinatus, and infraspinatus atrophy (possible peripheral nerve lesion)
❑ Muscle balling, particularly biceps and infraspinatus (probable rupture)
❑ Congenital anomalies such as syndactyly, polydactyly, Sprengle's deformity, and Klippel-Feil deformity (possible involvement of other systems including vertebral artery)
❑ Facial bruising (possible facial fracture)
❑ Mastoid bruising (Battle's sign; possible occipital or temporal fracture)
❑ Horner's syndrome signs (possible brainstem lesion or ganglion damage)
❑ Facial droop (possible brainstem lesion or facial nerve palsy)
❑ Pupil asymmetry (aniscoria; possible brainstem lesion)
❑ Squint (strabismus; possible brainstem lesion if paralytic)
❑ Nystagmus (possible vestibular or brainstem lesion)
❑ Wide-based ataxia (possible vestibular lesion)
❑ Lateral ataxia (possible brainstem lesion)

Sitting

1. *Changes in posture from standing*
2. *Articular*
   ❑ active flexion, rotations, side flexions, and extension
   ❑ traction
   ❑ compression
   ❑ quadrants

3. Muscular
   ❏ isometric tests in stretched position
   ❏ isometric tests in shortened position if positive in the stretched position
   ❏ palpation along suspect muscle-tendon unit

4. Dural
   ❏ neck flexion
   ❏ scapular retraction (T1)
   ❏ slump
   ❏ cough

5. Neurological
   ❏ motor
        C1 (short neck flexors)
        C4 (levator scapulae)
        C5 (shoulder abductors)
        C6 (elbow flexors)
        C7 (elbow extensors)
        C8 (extensor pollicis longus)
        T1 (hand intrinsics)
   ❏ sensory
        hypo- or hyperesthesia and distribution
   ❏ reflexes
        deep tendon reflexes
            C4 (levator scapulae)
            C5 (deltoid)
            C6 (biceps)
            C7 (triceps)
            C8 (extensor pollicis longus)
            T1 (thenar muscles)
        spinal cord reflexes
            extensor-plantar
            clonus
            lower limb tendon reflexes

6. Peripheral joint screening tests
   ❏ active, passive, and resisted movement tests of each upper limb joint

Supine-Prone

1. Palpation
   ❏ hypertonicity
   ❏ skin changes
   ❏ reactivity (myotactile response)
   ❏ tenderness

2. Posteroanterior pressure
- ❏ pain
- ❏ reactivity of the mobile segment

3. Craniovertebral ligament stress tests
- ❏ transverse ligament
- ❏ alar ligament
- ❏ transverse shear
- ❏ vertical (longitudinal ligaments)

Common Screening Tests

Quadrant Tests These are the end range combined movements of the neck and are described in Chapter 1. The indications for doing these tests are these:

- ❏ The pure movement tests (flexion, extension, rotation, and side flexion) were painless.
- ❏ Radicular pain is present.

Vertebral Artery Tests Technically speaking, vertebral artery sufficiency testing is a special test, but the indications are so numerous that it is almost always carried out unless there is a good reason not to do so. Almost any treatment we do will threaten the artery to some extent or another, and if the aim of our treatment is to increase range of motion, that aim, if fulfilled, also threatens the artery. It is easier to consider the contraindications to testing than the indications, and these include

- ❏ Cardinal signs or symptoms of potential vertebral artery origin
- ❏ The presence of a fracture (see "Fracture Tests")
- ❏ Recent trauma (strong caution)

Remember, however, that if it is not safe to test the artery, it is not safe to treat the patient.

For the straightforward nontraumatic, nondizzy patient, the so-called vertebral artery tests can be carried out in an abbreviated manner. Unless there is some indication to do so, the patient may be tested directly with the full-position Hautard's (Hauntant's) test. This is not appropriate in the patient who has suffered trauma or who relates a history of dizziness or any other symptoms that might be caused by vertebrobasilar compromise. In these patients, a much more detailed and graduated examination must be used, including cranial nerve testing, long tract testing, if necessary, and progressive stressing of the neck tissues. A more complete description of the tests for dizziness and the vertebral artery will be given in "The Examination of the Traumatic Neck Patient."

Upper Limb Neural Tension (Provocation) Tests An exercise in the constant-length phenomenon, these tests test the reactivity to movement and stretch of the neural tissues running from the spinal cord to the periphery. Cyriax described a diagnostic stretch for the ulnar nerve and its continuation into the brachial plexus and spinal nerve roots as early as 1970 (and possibly earlier).[54] Further work has been done by Elvey[55-57] since 1979 and by Butler[58,59] more recently. Butler classified responses into three:

> *Physiological,* which indicates normal sensations of tightness and discomfort that may come from a variety of sources and are not particularly relevant at that time.
>
> *Clinical Physiological* in which symptoms that are not exactly what brought the patient in for treatment are produced together with asymmetry in ranges in the tests. These may or may not be a relevant asymptomatic component of the patient's overall problem.
>
> *Neurogenic,* in which the reproduced symptoms arise from the peripheral nervous system. In the case of symptoms such as headache, which are not lancinating, causalgic, or paresthetic, the source is presumptive. However, because these symptoms must be alterable with changes in the test, it is reasonable to assume that they arise from the neuromeninges.

The head is placed into contralateral side flexion and rotation to maximally stretch the brachial plexus spinal nerve roots. The shoulder is abducted, extended, and laterally rotated to stretch the brachial plexus and its continuation into the upper arm. By flexing or extending the elbow and wrist in various combinations, a presumed differentiating stretch can be applied to the various parts of the neural tissues in the arm, and by eliciting symptoms specific to neurological distress, the affected component can be identified.

Structures Tested	Final Test Position
Median Nerve	1. Contralateral neck side flexion
• lateral cord	2. Shoulder girdle depression and
• C5, 6, 7 spinal nerves	retraction
• C5, 6, 7 roots	3. 90 degrees glenohumeral
• medial cord	abduction
• C8, T1 spinal nerves	4. Elbow extension and supination
• C8, T1 roots	5. Wrist extension
Ulnar Nerve	1. Contralateral neck side flexion
• Medial cord	2. Shoulder girdle depression and
• C7, 8, T1 spinal nerves	retraction
• C7, 8, T1 roots	3. 90 degrees glenohumeral
	abduction

Radial and Interosseus Nerves
- Posterior cord
- C5, 6, 7, 8, T1

4. Elbow flexion and supination
5. Wrist extension

1. Contralateral neck side flexion
2. Shoulder girdle depression and retraction
3. 90 degrees glenohumeral abduction
4. Elbow extension and pronation
5. Wrist flexion

It should be pointed out however, that regardless of the results of these tests, mechanical extraneural pathology must be accounted for prior to using these tests as stretches; otherwise, further damage may be done to the tissue. Among these mechanical pathologies would be

❑ Disk compression
❑ Osteophytic compression
❑ Humeral compression
❑ Ulnohumeral valgus instability caused by traction
❑ Carpal compression

These tests are useful in determining the presence of neural compromise when the more standard tests have failed or in demonstrating a double-crush syndrome. This syndrome occurs when there are two areas of nerve compression and each by itself is subthreshold, but together they produce signs and/or symptoms. An example of this is a form of carpal tunnel syndrome in which there is minor compression of the spinal nerve or root at one of the originating levels of the median nerve and compression further down the line. Often, the standard carpal tunnel tests, Phalen's maneuver, compression, Tinel's sign, and so on are negative, but when the full stretch position is attained, the symptoms are experienced.

The use of modifications of these test positions as treatment for neuromeningeal hypomobility is certainly useful in appropriate patients. However, extraneuromeningeal causes must be excluded before stretching; otherwise, a poor situation can be made considerably worse.

Vascular Tests The indications to carry out these tests are a history of coldness in the limbs, quadrilateral pain, color changes in the limbs, and any suggestion of intermittent claudication or demand ischemia. The tests include taking the proximal and distal pulses of the affected limb and its partner, and repetitive or sustained exercises for demand ischemia. Adson's test (diminution or obliteration of the pulse when the patient, seated and with the arm dependent, holds a full breath while tilting the head back and rotating it to the symptomatic side) and Wright's test (abduction and lateral rotation of the arm and strong retraction of the shoulder girdle) are tests for thoracic outlet syndrome. They should be carried out if the patient is complaining of color and temperature changes in the hands together with neurological signs and symptoms ascribable to the lower brachial plexus.[20] They are not particularly sensitive, affording both false positives and false negatives. However, if they are positive on the symptomatic side and the symptoms are appropriate, a diagnosis of thoracic outlet syndrome can be provisionally made.

Serious Disease Red Flags

Indications	Possible Condition
Dizziness	Upper cervical dysfunction, vestibular dysfunction vertebrobasilar ischemia, c/v (craniovertebral) ligament tear
Quadrilateral parasthesia	Cord compression, vertebrobasilar ischemia
Bilateral upper limb parasthesia	Cord compression, vertebrobasilar ischemia, syringomyelia
Hyperreflexia	Cord compression, vertebrobasilar ischemia
Babinski's or clonus sign	Cord compression, vertebrobasilar ischemia
Cardinal signs/symptoms	Cord compression, vertebrobasilar ischemia
Positive Sharp-Purser test	C1-2 instability
Consistent swallow on transverse ligament stress tests	C1-2 instability, retropharyngeal hematoma, RA (Rheumatoid Arthritis)
Nontraumatic capsular pattern	RA, AS (Ankylosing Spondylitis), neoplasm
Arm pain lasting more than 6 to 9 months	Neoplasm
Persistent root pain in patient under 30 years old	Neoplasm
Radicular pain with coughing	Neoplasm
Primary posterolateral pain	Neoplasm
Pain worsening after 1 month	Neoplasm
More than one segmental level involved	Neoplasm or neurological disease
Paralysis	Neoplasm or neurological disease
Trunk and limb parasthesia	Neoplasm
Bilateral root signs and symptoms	Neoplasm
Nontraumatic strong spasm	Neoplasm
Nontraumatic strong pain in the elderly patient	Neoplasm
Signs worse than symptoms	Neoplasm
Radial deviator weakness	Neoplasm
Thumb flexor weakness	Neoplasm
Hand intrinsic weakness and/or atrophy	Neoplasm, thoracic outlet syndrome, carpal tunnel syndrome

Horner's syndrome	Superior sulcus tumor, breast cancer, cervical ganglion damage, brainstem damage
Empty end feel	Neoplasm
Severe post-traumatic capsular pattern	Fracture
Sever post-traumatic spasm	Fracture
No ROM after trauma	Fracture
Post-traumatic painful weakness	Fracture

The Examination of the Traumatic Neck Patient

There are a number of concerns with post-traumatic neck patients that, in the nontraumatic patient, either are not factors or are considerably reduced. The possibilities of acute fracture and dislocation, rim lesions, pharyngeal and esophageal tears, brainstem and cerebral concussion or contusion, intracranial bleeding, traumatic brain injury, vertebral artery injury, ligament and muscle tearing, and litigation must all be considered and guarded against in the examination. Consequently, the sequencing of the examination and the initial examination's emphasis are altered and shifted respectively. The sequence of the examination must be designed to provide a measure of protection for the patient in case a serious injury is present. Systems have to be examined that in the nontraumatic patient can either be ignored, unless there is an indication to examine them, or explored superficially. A case in point is the brainstem. In nontraumatic neck patients, the chances of the cranial nerves being involved are remote, and they perhaps do not need to be examined unless something in the history suggests that they are a factor. However, central neurological damage is common in post-whiplash victims, and the most usual region involved is the brainstem.

Fracture Tests

Fracture tests are obviously important and must be carried out early in the examination, before any movement of the head and neck takes place. Studies have shown that about 30% of fractures either do not show up on initial x-rays or are missed when they do.[60,61] Add to this that many patients are not x-rayed after whiplash or the x-rays that are taken are inappropriate views and you have a potentially serious problem on your hands. Cadaveric studies support this view and have shown the frequency of small fractures in whiplash injuries to be very high.[10,62] The moral is, Do not rely on a negatively read x-ray to clear the patient.

A history of immediate severe pain is suggestive of profound structural damage. If this is followed by a severe loss of motion in most or all directions, the likelihood is that a fracture or some other profound tissue damage has occurred. With undisplaced dens fractures, patients may feel severely threatened and actually hold their head in their hands to prevent it "falling off." At least two cases have been related to me in which the physician has insisted that a patient take the hands away and move the head, whereupon the fracture displaced and the patient died because the lower medulla was compressed.

Inspect the patient. Is there bruising over the face? The raccoon mask, in which both eyes are bruised but often the lid and conjunctiva is spared, suggests a facial fracture. Mastoid bruising (Battle's sign) occurs with fractures of the temporal or occipital bones.

Gentle compression in the acute patient should not reproduce severe pain, even in the most inflamed. Although in the long-term patient it is one indication of chronic pain, in the acute patient, it must be considered as evidence of more structural damage.

Isometric contraction may be painful if a muscle is torn (the most common in whiplash injuries are the sternomastoid and longus colli), but the weakness should only be in one direction or perhaps two, depending on the muscle's actions and the extent of the tear. Multi- or omnidirectional painful weakness is more suggestive of a fracture than of a muscle tear. A note of caution: When testing isometrics in the recently injured patient, remember that there may be painful inhibition, in which case, the head could flip in the direction you are pushing. This may do more damage. Make sure that you are ready to support the other side of the head should this occur.

Motion in the most inflamed neck is present to a greater or lesser extent. When you are testing for motion early in the course of the posttraumatic patient, the purpose is not to see how much movement is present but rather how much is missing. To this end, I position my hands so as to block any movement of more than about 20 degrees. This safeguards the vertebral artery. If there is no movement, or if there is severe multidirectional restriction, there may be a fracture present. If severe restriction is present, apply very gentle overpressure in the limited ranges and assess the end feel. If the end feel is spasm in all or most directions, a fracture is possible.

A low-frequency vibrating tuning fork applied to the occiput, temporal region, facial bones, and vertebral transverse and spinous process tips may help identify fractures. Severe pain would indicate a fracture, although the test may also be positive in the presence of severe inflammation.

None of these tests have, as far as I know, been checked against a gold standard, but there does not seem to be any pathology other than a fracture or bone cancer that would generate a positive result in all of these tests. Consequently, if only one or two tests reproduce pain, they are weakly positive for fracture, but if all are painful, they are very strongly positive for a fracture.

Fracture Tests and Results

Test	Positive Finding
Light compression	Severe pain
Range of movement	None or severely restricted in all directions
End feel	Spasm in all or most directions
Isometric	Painful weakness in multiple directions
Observation	Mastoid or facial bruising
Tuning fork	Pain

Neurological Examination

It is important to examine for neurological and neurovascular signs and symptoms on patients attending for cervical treatment or who have been involved in significant neck and head trauma. It is estimated from sample studies that about 50% of whiplash patients have central nervous system damage to some extent,[63,64] although another researcher refuted this finding, stating that there was little if any difference between traumatized and nontraumatized subjects in this regard.[65,66] An EEG and clinical examination study on whiplash patients found about the same level of EEG abnormality (approximately 50%), and on otolaryngological examination a little over 50% had clinical manifestations of dysfunction in the brainstem. Generally the level of damage is very low and tends to affect the brainstem, particularly the vestibular nucleus.

However, in some patients damage is much more extensive and may involve the cerebrum as well as the brainstem. The percentage of patients suffering cognitive deficiency may be as high as 61% immediately after whiplash and 20% at one year.[59] More serious yet is the possibility of damage to the vertebral artery. The earliest and most sensitive signs and symptoms of this seem to be cranial nerve deficits. However, these tend to be transient and depend on the position of the head, so testing in the neutral position will probably be fruitless if this condition is present. Testing in the neutral position, however, will give us a baseline when we retest some of the cranial nerves and test the functions of the structures supplied by the vertebrobasilar system.

The tests described here are those that test the function of the following:

- ❏ Cranial nerves
- ❏ Long tracts
- ❏ Temporoparietal area
- ❏ Visual cortex

Cranial Nerve Signs, Symptoms, and Tests

Most of the following cranial nerve tests, which are simple and instrument-free, are taken from Goldberg's excellent short, inexpensive, and clinically oriented book *The Four Minute Neurological Examination.*[67]

First Cranial Nerve The olfactory bulbs and tracts are the only cranial nerves not vascularized by the vertebrobasilar system but by the anterior cerebral artery. However, facial impact may damage this system. The patient may completely lose the sense of smell (anosmia) or may retain a distorted sense of smell (paraosmia), in which case, the patient complains of a foul smell. As an aside, a patient suffering facial impact may fracture one or more facial bones, which may result in cerebrospinal fluid leaking out through the nose, so if a patient talks about a runny nose after a facial impact, it may well be cerebrospinal fluid rather than mucus. To test the function of this system, a piece of soap is held under one of the blindfolded patient's nostrils while the other is closed. The patient is asked to identify the smell, not simply, Can you smell this? The patient is then told the smell is going to be changed and the soap is held under the other nostril with the same question. Unfortunately, a large percentage of the population is functioning with chronic upper respiratory tract infections or allergy reactions in the nose and may have trouble smelling at any time.

Second Cranial Nerve Visual fields can be affected by neurovascular problems because the vertebrobasilar system vascularizes the lateral geniculate body as well as the optic radiation (geniculocalcerine tract) and the visual cortex of the occipital lobe. From the perspective of the orthopedic therapist, the vision problem that will be most significant will be hemianopia or quadranopia. This will be bilateral because the lesion will lie posterior to the optic chiasm, and if it is caused by vertebrobasilar compromise, the deficit will be homonymous; that is, the visual fields affected will be both right or both left but not right and left. The patient may complain of hemianopia or quadranopia if there is scintillation within the deficit but may not be aware of any visual loss if there are no flashing lights because the blind spot moves with the head. As a result, it may not be noticed until objective testing is undertaken. The definitive testing method for visual field deficits is computerized perimetry testing, but in the clinic, the confrontation test can be utilized to determine if more sophisticated tests should be employed.

During the confrontation test, the patient and therapist stand or sit opposite each other, making sure that the eyes of each are level. The patient is instructed to look only into the therapist's eyes. The therapist brings colored targets into the two lateral visual fields, asking the patient to indicate when the targets are seen. The therapist looks only into the patient's eyes and checks the patient's visual field against his or her own. The entire lateral perimeter is tested, and if the patient notes a deficit, the area of vision loss is mapped out with the targets. To test the medial field, the patient covers up one eye and the therapist follows suit, covering the eye directly (not diagonally) opposite. A target is then gradually introduced into the medial field by the therapist who gives the same instructions to the patient. The medial perimeter is covered, and any deficits are mapped out.

Third Cranial Nerve The oculomotor nerve is unique among the extraocular nerves in that it supplies a facial muscle, the levator palpebrae, and intraocular muscles, the pupil constrictors. The oculomotor nucleus is actually a collection of subnuclei, one for each of the four extraocular muscles (superior rectus, inferior rectus, medial rectus, and inferior oblique) it innervates, one for the levator palpebrae, and the Edinger-Westphal nucleus for the parasympathetic supply to the pupil. Testing is in two parts, the test for the pupil's ability to react to light and a second test, which is shared by the fourth and sixth cranial nerves, for the ability of the eye to track a moving object. Symptoms of oculomotor paresis or paralysis include diplopia, caused by reduced ability to fix the eyes on an object correctly and fuse the two images, and photophobia, caused by the dilated pupil.

Consensual Test The test is based on the principle of agreement between the two pupils. That is, the other reflects what the one pupil does providing light conditions are not too intense. Sitting in front of the patient, first observe the pupil for symmetry. Cover one of the patient's eyes while holding the other open to prevent the patient from blinking. Watch the uncovered eye. It should undergo the same changes as the covered. It first dilates, and then, as the covered eye is uncovered, it constricts. The test is repeated for the opposite eye. The therapist looks for aniscoria (asymmetric pupils), dilation on covering, and constriction on uncovering. Failure to dilate may indicate a fixed constricted pupil, and a dilated pupil that does not constrict normally may indicate an oculomotor lesion.

Tracking Test Sitting opposite the patient, the therapist holds a target about 18 inches in front of the patient and asks the patient to follow the target with the eyes while keeping the head still. The standard test is to smoothly and at moderate speed move the target in a H configuration and then in the midline just above eye level toward the base of the patient's nose. The target must stay within about 45 degrees of midline to limit the appearance of normal end-point or physiological nystagmus. The patient should be able to track the target smoothly. Look for nystagmus and paresis or paralysis. The ability to converge is often affected, and either the patient will not be able to converge at all or it will not be able to maintain the convergence on one side. Paralysis or paresis of one or more extraocular muscles may result in diplopia. The patient may be able to tell the examiner this or may have unconsciously accommodated to it by tilting the head appropriately. If paresis or paralysis is present or the patient has a correctable painless torticollis, test for diplopia by presenting the target to the patient and ask how many targets are present. Move the target around the patient's visual field, or if the patient is not acute, have the patient move his or her head, asking all the time how many targets are seen. If the movement produces one target on some movements and two on others, the patient almost certainly has diplopia and more sophisticated testing is indicated. Distance diplopia is more difficult to test. The patient is asked to look at a distant object and then move his or her head around. The same significance is placed on this test as on near vision testing.

Fourth Cranial Nerve   The trochlear nucleus and nerve supply the superior oblique muscle, which depresses the eye. Again, paresis or paralysis will result in diplopia. The tracking tests for this nerve are carried out simultaneously with those for the third nerve.

Fifth Cranial Nerve   The trigeminal nucleus and nerve are responsible for all of the sensation of the head and the posterior upper cervical spine except for the skin of the neck. Symptoms of deficit from this nerve include facial paresthesia, often patchy and usually over the areas innervated by the maxillary and mandibular branches. The nerve's innervation of tensor tympani may cause hyperacusia when this muscle is paretic or paralyzed. Sensation is tested with pinprick close to the midline of the face, because the skin that is more lateral is overlapped by the nerves from the face. Anesthesia or hypoesthesia is positive. The jaw deep tendon reflex is assessed by hyperreflexia.

Sixth Cranial Nerve   The abducens nucleus and nerve supply the lateral rectus, which turns the eye laterally. Paresis or palsy results in an inability to diverge the eye and diplopia. The tracking tests for this nerve are carried out simultaneously with those for the third nerve.

Seventh Cranial Nerve   The muscles of facial expression, the stapedius and the anterior part of the tongue, are supplied by the facial nerve. Symptoms of deficit could include a persistent bitter or metallic taste and/or painful hyperacusia to loud sounds caused by stapedius paralysis. The nerve is partially decussed, with the muscles above the eyes having partial innervation from the other side. Consequently, a supranuclear lesion will cause loss of function of the lower facial muscles but not the upper. A facial nerve palsy such as Bell's palsy will cause paralysis of all of the facial muscles. The test is to ask the patient to smile. If there is asymmetry, the patient is asked to frown or wrinkle the forehead. Loss or reduced ability to smile and frown is caused by a peripheral palsy; the loss of the smile only is caused by a supranuclear lesion.

Eighth Cranial Nerve Dizziness is the most common sign of vertebrobasilar compromise and as such requires careful attention. Dizziness is a sense of imbalance and is a nonspecific term. It may include wooziness, giddiness, lightheadedness, nausea, vomiting, disequilibrium, and so on. Vertigo is a form of dizziness but is defined as an illusion of rotatory movement. Oscillopsia is akin to vertigo but is an illusion of linear motion. Both vertigo and oscillopsia are caused by disturbances in the vestibular system. This system includes the vestibular apparatus, the eighth cranial nerve, the vestibular nuclei, and their neural projections, the exteroceptors throughout the body but particularly in the upper cervical spine and the eyes. Although all of these structures may cause vertigo/oscillopsia, except for the vestibular apparatus, the vestibular nuclei, and their projections, they usually do not, and when they do, the resulting illusion of motion is generally mild. For the most part, then, it is not too bad an assumption that moderate to severe vertigo/oscillopsia is caused by one of the many dysfunctions of the vestibular apparatus or by a deficit in its neurological projections. Certainly, moderate to severe vertigo or oscillopsia should be referred to the physician whether or not the patient is to undergo concurrent treatment. Even if the cause is benign, and it usually is, it needs to be assessed and addressed by somebody other than the orthopedic therapist (unless the therapist is also a vestibular rehabilitation therapist) because treating the musculoskeletal system is unlikely to help this degree of vertigo.

One method of classifying dizziness is based on the patient's complaints rather than the cause of the dizziness. This classification is of more value to the clinician in that it helps to determine the cause rather than deriving from the artificial situation in which the cause has already been determined. The symptom-based classification is as follows:

Type 1	Vertigo/oscillopsia
Type 2	Presyncope (lightheadedness, nausea, giddiness, wooziness, etc.)
Type 3	Disequilibrium

The main concern of the orthopedic therapist is not to definitively diagnose the cause of the dizziness but to ensure that it is not being caused by a serious condition such as vertebrobasilar compromise. When taking the history from a cervical or headache patient, if the patient does not volunteer information about dizziness, the therapist must ask directly. If there is dizziness in the history, the therapist must then ask the patient to describe it, if necessary prompting the patient with questions such as, Do you feel that you or the room is spinning or bobbing? The onset is important, so was it traumatic and how sudden was it? An immediate onset related to trauma could indicate labyrinthine concussion or vertebral artery damage and spasm. A delayed onset, especially if it is associated with increasing cervical pain, is likely to be caused by cervical segmental injury. If a delayed onset coincides with decreasing pain, it is probable that the cause is not cervicogenic but may be related to increasing range and could be vertebral artery compromise from the increased range of motion or vestibular for the same reason. If there is any doubt that the cause is benign and/or within the scope of practice of a particular therapist, the patient should be referred back to the physician for further testing.

The main clinical test for vestibular function is the Hallpike-Dix test. This involves having the patient suddenly lie down from a sitting position with the head rotated in the direction that the examiner feels is the provocative position. The end-point of the test is where the head overhangs the end of the bed so that the neck is extended. Certainly, this test applies considerable stress to the vestibular apparatus but cannot be utilized in the acute neck patient for obvious reasons, nor can it be used when the vertebral artery has not been cleared. A less exhaustive but more appropriate test for the acute patient is body and head tilting. The patient sits at the end of the bed, and the therapist stabilizes the head and neck by holding the forehead and the posterior neck and then tilts the patient backward and forward and side to side. A positive result is one that reproduces dizziness and/or nystagmus.

Hearing Post-traumatic hypoacusia can be either conduction or sensorineural in nature. Fracture and/or dislocation of the auditory ossicles or rupture of the tympanic membrane by sudden changes in middle ear pressure may cause mechanical impairment of sound waves such that the patient becomes hypoacusic. Sensorineural deafness is of course more significant to the orthopedic therapist, because it can be caused by vertebrobasilar compromise.

Hearing loss can be straightforward, the patient recognizing it for what it is, but it may also be unrecognized if it is relatively minor. In this case, ask the patient about tinnitus, difficulty hearing conversations in noisy rooms, and changing the ear that the telephone is held to.

Hearing can be tested in the clinic without the use of tuning forks. The first step is to establish that there is a difference in hearing from side to side. This is done by rustling paper or rubbing your fingers equidistant from each ear simultaneously and asking the patient to identify in which ear the noise is mostly heard. Having established a difference (if there is no difference, you can go no further with this method) the type of deafness must be determined. When conduction deafness is present, bone conduction is enhanced. (You can demonstrate this to yourself by plugging one ear and humming. The sound will be heard in the plugged ear.) If sensorineural hypoacusia exists, the patient has reduced hearing no matter how the sound reaches the cochlea. The patient closes both ears with his or her fingers and hums. If the hum is heard louder in the deaf ear, conduction hypoacusia is present, if in the ear that heard better, sensorineural.

Ninth Cranial Nerve The glossopharyngeal nerve supplies most of the pharyngeal muscles, one of the tongue muscles, and the posterior part of the tongue's special sense. Dysarthria, dysphagia, and taste disturbances are among the possible symptoms that the patient might experience if this nerve or nucleus is damaged. The gag reflex is used to test this nerve in severely affected patients, but in the patients coming into the clinic, this reflex will be unaffected and it is unnecessary to test it.

Tenth Cranial Nerve The vagus nerve and its accessory nerve component innervate the viscera and the laryngeal, soft palate, and uvularis muscles. Symptoms include nausea and vomiting, although these are rarely caused by vagus nerve deficit. More commonly, the patient will complain of voice changes (dysphonia) such that the voice becomes hoarse and rasping because of laryngeal muscle paresis.

   To test the function of this nucleus, have the patient open the mouth and visualize the uvula and soft palate. Occasionally the tongue blocks the view of the uvula and palate, but it generally descends as the test proceeds. As you watch these structures, ask the patient to say "ah." The uvula and soft palate should elevate symmetrically. Weakness on one side results in the uvula and soft palate being drawn to the strong side.

Eleventh Cranial Nerve There is no sensory component to the accessory nerve and so no symptoms. The nerve is the motor supply to the sternomastoid and trapezius. The sternomastoid innervation is partially decussed, so weakness is less common in this muscle than in the trapezius. Look for atrophy and fasciculation. The presence of rapid severe wasting and/or coarse fasciculation is indicative of a lower motor lesion and if present in the nontraumatic patient suggests neuroma. If it is found in a post-traumatic patient, there is the possibility of an occipital fracture near where it exits at the jugular foramen. Supranuclear lesions cause gradual and mild wasting and fine if any fasciculation. This trapezius is tested for strength by having the patient shrug his or her shoulder against the therapist's resistance. The therapist should not be able to break the patient's contraction.

Twelfth Cranial Nerve The hypoglossal nerve is the motor supply for all of the intrinsic and extrinsic tongue muscles except the palatoglossus. Symptoms of deficit can include dysphagia and dysarthria (usually slow and slurred speech). Observe the tongue for atrophy. If there is any, the lesion is likely to be at the nerve as it exists the hypoglossal foramen. The cause for this may be an occipital fracture. The clinical test is to have the patient protrude the tongue while the therapist looks for deviation. If there is weakness, the tongue deviates to the weak side.

Vertebral artery insufficiency is a concern with all neck patients, but injury to the vessel is particularly common in trauma to the neck. Fortunately, the vast majority of cases do not become dysfunctional, and only a few demonstrate minor symptoms. However, our treatments often pose a threat, albeit a very small one, to the artery, and it is in the patient's best interests if we try to ascertain that it is safe to treat him or her. This is, of course, a concern with the nontraumatic patient but a smaller one, and in addition, we do not have to worry too much about a careful examination increasing the damage to the artery. Previously damaged arteries have been worsened during positioning for x-rays and angiographs; consequently, the clinical testing of potentially damaged arteries must be gradual and progressive. Although in the nontraumatized patient, we may be able to go straight to the positions of maximal stress with confidence, this could prove dangerous in the injured neck patient. The other question is, When do you test this structure? If it has been damaged, even careful testing has the potential to inflict further damage to the artery (although to my knowledge this has never occurred in a physical therapy examination). Certain types of arterial damage seem to self-heal in about 6 weeks, so ideally this is the period that should be waited before testing the artery. However, this is not practical, because if the artery is not tested, no attempt should be made to actively regain the range.

Long Tract Tests

Some of these tracts are nondifferentially tested during the routine examination, including deep tendon reflexes, clonus, and extensor-plantar responses. However, when a lesion to the brainstem or higher is suspected, the tracts that carry inhibition for these reflexes may not be among those affected. In this case, a more extensive examination needs to be undertaken. However, these tests need only be carried out if the patient is experiencing signs and symptoms suggestive of such a lesion or if the cranial nerve tests are thought to be positive.

The tests are

1. Sensation
   ❑ Light touch
   ❑ Pinprick (temperature)

2. Mechanoreception
- ❏ Proprioception
  a. Finger to nose
  b. Finger tips to thumb
  c. Heel to knee to ankle
- ❏ Vibration
  a. Tuning fork
- ❏ Stereognosis
  a. Letter or number skin scribing recognition
  b. Shape identification (not done in orthopedic patients)

3. Motor
- ❏ Strength
- ❏ Spasticity
- ❏ Coordination with proprioception tests

4. Dynamic stretch reflexes
- ❏ Deep tendon reflexes
- ❏ Clonus
- ❏ Scapulohumeral (Shimizu)

5. Nociceptive reflexes
- ❏ Extensor-plantar
- ❏ Oppenheimer
- ❏ Hoffman
- ❏ Dynamic Hoffman's reflex

By assessing the location of the discrepancies in the tests, any lesion can be ascertained as being bilateral, hemilateral, or quadrilateral. Assessment of the losses will give an idea of the tracts involved and what brainstem lesion is present. However, this is food for the neurologist; all we have to do is recognize patterns of disturbance of these tests and refer them out. However, the most common brainstem lesion from vertebrobasilar compromise is lateral medullary (Wallenberg's) syndrome, and some idea of the components of this are in order for the orthopedic therapist.

The lesion is most commonly caused by damage to the vertebral artery and impairment of vascularization of the lateral medulla, lower pons, and cerebellum. The result is deficits in the eighth through twelfth nerves and the lateral spinothalamic tract. The patient experiences dizziness (usually including vertigo), nystagmus, dysphagia, dysphonia, dysarthria, lateral ataxia, contralateral paresthesia, and reduced or lost pain and temperature sensation. Of course, the problems that we see are transitory and may not be present until the patient has provoked them, and then they are likely to be patchy.

Summary of the Neurological Tests

Nerve	Test	Positive Symptoms	Positive Test Result
1	Soap smell	Anosima/parosmia	Anosmia
2	Confrontation	Scintillating hemi- or quadranopia	Hemi- or quadranopia
3 E-W	Consensual light reflex	None	Aniscoria, absent, sluggish, or oscillating constriction
3, 4, 6	Tracking, convergence	Diplopia	Paresis/paralysis, nystagmus
5	Facial sensation, jaw jerk, jaw clonus	Hemifacial parasthesia, taste disturbance	Hypo-anesthesia, hyperreflexia, clonus
7	Smile frown	Taste disturbance, facial droop	Facial droop, loss of smile, retention of frown (CNS)
8 V	Tilt, hallpike-dix, Rhomberg's, stance, tilt board, foam/dome	Types 1, 2, and/or 3 dizziness	Types 1, 2, and/or 3 dizziness, nystagmus
8 C	Finger rustle, hum	Tinnitus, deafness	Hypoacusia, hum heard in better ear
9	Gag	Dysphagia, dysarthria	Not tested
10	Uvula displacement	Dysphonia, nausea	Uvula displaces to strong side
11	Sternocleidomastoid, trapezius strength, trapezius reflex/clonus	None	Weakness of sternocleidomastoid and trapezius, hyperreflexia, clonus
12	Tongue protrusion	Dysarthria, dysmastication	Tongue deviates to weak side

Long Tract Tests

Test	Positive
Deep tendon reflexes	Hyperreflexia
Light touch	Anesthesia
Pinprick	Hypo- or anesthesia
Vibration	Reduced or absent
Proprioception	Reduced or absent
Muscle tone	Hypertonicity or spasticity
Strength	Weakness

Summary of the Neurological Conditions

Condition	Type	Possible Cause
Scotoma, hemianopia, quadranopia	1. Unilateral	Anterior to optic chiasm • ophthalmic (amblyopia, papilloedema, etc. • retinal • macular • optic neuropathies (multiple sclerosis, retrobulbar neuropathy, ischemia, syphilis, glaucoma)
	2. Bilateral	At or posterior to the optic chiasm
	• homonymous hemianopia or quadranopia	Arterial infarction, damage, or tumors of one or more of the following structures: • visual (calcerine) cortex • optic tract • optic (calcerine) radiation • lateral geniculate body
	• heteronymous hemianopia or quadranopia	Suprasellar tumors, angiomas, and arachnoiditis affecting one or both of the following: • optic chiasm • optic tract
	• central scotoma (concentric constriction, tunnel vision)	• hysteria • optic neuropathies (multiple sclerosis, ischemia, syphilis, glaucoma, papilloedema)
Diplopia	1. Nonparalytic strabismus	Ophthalmic (squint)
	2. Paralytic strabismus	Neurological; paresis or paralysis of one or more of the extraocular muscles caused by • vasculopathy of the brainstem • petechial hemorrhaging of the brainstem • tumors of the brainstem affecting the third, fourth, or sixth cranial nerve
Nystagmus	1. Pendular	• loss of central visual field (caused by albinism, retinal disease, miner's nystagmus) • Multiple sclerosis • congenital
	2. Jerk • rotatory (torsional) • vertical (downbeat or upbeat) • horizontal	Various causes both central and peripheral including: • physiological (caloric, rotatory, end-point optokinetic) • vestibular

Summary of the Neurological Conditions (continued)

Condition	Type	Possible Cause
	• retractive • vergent • mixed • end-point	• drug-induced (alcohol, barbiturates, phenytoin) • brainstem lesions • cerebellum diseases and lesions • cerebellopontine tumors
Absent or diminished pupil light reflexes	1. Direct 2. Consensual	• ophthalmic (direct and contralateral consensual absent) • optic nerve (direct and contralateral consensual absent • third cranial nerve lesions (direct and contralateral consensual absent) • sympathetic paralysis (direct and consensual absent)
Facial hypoesthesia or anesthesia	1. Pain and temperature only (usually with same sensation loss over contralateral body and limbs	• medullary or lower pontine lesion
	2. Pain, temperature, proprioception and touch (usually produces anesthesia in face, and contralateral body, and limbs)	• upper pontine or midbrain lesion
Jaw jerk	1. Hyperreflexia 2. Hyporeflexia 3. Clonus	• pontine or midbrain lesion • mandibular nerve palsy • pontine or midbrain lesion
Facial paresis or paralysis	1. Complete 2. Incomplete (lower facial only)	• facial nerve palsy • supranuclear (brainstem or cortex) lesion
Hyperacusia	Especially sensitive to high-decibel sound levels	Stapedius or tensor tympani paresis or paralysis: • facial or trigeminal nerve palsy • supranuclear lesion
Hypoacusia	1. Conduction	Mechanical impairment of sound: • tympanic membrane rupture • tensor tympani hypertonicity • tensor veli palatini hypertonicity • auditory ossicle damage • otitis media

		• otosclerosis
		• wax buildup
	2. Sensorineural	Impairment of neural conduction:
		• congenital/hereditary
		• prenatal measles
		• mumps
		• otitis intima
		• prolonged exposure to high-decibel conditions
		• drugs (streptomycin, gentomycin, quinine, aspirin)
		• age
		• cerebellopontine tumors
		• auditory neuroma
		• internal auditory artery infraction
		• vertebrobasilar infarction
Tinnitus	1. Objective (vibratory)	• tensor veli palatini crepitus
		• tensor tympani crepitus
		• stapedius crepitus
		• palatal myoclonus
		• suprahyoids
		• cervical vascular bruit
		• intracranial arteriovenous malformations
	2. Subjective (nonvibratory)	• hypoacusia
		• otosclerosis
		• tympanic membrane damage
		• cochlear dysfunction
		• auditory neuropathy
		• Meniere's disease
		• pontine and temporal lobe lesions
Dizziness	1. Vertiginous	• benign paroxysmal positional vertigo
		• head trauma
		• positioning vertigo
		• migraine
		• Meniere's disease
		• perilymph fistulas
		• acute peripheral vestibulopathy (labyrinthitis)
		• multiple sclerosis
		• vertebrobasilar insufficiency
		• acoustic neuroma
		• medication (antibiotics, barbiturates)
	2. Nonvertiginous	• orthostatic hypotension
		• alcohol
		• hyperventilation

Summary of the Neurological Conditions (continued)

Condition	Type	Possible Cause
		• vasovagal attacks
		• cardiopathies
		• ophthalmic problems
		• vestibular degenerative disease
		• medication (antibiotics, anti-inflammatories, muscle relaxants, aspirin, quinine, sedatives, etc.)
		• head trauma
		• cervical joint dysfunction
		• temporomandibular joint dysfunction
		• metabolic conditions (diabetes, anemia, hypoglycemia)
		• migraine
		• (central nervous system diseases (multiple sclerosis, Parkinson's disease, dementia, pyramidal and extrapyramidal)
		• vertebrobasilar insufficiency
		• dementia
		• slow-growing acoustic neuromas
		• psychiatric
Dysphasia (work formation OK, syntax and comprehension affected)	1. Palilalia	• bilateral upper brainstem lesions (vertebrobasilar insufficiency) • supranuclear palsies
	2. Echolalia	• transcortical lesions (parietal-occipital isolation syndromes)
Dysarthria (word formation affected with slurring, stuttering etc.; comprehension depends on other tissues affected)	1. Lower motor neuron	• glossopharyngeal nucleus or nerve palsy • vagal nucleus or nerve palsy • hypoglossal nucleus or nerve palsy
	2. Spastic and rigid	• corticobulbar tract lesions (vertebrobasilar insufficiency, Parkinson's disease, myoclonus, chorea)
	3. Ataxic	• acute and chronic cerebellar lesions
Dysphonia (word formation and	1. Whispering	• stupor • concussive injuries

comprehension OK but voice sound affected)

		• laryngeal muscle paresis or paralysis
	2. Hoarse (rasping and nasal)	• vagal nerve palsy • laryngeal structural changes caused by smoking, etc.
Horner's syndrome (ptosis, enophthalmos, anhydrosis, facial flushing, mitosis)		Sympathetic interruption at the hypothalamus, reticular formation, descending sympathetic nerve, superior, middle, or inferior cervical ganglia, or sympathetic outflow in the upper thoracic region of the cord • vertebrobasilar insufficiency • tumors • neurological disease • spinal cord lesions
Pancoast's syndrome (Horner's syndrome plus evidence of a lower brachial plexus palsy)		Invasion of the lower brachial plexus and stellate ganglion • apical lung (superior sulcus) tumor • breast cancer
Wallenberg's (lateral medullary) syndrome (ipsilateral facial and contralateral body hyposensitivity to pain and temperature, hemihypotonia, dizziness, ataxia, Horner's syndrome, dysphagia, dysphonia, dysarthria)		• vertebrobasilar insufficiency
Trapezius/ sternomastoid weakness	• atrophic (lower motor lesion) • nonatrophic (upper motor lesion)	• occipital fractures • accessory neuromas • occipital metastases • polymyositis • muscular dystrophy • spinal cord lesions • vertebral artery insufficiency
Tongue weakness	• atrophic (lower motor lesion) • nonatrophic (upper motor lesion)	Hypoglossal nucleus or nerve palsy • occipital fractures • bulbar palsy syndrome • vertebral artery insufficiency

Craniovertebral Ligament Stress Tests

Testing craniovertebral stability can be important. Rheumatoid arthritis, ankylosing spondylitis, Reiter's disease, Grisel's syndrome, and Down's syndrome can destabilize the atlantoaxial segment in particular and lead to lower medulla, cord, and/or vertebral artery compression.[68-72] In addition to pathology, children present a special problem because before the age of 10 or 11, the bony dens does not even reach the arch of atlas, being comprised of cartilage.[73]

These stress tests are considered important enough to be carried out routinely by many therapists. Certainly they are done quickly enough that there is no reason why they should not be carried out in all cervical patients. Trauma only unusually results in isolated transverse ligament damage. More commonly it will fracture the odontoid or arch of atlas and occasionally avulse the ligament simultaneously.[74-76] The more common mechanism for destabilization of the area is disease. All patients with a history of one of the conditions listed must have the craniovertebral joints tested for stability, as must patients complaining of dizziness, because dysfunction of this area can be the cause of the dizziness.

Transverse Ligament Stress Test

The function of the transverse ligament is to limit anterior displacement of the atlas during flexion, preventing spinal canal stenosis and compression of the spinal cord. The tolerance for displacement is about 3 mm in the normal population and 4 mm in the rheumatoid arthritic population. Anything greater than these values may be an indication for surgical stabilization. Only one clinical test has been validated for anterior stability, the Sharp-Purser test.[77]

The original test was described by Sharp as follows:

> The palm of one hand was placed on the patient's forehead and the thumb of the other on the tip of the spinous process of the axis. The patient was then asked to relax the neck in a semi-flexed position. By pressing backward with the palm a sliding motion of the head backwards in relation to the spine of the axis could be demonstrated.

More recently the test has been modified for use in the patient experiencing cardinal signs of cord or vertebrobasilar compromise, particularly spinal cord symptoms of paresthesia. Here the object of the test is to reduce or eliminate the symptoms.[78] However, the presence of the symptoms themselves is sufficient to make a provisional diagnosis of cord compression and get the patient back to the physician for more objective testing.[79]

The *anterior shear* test is the one commonly in use among physical therapists. The patient lies supine with the head supported by a pillow in the neutral position. The therapist supports the occiput in the palms of the hands and the third, fourth, and fifth fingers while the two index fingers are placed in the space between the occiput and the C2 spinous process, thus overlying the neural arch of the atlas. The therapist's thumbs lie alongside the patient's cheeks on either side to maintain the neutral head position. The head and C1 are then sheared anteriorly as a unit while the head is maintained in its neutral position and gravity fixes the rest of the neck. The patient is instructed to report any symptoms other than local pain and soreness.

Only the transverse ligament can resist the shear because the ligamentum nuchae is slackened off by the neutral starting position. This shear is held until no further motion is detected or until a positive sign or symptom is elicited. The therapist watches the eyes for changes in the pupils and for nystagmus. Other positives include spasm, an abnormally soft capsular end feel, a slip, the production of dizziness, nausea, facial or limb paresthesia, parasthesia of the lips, nystagmus, a sensation of a lump in the throat, or consistent reflex swallowing. If there is an abnormal end feel but no symptoms, maintain the shear, as this then becomes an ischemic test of the vertebral artery. Ask the patient to count backward from 15 and listen for speech or language changes as well as any symptoms the patient might describe or signs that you might see. The sensation of a lump in the throat or the presence of a consistent swallow during the test has been ascribed to an anterior instability irritating the posterior aspect of the pharynx. However, a more probable explanation when this is experienced in the post-traumatic patient during a test with a normal end feel and no slip is that the pharynx has been injured and there is a small retropharyngeal hematoma.

Dizziness and other noncardinal symptoms will in all probability be false positives for transverse ligament instability, but all must be taken seriously because tearing of this ligament can have serious consequences for the patient. The reproduction of the more definite signs and symptoms, such as parasthesia in any area, vertigo, or nystagmus, as opposed to nausea or wooziness, should immediately be reported to the physician after the patient has been put into a hard collar until it has been established to the therapist's satisfaction that further testing and treatment is safe. Other, less definite symptoms may be from other causes, and further testing can be carried out, provided that it is done with caution.

Alar Ligament Tests

The major part of the alar ligament runs mainly from the posterior aspect of the upper two thirds of the dens to the medial nonarticular part of the occipital condyle. Its function is to tighten during contralateral rotation and contralateral side flexion, initially transferring rotational forces to the axis from the head, and then to limit rotation and side flexion of the atlanto-occipital and atlantoaxial segments.

The *alar ligament kinetic test* based on the effect of side flexion on the axis as a result of the ligament tightening. Because the occiput and the axis are directly connected by the ligament, induced rotation of the axis should be immediate and in the same direction as the side flexion. The test is carried out with the patient lying supine or seated and the therapist palpating the spinous process of the axis. The head is side flexed around the axis of the craniovertebral joints (around the nose), and the therapist feels for immediate contralateral motion of the spinous process as the axis rotates to the same side. A positive test is one in which there is a delay between the side flexion and the spinous process movement.

The advantage to this test is that it is not very stressful and can be done in all but the most acute patients, in whom spasm intervenes and prevents the test being useful. The disadvantage is that it is not a stress test, and if there is mild spasm or of the rectus capitus posterior major, a false negative can occur.

The *alar ligament stress test* is carried out in the same position, but is now gripping the spinous process and the lamina in a wide pinch grip that stabilizes the axis. The head and atlas are then side flexed around the coronal axis for the atlantoaxial joint. The ipsilateral rotation of the axis is prevented by the fixation. If the alar ligament is intact, no side flexion can occur and the end feel will be normal capsular. If there is any laxity in the ligament, some side flexion will result until the laxity is taken up. This motion and soft capsular end feel are appreciated by the examiner and considered to be an indicator of alar ligament instability. When the ligament is irritable, pain occurs as the test is carried out. If the pain is associated with no instability, a grade 1 tear may be present; if there is pain and moderate instability, a grade 2 tear; and if there is pain with severe instability, a grade 3 tear. In addition to excessive motion, symptoms ascribable to disorders of the balance mechanism are noted. This ligamentous instability is not the life-threatening hazard that atlantoaxial instability can be, and the finding of instability without cardinal symptoms does not prevent careful and appropriate treatment. For a more complete description of these techniques that purport to test the stability of the craniovertebral region, read Pettman.[78]

If the therapist is at all concerned about the anteroposterior stability of the craniovertebral region, the patient should not be treated until open mouth and flexion-extension radiographs are taken and found to be negative. It should be noted that false negatives with the radiographic results could be a potential problem. If muscle spasm is a factor when the region is moved, it will splint the joints and the x-rays will look negative. The other problem lies with the axis of the motion during the radiographic procedure. The motion must occur around the craniovertebral axis and not about a midcervical axis. For flexion and extension, the axis is roughly through the external auditory meatus; for side flexion it is through the nose. If motion occurs around other axes, a false negative may result because such motion may preclude movement at the craniovertebral joints. As a consequence of these false positives, it essential that the therapist not undertake any treatment that will put the patient at risk for as long as the tests appear positive. If they do prove negative and there is still real concern, then CT and bone scans and MRIs can be taken. In those patients who have dizziness, a history of trauma, or one of the collagenous diseases listed earlier, no mechanical evaluation or treatment of the region should be undertaken until either the clinical tests or the correctly taken imaging tests prove negative.

Insufficiency of the alar ligament will produce and increase the average contralateral rotation at the atlantoaxial joint by up to 30%, or 10 degrees, and flexion by almost 28%.[79,80] Hypermobility of this region caused by alar ligament, odontoid process, or transverse ligament insufficiency has been shown to be a factor in the production of vertigo and associated symptoms by occlusion of the vertebral artery or by disturbance of afferent input to the vestibular nuclei.

Vertebrobasilar Insufficiency

The vertebral artery is subject to occlusion from internal and external causes. Causes of stenosis to the vertebrobasilar arteries include[82]

- ❏ Atherosclerosis
- ❏ Trauma
- ❏ Motion-related and spontaneous dissection
- ❏ Vasospasm
- ❏ Fibromuscular dysplasia
- ❏ Atheroma
- ❏ Thrombosis
- ❏ Embolus
- ❏ Arteriovenous fistula
- ❏ Compression by fibrous bands, disk, osteophyte, bone, or tumor
- ❏ Traction from trauma
- ❏ Traumatic dissection
- ❏ Transection
- ❏ Pseudoaneurysm
- ❏ Intramural tears

Assessment of the Vertebrobasilar System

Clinical testing for vertebrobasilar ischemia is based on construct validity and not criterion validity, so the tests are only assumed to be effective because they make sense in the light of the understood anatomy, physiology, pathology, and pathophysiology. Their sensitivity and specificity is unknown, so it is not possible to say that a negative test categorically clears the patient's vertebrobasilar system. Rather, if the tests do demonstrate a problem, there is a greater or lesser degree of probability that there is a vertebral artery defect, depending on the sign or symptom elicited (that is whether it is cardinal or noncardinal). One study on one patient found that the objective clinical tests commonly used in the investigation of vertebrobasilar insufficiency (Hautard's, Maine's, Smith and Estridge's, and Underberg's) failed to demonstrate a problem on a patient who was known to have an occluded artery.[83] However, even with the lack of research evidence, testing the vertebral artery is a resonable procedure provided certain precautions are taken. It should be understood that testing the integrity of the artery is not simply carrying out Hautard's or one of the other tests but also including such tests into the overall neurological examination, including the history. In the case study in which the so-called vertebral artery tests failed to predict the presence of vertebrobasilar pathology, the overall examination did. Although the examination is principally for the vertebrobasilar system, the therapist is using central nervous system function as a monitor. It has been established that damage to the central system is relatively common in motor vehicle accidents (discussed earlier), and the therapist will more likely pick up signs of concussion or possibly more serious neurological damage than vertebrobasilar ischemia in this examination. Contraindications for testing the vertebral artery include

- ❏ A history of cardinal signs and/or symptoms
- ❏ The presence of a fracture
- ❏ The presence of craniovertebral instability

A very careful and graduated examination sequence would be demanded by the presence of suspect symptoms or by recent trauma (less than 6 weeks) to safeguard the patient from the possible adverse effects of the examination itself.

The purpose of testing is

1. To reproduce signs and/or symptoms potentially attributable to vertebrobasilar insufficiency either by testing or from the patient's history

2. To differentiate those signs and/or symptoms if they are noncardinal

3. To determine the risk to the patient of treating his or her neck with any treatment that threatens the vertebral artery

The main causes of signs and symptoms potentially sourced from the vertebrobasilar system are

- ❏ The tissues vascularized by the system itself
- ❏ The cervical nonvascular tissues (which we know from clinical and experimental evidence can cause many of these signs and symptoms[84-88])
- ❏ The vestibular apparatus and neurological projections

The testing sequence outlined in this chapter will gradually increase the stress on the vertebral artery so that the examination can be curtailed at the first sign of ischemia. It begins with the least stressful of tests, the history, and progresses gradually to the most stressful, the full occlusion position of extension and rotation. A number of clinicians have suggested that the full occlusion position and even extension be left untested as a safety consideration, especially because our treatment techniques should not be going into that range. However, our responsibility to the patient goes a little further than our own clinic. We must ensure that the function of the patient is safe. Combined rotation and extension is a functional movement, and if the patient is capable of going into that position, it must be tested.

History If indirect open-ended questions do not elicit useful responses, direct questions must be asked about central nervous system symptoms. Has the patient had any dizziness? If so, what type? Was the onset of dizziness immediate or delayed? Is it still present? If so, is its onset/offset related to head or body position and movements, medication, intake, and so forth? Are there any visual disturbances such as blurred vision or field defects, and are these related to head position and movements? Do you experience any paresthesia or anesthesia, and if so, where? Do you have ataxia, drop attacks, problems waking, clumsiness, tendencies to stumble or fall, or any other movement problems? Do you faint episodically or have problems concentrating or staying alert? Is there any amnesia? If so, is it postconcussion or is it ongoing? The latter indicates something more than concussion, and the patient needs to get back to the physician. Has the patient noted recent deafness, speech defects, swallowing difficulties, or tinnitus?

Observation The therapist should be making observations while taking the patient's history. For the central nervous system function part of the examination, look and listen for the following:

- ❏ Nystagmus
- ❏ Dysphasia
- ❏ Dysarthria
- ❏ Dysphagia

- ❏ Ataxia
- ❏ Unsteadiness
- ❏ Loss of concentration
- ❏ Sternomastoid/trapezius atrophy
- ❏ Horner's signs
  - a. Enophthalmos
  - b. Ptosis
  - c. Miosis
  - d. Anhydrosis
  - e. Facial flushing

Objective Tests *Carotid Pulses* The assessing of the carotid pulses is the first step in the assessment of the vertebral artery. Atherosclerosis, being a systemic condition, has the potential to affect all arteries, and there is a good chance that if the carotid arteries are occluded, the vertebrals will be, too. Absence or a severe reduction in the strength of the carotid pulse should require caution from the examining therapist. Various studies have determined that a decrease in flow through the vertebral artery results in an increased flow through the common carotid, particularly in the contralateral artery.[89,90] Accordingly, the carotid pulse should be taken and the sides compared for gross differences. This should be done in the rotated, extended, and combined rotated and extended positions, as well as in the neutral position. The therapist looks for an increase in the strength of the pulse over that found in the neutral position. A side to side difference in carotid pulse strength with a change in head position may indicate hypoplasia, aplasia, atresia, or occlusion. If a side to side difference is associated with a history of blatant neurological symptoms or if the pulse changes with a position change, the patient should be referred back to the physician. If the patient's complaints are of a vaguer nature and if the resting pulse is different from side to side, further testing can be carried out, but with caution.

Neurological Examination The neurological examination can be carried out without stressing the spine or the arterial system. The cranial nerves and long tracts are examined and assessed as discussed earlier. Multisegmental hypotonia, hypertonia, and weakness can also be tested using palpation, passive movements of the limbs, and strength testing.

Early Vestibular Tests Parts of the vestibular system can be examined without stressing the cervical spine and its arteries. However, the need to protect the potentially damaged vertebral artery or severe musculoskeletal damage limits just how much you can do. The Hallpike-Dix test, probably the most stressful clinical test available for the vestibular apparatus, is contraindicated until the vertebral artery is excluded as a possible source of the patient's symptoms. A modified test based on an observation made by Cope and Ryan can be utilized. They observed that the wearing of a soft collar effectively eliminates the neck (joints or arteries) as a cause of dizziness or vertigo.[91] A hard collar can be used, or the therapist can fix the patient's head and neck and then rock the patient backward and forward, side to side, and in circles in ever larger amplitudes until symptoms or signs are reproduced or until maximum safe excursions have been reached. If symptoms are reproduced during this test, the neck has been eliminated as the source of symptoms, so it is unlikely that the vertebral artery or the cervical musculoskeletal structures are playing in a role in any dizziness that the patient may be experiencing.

If the test is positive for noncardinal symptoms, the cause is unlikely to be cervical in origin, because the position of the spine has remained constant during the test. The patient is asked about any symptoms that occur during the test, and the eyes are monitored for nystagmus and pupil changes.

The so-called vertebral artery tests obviously test many things other than the vertebral artery, but this is the main concern. To try to clarify the thinking behind neurovascular or dizziness testing, the tests can be divided in two categories, tests that reproduce the patient's symptoms and those that differentiate them.

Reproduction Tests The purpose of this part of the examination is to see if the therapist can reproduce the dizziness by moving the head, body, and neck. The reproduction of cardinal symptoms requires an immediate referral to the physician because the reproduction of central neurological signs or symptoms with changes in head position must be considered to be a result of neurovascular compromise until proven otherwise by exhaustive objective testing such as magnetic resonance angiography, Doppler ultrasonography, or angiograms. The reproduction of dizziness or any other noncardinal sign or symptom indicates the need for the therapist to carry out differentiation tests to try to determine the source. Dizziness in itself is not a contraindication to treatment and is frequently the indication to perform manual techniques if it is believed that the cervical spine is the source of the dizziness. From cadaveric experiments,[92,93] the fully stressed position for one vertebral artery is cervical extension, rotation, and traction. This is often called the *vertebral artery stress test,* but it must be understood that although this position is most likely to occlude the vertebral artery, it also puts other tissues under stress and is therefore not specific to the vertebral artery. The position simply tests whether or not cervical movement causes dizziness, not what tissue causes it.

At least 30 degrees of rotation is required for partial occlusion of the artery in cadavers, and in the living the critical angle for blood flow disturbance in the vertebral artery was less than 45 degrees, with at least another 10 to 15 degrees required before complete obstruction occurred in some subjects. It is therefore of little use to do these tests in patients who do not have the required amount of cervical motion.[87]

Testing in patients who are experiencing noncardinal symptoms (remember that the presence of cardinal symptoms contraindicates these tests) is carried out in stages. The cadaveric studies quoted earlier suggest that traction is occlusive but minimally so, extension is less occlusive than rotation, and rotation combined with extension is more occlusive than either alone. The addition of traction on the combined rotation and extension position is maximally occlusive, and 50% of body weight traction (which is not difficult to achieve in a 120-lb person) will occlude every artery tested. This last maneuver is unnecessary because it is not functional, will not be a treatment, and is potentially dangerous.

The test position must be sustained for a set period or until signs or symptoms are provoked. The time each position is held for varies from one authority to another from 10 seconds to a minute. Grant[94] and the Australian Physiotherapy Association's protocol for premanipulative testing[95] suggest 10 seconds as a compromise that takes into consideration clinical logistical requirements, patient safety, and physiological needs. There is some experimental evidence that changes in evoked potentials in hearing occur within 15 seconds of vertebrobasilar occlusion.[96]

I suggest that certain cranial nerves be tested while holding the patient's position and that this testing be started at around the 10-second mark in the test. It will take about 5 or 6 seconds to run through the selected cranial nerve tests, taking the duration of the position to about 15 or 16 seconds.

The cranial nerves that lend themselves to being tested in these occlusive positions are

❑ Oculomotor, trochlear, and abducens (horizontal and vertical gaze and convergence)
❑ Edinger-Westphal (consensual light reflex)
❑ Vagal/accessory (phonation and uvular movement)
❑ Hypoglossal (tongue protrusion)

It is especially important that the cranial nerves are re-tested if symptoms such as dizziness are provoked while the patient is still experiencing the evoked symptoms. Language, speech, and voice changes can be detected by having the patient act as the timer for each position by counting backward from 15.

Take the carotid pulses during the tests and look for an increase in their strength. This could indicate increased flow through the anterior circulation to compensate for decreased flow through the posterior, as has been demonstrated.[82,86]

If cardinal signs or symptoms are provoked with any of the following tests, no further testing should be carried out and the patient must be returned to the physician or the emergency room. The reproduction of cardinal signs or symptoms with changes in head position is far more urgent than the same signs or symptoms being present in the resting position of the head. The patient should be in supine lying so that if loss of consciousness does occur there is no danger of further damage from a fall.

Consistent with the concept of testing with least risk, the full-stress position of combined rotation and extension is attained in stages, with progression to the next most occlusive position occurring only if the previous stage had proven negative. Traction in neutral is tested initially. This has very little effect on the vestibular system because the movement is linear, so it does not disturb the semicircular canals or change the head relative to gravity and therefore does not stimulate the utricle or saccule. Consequently, if this position produces symptoms, they cannot be caused by vestibular problems but must be caused by the cervical joints (not very likely) or the vertebral artery. Be extremely cautious with further testing.

Rotation is tested next. Rotation is used as the second position rather than the less occlusive extension because extension symmetrically affects both arteries, thereby reducing the ability of the healthy side (if there is a lesion) to compensate. The head is rotated as far as is compatible with comfort. It is held in this position until the patient complains, symptoms potentially attributable to arterial occlusion become apparent, or 15 seconds have passed, whichever is the sooner. The opposite rotation is tested if the previous rotation was negative. The same protocol is repeated for extension and then for combined rotation and extension in both directions, providing the previous tests are negative. If all of these tests are negative, only the addition of traction will further reduce its diameter, and there are good arguments for avoiding this much stress (discussed earlier).

While the tests are being carried out, the patient is asked to keep the eyes open. This is done for two reasons: first, to make sure that the patient retains consciousness during the test; second, to observe the onset of nystagmus, which, if it is central in origin (which is what we are interested in), will be asymmetrical, gaze evoked (that is, it will appear when the patient is asked to look in the nystagmatic direction), and not suppressible.[34]

It is as well to note that at least one patient who had angiographic evidence of and symptoms ascribable to vertebral artery occlusion did not demonstrate any signs or symptoms when the stress tests for the vertebral artery were carried out.[77]

The common practice of testing with the head overhanging the bed (De Kleyne's Test) is not recommended because the severe stress that is likely to be generated by stretching from top and bottom and the weight of the head, applying traction to all simultaneously, is potentially dangerous. In addition, the problem of repositioning the patient should consciousness be lost could be considerable. How do you push somebody down the bed when you are supporting the head?

Differentiation Tests If any of the reproduction tests were positive, the problem now becomes one of differentiation. The head position that reproduced the patient's noncardinal sign(s) and/or symptom(s) is retested differently to try to differentiate the source of those signs or symptoms.

The vestibular system must be retested because only parts of it were excluded by the body tilt tests. The patient sits over the end of the bed while the therapist holds the head still. The patient is asked to reproduce the position that makes him or her dizzy by moving the body under the stabilized head. For example, if right rotation reproduced dizziness, the patient is asked to left-rotate the trunk and neck under the fixed head. The vestibular labyrinth consequently remains undisturbed during the test whereas the cervical articular receptors and the vertebral artery are stressed. Any dizziness produced during the test is unlikely to be of vestibular in origin. If extension is the movement that is to be retested, the head is fixed by the therapist and the patient slumps forward or very carefully juts the chin out, simulating extension. If combined right rotation and extension is retested, the patient extends the neck (this has been cleared already) and then left-rotates the body under the fixed and extended head.

If symptoms are reproduced during these differentiation tests, the vestibular system is unlikely to be the cause because it is not disturbed during these tests. If symptoms are reproduced, then the cause is almost certainly in the neck. Either the vertebral arteries are being occluded to the point of ischemia or the musculoskeletal tissues are causing the symptoms.

One concern, however, must be that the body movement tests (under the fixed head) do not completely simulate the effects on the vestibular system that head movements in lying do. It is therefore worthwhile repeating the reproduction tests with the patient sitting. If the patient does not now experience the previous symptoms, it is reasonable to assume that the vestibular apparatus is at fault and that the sitting test was not stimulating the affected part.

Hautard's Test   Hautard's (Hautant, Hautart, and Hautarth appear to be alternative spellings) test may assist in differentiating articular and vascular vertigo. Hautard's test is a modification of Rhomberg's test for cerebellar disease. The principle difference between the two is that in Rhomberg's test, shutting the eyes and so closing off their stabilizing effect on balance is sufficient to cause proprioceptive disturbance, whereas Hautard's test produces the disturbance by reducing blood flow to the cerebellum.[97]

Proprioceptive loss, not dizziness, is sought in Hautard's test. The patient sits on a treatment table, elevates both arms to 90 degrees, and supinates the forearms. The eyes are then closed for a few seconds while the therapist watches for a loss of position of one or both arms for a few seconds. This initial phase, which does not include head positioning, tests for nonvascular proprioception loss. If this part of the test is negative, the patient then stresses the vertebral artery, positioning the head in the position that reproduced the dizziness in the reproduction tests. The arms are observed for wavering from the original position. Usually supination is lost first, but the patient may also lose trunk position sense and tend to fall, so be in a position to catch him or her. Because the dysfunction did not occur until the head was moved and the artery stressed, it must be vasculogenic or vestibular, but the vestibular system has already been cleared. Dizziness reproduced during this test is not a positive sign. It is already known that the stress position will reproduce dizziness; it is the proprioceptive loss characterized by displacement of the arm that is the criterion.[54] A false positive may be caused by cervical joint dysfunction, causing proprioception loss in the arms. However, it is likely that the arm position loss will be smaller under these circumstances, so if it is considerable, assume that the cause is neurovascular.

A large percentage of patients presenting with cervicogenic dizziness will be post-traumatic, usually as a result of a motor vehicle accident. A proportion of these patients will be impossible to differentiate as to cause. The most confusing will be the differentiation between arterial occlusion and cervical articular dysfunction. Both causes of dizziness are related to cervical motion, and they produce very similar signs and symptoms. If these tests do not assist in evaluating the cause, the patient may be put into a cervical collar for a short period (a week or two). This will promote resolution of any zygapophyseal joint inflammation as well as maintain stability with a consequent lessening of the proprioceptive dysfunction, providing the musculoskeletal tissues of the neck are causing this dysfunction. When the patient is examined about a week later, if the upper cervical joints are the cause, the dizziness will have disappeared or reduced considerably. If the dizziness remains the same but the pain has improved, it is unlikely that the dizziness is a result of joint dysfunction.

Even if the formal tests prove negative, it is advisable to put the neck in the treatment position and maintain this position for 15 seconds prior to any treatment actually being given. If there is considerable loss of range of motion in the neck, the artery cannot be fully stressed and treatment must be given only in the available ranges; high-velocity, low-amplitude techniques should only very carefully be carried out, with an emphasis on the low amplitude. Gross rotational techniques should be avoided in both manual and exercise treatment programs. The reproduction tests should be repeated at every session if manipulation is being utilized, because many case reports indicate that it is not necessarily the first one or two manipulations that cause problems but often subsequent treatments.

Finally in those nontraumatic patients who have not experienced any symptoms potentially attributable to vertebrobasilar compromise, a shortened examination can be undertaken. A full Hautard test is carried out in the sitting position, and if the results are negative, the manipulation position is sustained for 10 or 15 seconds. If either of these produce noncardinal symptoms, the full testing protocol should be carried out.

Neurovascular Examination Summary

Subjective

Dizziness type	Type 1, 2, or 3	• All may be due to vertebrobasilar ischemia, but severe vertigo or oscillopsia is more likely to be peripheral vestibular and

(continued)

		isolated disequilibrium is more likely to be caused by neurological disease
Onset	Immediate	• Severe transection will not reach the Physical Therapy clinic and will rapidly progress. • Pseudoaneurysm dizziness may be from vasospasm and may disappear in reasonable time. • Most peripheral vestibular vertigo will be severe and long-lasting (24 h).
	Delayed	• Associated with decreasing pain and increasing ROM may be a result of occluding the artery • Arthrogenic • Embolus • Pseudoaneurysm dissection
Other symptoms	Hemianopia; quadranopia; scotoma; drop attacks; hemianesthesia; quadranesthesia; bilateral, facial, or perioral anesthesia; dysarthria; dysphasia; dysphonia; painless dysphagia; tinnitus; hypoacusia	• All must be assumed to be vertebrobasilar ischemia until proven otherwise, but other causes include: • postconcussion syndrome • intracranial hemorrhage • direct brainstem damage from petechial hemorrhages • intracranial nerve injury

Objectives

Test Type	Results	Action
Reproduction tests positive	Cardinal signs Noncardinal signs	• Refer out. • Move to differentiation tests.
Reproduction tests negative		• Do Hautard's test, and if negative, begin treatment or move to another part of the examination.
Carotid pulses	Absent or seriously unequal	• May indicate sclerosis of vertebral arteries • Will also be used as baseline measurement for strength
Cranial nerve examination	Deficit	• Probably nonvascular in origin and if unchanged during vertebrobasilar testing likely not significant for vertebrobasilar ischemia. If there is definite evidence of cranial nerve deficit refer to the physician.
	No deficit	• Any deficit produced during vertebrobasilar testing is likely to be vasculogenic.

Traction	Cardinal signs and symptoms	• Refer out.
	Noncardinal signs and symptoms	• Likely vertebrobasilar ischemia. Use best judgment but it would be prudent to refer out.
Rotation right then left	Cardinal signs and symptoms	• Refer out.
	Noncardinal	• Move to differentiation tests.
Extension	Cardinal signs	• Refer out.
	Noncardinal	• Move to differentiation tests.
Rotation/extension right then left	Cardinal signs and symptoms	• Refer out.
	Noncardinal	• Move to differentiation tests.
Body rotation	Symptomatic	• Nonvestibular
	Asymptomatic	• Vestibular
Hautard's test	Severe proprioception loss	• Assume vertebrobasilar ischemia.
	Minor proprioception loss	• May be vertebrobasilar ischemia or arthrogenic; use judgment.

Sequencing the Examination of the Post-Traumatic Neck Patient

The sequencing is based on progressive stressing of the tissues so that testing can be discontinued if any serious signs or symptoms appear.

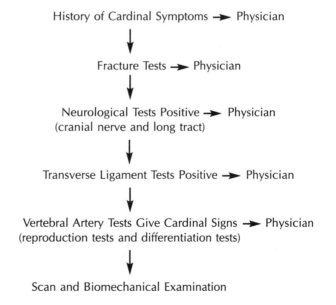

Cervical Disk Prolapse

Disk prolapses tend to be less common in the cervical than in the lumbar spine, perhaps because of a number of differences between the cervical and lumbar spine, which could include the forces acting on the neck, the makeup of the cervical disk, with its smaller nucleus, the differences in the degenerative processes (the disappearance of the cervical nucleus), and the presence of the uncinate processes protecting the posterolateral corner of the segment (especially in the higher segments). When cervical disk herniations do occur (exclusive of traumatic herniations), they tend to affect the lower levels, particularly C5, 6, and 7. The horizontal orientation of the cervical spinal nerves and roots makes it difficult for a disk prolapse to hit two of them. It will generally compress the nerve at one level lower, so a fourth disk will compress the fifth nerve. If two levels are found to be affected, some pathology other than a disk herniation may well be present, and this may include neoplastic disease. These cases need extra care in both examination and treatment. Be very critical of the results of your treatment.

The following table describes the muscles, area of skin, and tendon reflexes affected. These are, of course, approximate and depend entirely on which text you read. The variations probably reflect normal anatomic variances.

Level	Myotome Test	Dermatome	Reflex
C2	None*	Occiput Posterior to ear and the upper posterolateral neck	Sternomastoid
C3	Elevation of the superior scapular angle (not shoulder girdle elevation)	Suboccipital and occipital Posterior neck and upper trapezius	Levator scapulae
C4	Elevation of the superior scapular angle (not shoulder girdle elevation) Inspiration, feeling for descent of diaphragm (not an easy test and generally unnecessary)	Upper trapezius to point of shoulder and upper deltoid Supra- and infraclavicular	Levator scapulae
C5	Shoulder abduction and lateral rotation Elbow flexion (lesser)	Deltoid Lateral upper and lower arms to wrist	Deltoid Biceps Rhomboid
C6	Elbow flexion Wrist extension	Lateral and lower arm Thumb and radial aspect of index finger	Brachioradialis

C7	Elbow extension	Posterior upper and lower arms	Triceps
	Wrist flexion	Middle three fingers	
C8	Finger flexion	Ulnar border of hand	Flexor pollicis
	Thumb extension	Ulnar digit(s)	Abductor pollicis
T1	Abduction and adduction of the fingers		
	Lumbrical action of fingers		

Gray's Anatomy states that there is evidence that the nerve from this segment carries some motor fibers to the sternomastoid with it and that it is not, as had been thought, purely proprioceptive. However, the bulk of the muscle is innervated by the accessory nerve and so is not tested as a spinal myotome.

Red Flags for Potentially Serious Disease

Indications	Possible Condition
Dizziness	Upper cervical dysfunction, vertebrobasilar ischemia, c/v craniovertebral ligament tears
Quadrilateral parasthesia	Cord compression, vertebrobasilar ischemia
Bilateral upper limb parasthesia	Cord compression, vertebrobasilar ischemia
Hyperreflexia	Cord compression, vertebrobasilar ischemia
Babinski or clonus sign	Cord compression, vertebrobasilar ischemia
Cardinal signs/symptoms	Cord compression, vertebrobasilar ischemia
Consistent swallow on transverse ligament stress tests	Instability, retropharyngeal hematoma, RA Rheumatoid Arthritis
Nontraumatic capsular pattern	Rheumatoid Arthritis, Ankylosing Spondylitis, neoplasm
Arm pain lasting more than 6 to 9 months	Neoplasm
Persistent root pain in patient under 30 years of age	Neoplasm
Radicular pain with coughing	Neoplasm
Primary posterolateral pain	Neoplasm
Pain worsening after 1 month	Neoplasm
More than one level involved	Neoplasm
Paralysis	Neoplasm or neurological disease
Trunk and limb paresthesia	Neoplasm
Bilateral root signs and symptoms	Neoplasm
Nontraumatic strong spasm	Neoplasm
Nontraumatic strong pain in the elderly patient	Neoplasm
Signs worse than symptoms	Neoplasm

Red Flags for Potentially Serious Disease (continued)

Indications	Possible Condition
Radial deviator weakness	Neoplasm
Thumb flexor weakness	Neoplasm
Hand intrinsic weakness and/or atrophy	Neoplasm, thoracic outlet syndrome, carpal tunnel syndrome
Cranial nerve signs	Brainstem lesion
Long tract signs	Spinal cord, cerebral, or brainstem lesions
Horner's syndrome	Superior sulcus tumor, breast cancer, cervical ganglion damage, brainstem damage
Empty end feel	Neoplasm
Severe post-traumatic capsular pattern	Fracture
Severe post-traumatic spasm	Fracture
No ROM after trauma	Fracture
Post-traumatic painful weakness	Fracture

Notes

1. Sherk HH: Atlantoaxial instability and acquired basilar invagination in rheumatoid arthritis. Orthop Clin North Am 9:1053, 1978.

2. McNab I: Acceleration injuries of the cervical spine. J Bone Joint Surg Am 46:1797, 1964.

3. McNab I: The whiplash syndrome. Clin Neurosurg 20:232, 1973.

4. Forsyth HF: Extension injury of the cervical spine. J Bone Joint Surg Am, 1792, 1964.

5. Taylor AR, Blackwood W: J Bone Joint Surg Br 30:245, 1948.

6. Ommaya AK: Whiplash injury and brain damage: an experimental study. JAMA 204:285, 1968.

7. Davis SJ et al: Cervical spine hyperextension inujries L MR findings. Radiology 180:245, 1991.

8. Toglia JU: Acute flexion/extension injury of the neck. Neurology 26:808, 1976.

9. Sturzzenegger M et al: The effect of accident mechanisms and initial findings on the long-term course of whiplash injury. J Neurol 242:443, 1995.

10. Taylor JR, Twomey LT: Acute injuries to the cervical joints: an autopsy study of neck sprain. Spine 18:1115, 1993.

11. Taylor JR et al: Road accidents and neck injuries. Proc Austr Soc Hum Biol 5:211, 1992.

12. Showalter W et al: Vertebral artery dissection. Acad Emerg Med 4:991, 1997.

13. Jerome M et al: Vertebral artery injuries associated with cervical spine trauma: a prospective analysis. Comp Orthop 11:12, 1996.

14. Barnsley L et al: The prevalence of chronic cervical zygapophyseal joint pain after whiplash. Spine 20:20, 1995.

15. Norris SH, Watt I: The prognosis for neck injuries resulting from rear end collisions. J Bone Joint Surg Br 65:608, 1983.

16. Gargan MF, Bannister GC: Long term prognosis of the neck. J Bone Joint Surg Br 72:901, 1990.

17. Hohl M: Soft tissue injuries of the neck in automobile accidents: factors influencing prognosis. J Bone Joint Surg Am 56:1675, 1974.

18. Adams RD et al: *Principles of Neurology,* 6th ed., Part 5 (CD-ROM version). New York, McGraw-Hill, 1998.

19. Hicks PA et al: Ophthalmic manifestations of vertebral artery dissection. Ophthalmology 101:1786, 1994.

20. Adams RD et al: *Principles of Neurology,* 6th ed., Part 2 (CD-ROM version). New York, McGraw-Hill, 1998.

21. Husni EA et al: Mechanical occlusion of the vertebral artery: a new concept. JAMA 196:475, 1966.

22. Adams RD et al: *Principles of Neurology,* 6th ed., Part 4 (CD-ROM version). New York, McGraw-Hill, 1998.

23. Rolak LA: *Neurology Secrets,* pp 21–23. Philadelphia, Hanley & Belfus, 1993.

24. Milandre L et al: Lateral bulbar infarctions. Distribution, etiology and prognosis in 40 cases diagnosed by MRI. Rev Neurol (Paris) 151:714, 1995.

25. Nagahata M et al: Arterial dissection of the vertebrobasilar systems: a possible cause of acute sensorineural hearing loss. Am J Otol 18:32, 1997.

26. Sismanis A, Smoker WR: Pulsatile tinnitus. Recent advances in diagnosis. Laryngoscope 104:681, 1994.

27. Koyuncu M et al: Doppler sonography of vertebral arteries in patients with tinnitus. Auris Nasus Larynx 22:24, 1995.

28. Mullen DA: Physical complaints of the aging. Geriatr Marketer 4: 1965.

29. Grant R: Dizziness testing before cervical manipulation: can we recognise the patient at risk? Proc Manip Ther Assoc Austr 5th Biennial Conf, pp 123–136, Melbourne, 1987.

30. Terrett AGJ: Vascular accidents from cervical spine manipulation: the mechanisms. J Austr Chiro Assoc 17:131, 1987. (Reprinted in J Chiro 22:59, 1988.)

31. Meadows J, Magee DJ: An overview of dizziness and vertigo for the orthopedic manual therapist, in JD Boyling, N Palastanga (eds), *Grieve's Modern Manual Therapy,* 2d ed. Edinburgh, Churchill Livingstone, 1994.

32. Jenson JM: Vertigo and dizziness, in WJ Weiner, CG Goetz, *Neurology for the Non-Neurologist,* 3d ed. Philadelphia, JB Lippincott, 1994.

33. Thomas CL (ed). *Taber's Cyclopedic Medical Dictionary.* Philadelphia, FA Davis, 1979.

34. Honrubia V: Quantitative vestibular function tests and clinical examination, in SJ Herdman (ed). *Vestibular Rehabilitation.* Philadelphia, FA Davis, 1994.

35. Leigh RJ: Pharmacologic and optical methods of treating vestibular disorders and nystagmus, in SJ Herdman (ed). *Vestibular Rehabilitation.* Philadelphia, FA Davis, 1994.

36. Ballantyne J, Ahodhia J: Iatrogenic dizziness, in MR Dix, JD Hood (eds). *Vertigo.* Chichester, John Wiley & Sons, 1984.

37. Sevy RW: Drugs as a cause of dizziness and vertigo, in AJ Fineston (ed). *Dizziness and Vertigo.* Boston, John Wright, 1982.

38. Giacobetti FB: Vertebral artery occlusion associated with cervical trauma: a prospective analysis. Spine 22:188, 1997.

39. Coman WB: Dizziness related to ENT conditions, in GP Grieve (ed). *Modern Manual Therapy of the Vertebral Column.* Edinburgh, Churchill Livingstone, 1986.

40. Ross Russell RW: *Vascular Disease of the Central Nervous System,* 2d ed. Edinburgh, Churchill Livingstone, 1983.

41. Rigueiro-Veloso MT et al: Wallenberg's syndrome: a review of 25 cases. Rev Neurol 25:1561, 1997.

42. Appenzeller O: Getting a sore head by banging it on the wall (editorial). Headache 13:77, 1973.

43. Bogduk N: Cervical causes of headache and dizziness, in JD Boyling, N Palastanga (eds). *Grieve's Modern Manual Therapy,* 2d ed. Edinburgh, Churchill Livingstone, 1994.

44. Jull GA: Cervical headache: a review, in JD Boyling, N Palastanga (eds). *Grieve's Modern Manual Therapy,* 2d ed. Edinburgh, Churchill Livingstone, 1994.

45. Chirls M: Retrospective study of cervical spondylosis treated by anterior interbody fusion (in 505 patients) performed by the Cloward technique. Bull N Y Hosp Joint Dis 39:74, 1978.

46. Braff MM, Rosner S: Trauma of the cervical spine as a cause of chronic headache. J Trauma 15:441, 1975.

47. Jones R: Osteoarthritis of the paravertebral joints of the second and third cervical vertebrae as a cause of occipital headaches. S Afr Med J 38:392, 1964.

48. Calliet R: *Head and Face Pain Syndromes,* pp 125–134. Philadelphia, FA Davis, 1992.

49. Miller H: Accident neurosis. BMJ 9:19, 1961.

50. Friedman AP, Merritt HH: Relationship of intracranial pressure in the presence of blood in the cerebrospinal fluid to the occurrence of headache in patients with injuries to the head. J Nerv Ment Dis 102:1, 1945.

51. Ommaya AK, Yarnell P: Subdural hematoma after whiplash injury. Lancet 2:237, 1969.

52. Calliet R: *Head and Face Pain Syndromes,* 1st ed. pp 25–38. Philadelphia, FA Davis, 1992.

53. Saper JR: Chronic headache: current concepts in diagnosis and treatments, in WJ Weiner, CG Goetz (eds). *Neurology for the Non-Neurologist,* 3d ed. Philadelphia, JB Lippincott, 1994.

54. Cyriax J: *Textbook of Orthopedic Medicine,* vol. 1, 8th ed. London, Bailliere Tindall & Cassell, 1982.

55. Elvey RL: Brachial plexus tension tests and the pathanatomical origin of arm pain, in EF Glasgow, LT Twomey (eds). *Aspects of Manipulative Therapy.* Melbourne, Lincoln Institute of Health Sciences, 1979.

56. Elvey RL: Abnormal brachial plexus tension and shoulder joint limitation. Proc IFOMT Conf, Vancouver, 1984.

57. Elvey RL: The investigation of arm pain: signs of adverse responses to the physical examination of the brachial plexus and related neural tissues, in JD Boyling, N Palastanga (eds). *Grieve's Modern Manual Therapy,* 2d ed. Edinburgh, Churchill Livingstone, 1994.

58. Butler DS: *Mobilization of the Nervous System.* Edinburgh, Churchill Livingstone, 1991.

59. Slater H et al: The dynamic central nervous system: examination and assessment using tension tests, in JD Boyling, N Palastanga (eds). *Grieve's Modern Manual Therapy,* 2d ed. Edinburgh, Churchill Livingstone, 1994.

60. Dalinka MK et al: The radiographic evaluation of spinal trauma. Emerg Med Clin North Am 3:475,

61. Reid DC et al: Etiology and clinical course of missed spinal fractures. J Trauma 27:980, 1987.

62. Taylor JR et al: Road accidents and neck injuries. Proc Austr Soc Hum Biol 5:211, 1992.

63. Fischer D, Palleske H: EEG after so-called whiplash injury of the cervical vertebral column (cervicocesphalic trauma) Zentrabl Neurochir 37(1)25–35, 1976.

64. Ettlin TM et al: Cerebral symptoms after whiplash injury of the neck: a prospective clinical and neuropsychological study of whiplash injury. J Neurosurg Psych 55:943, 1992.

65. Jacome DE: EEG in whiplash: a reappraisal. Clin Electroencephalogr 18:41, 1987.

66. Jacome DE, Risko M: EEG features in posttraumatic syndrome. Clin Electroencephalogr 15:214, 1984.

67. Goldberg S: *The Four Minute Neurological Examination.* Miami, Medmaster Inc., 1992.

68. Park WW et al: The pharyngovertebral veins: an anatomic rationale for Grisel's syndrome. J Bone Joint Surg Am 66:568, 1984.

69. Sharp J, Purser DW: Spontaneous atlantoaxial dislocation in ankylosing spondylitis and rheumatoid arthritis. Ann Rheum Dis 20:47, 1961.

70. Matthews JA: Atlanto-axial subluxation in rhematoid arthritis. Ann Rheum Dis 28:260, 1969.

71. Stevens JC et al: Atlantoaxial subluxation and cervical myelopathy in rheumatoid arthritis. Q J Med 40:391, 1971.

72. Pueschel SM et al: Computerized tomography in persons with Down's syndrome and atlantoaxial instability. Spine 17:735, 1992.

73. Elliot S: The odontoid process in children—is it hypoplastic. Clin Radiol 39:391, 1988.

74. Greene KA et al: Transverse atlantal ligament disruption associated with odontoid fractures. Spine 19:2307, 1994.

75. Dickman CA et al: Injuries involving the transverse atlantal ligament: classification and treatment guidelines based on experience with 39 injuries. Neurosurgery 38:44, 1996.

76. Heller JG et al: Jefferson fractures: the role of magnification artifact in assessing transverse ligament integrity. J Spinal Disord 6:392, 1993.

77. Uitvlugt G, Idenbaum S: Clinical assessment of atlantoaxial instability using the Sharp-Purser test. Arthritis Rheum 31:918, 1988.

78. Pettman E: Stress tests of the craniovertebral joints, in JD Boyling, N Palastanga (eds). *Grieve's Modern Manual Therapy* 2d ed. Edinburgh, Churchill Livingstone, 1994.

79. Meadows J: The Sharp-Purser test: a useful clinical tool or an exercise in futility and risk? J Man Manipulative Ther 6:97, 1998.

80. Dvorak J et al: CT-functional diagnostics of the rotatory instability of the upper cervical spine. I. An experimental study on cadavers. Spine 12:197, 1987.

81. Panjabi MM et al: Instability in injury of the alar ligament. A biomechanical model. Orthopade 20:112, 1991.

82. George B, Laurian C: *The Vertebral Artery: Pathology and Surgery.* New York, Springer-Verlag, 1987.

83. Bolton PS et al: Failure of clinical tests to predict cerebral ischemia before neck manipulation. J Manip Physiol Ther 12:304, 1989.

84. Wing LW, Hargrave-Wilson W: Cervical vertigo. N Z J Surg 44:275, 1974.

85. de Jong PTVM et al: Ataxia induced by injection of local anesthesia in the neck. Ann Neurol 1:240, 1977.

86. Cohen LA: Role of the eye and neck proprioceptive mechanisms in body orientation and motor coordination. J Neurophysiol 24:1, 1961.

87. Biemond A, de Jong JMBV: On cervical nystagmus and related disorders. Brain 92:437, 1969.

88. Hikosaka O, Maeda M: Cervical effects on abducens motorneurons and their interaction with vestibulo-ocular reflex. Exp Brain Res 18:512, 1973.

89. Smith GA, Stern WE: Experiments on carotid artery flow increase as a result of contralateral vertebral occlusion. Acta Neurochir 23:221, 1970.

90. Hardesty WH et al: Studies on vertebral artery blood flow in man. Surg Gynecol Obstet 116:662, 1963.

91. Cope S, Ryan GMS: Cervical and otolith vertigo. J Laryngol Otol 73:113, 1959.

92. Toole JF, Tucker SH: Influence of head position upon cerebral circulation: studies in blood flow in cadavers. Arch Neurol 2:616, 1960.

93. Brown BSJ, Tatlow WFT: Radiologic studies of the vertebral artery in cadavers. Radiology 81:80, 1963.

94. Grant R: Clinical testing before cervical manipulation—can we recognize the patient at risk? Proc 10th Int Congr World Confed Phys Ther, Sydney, 1987.

95. Australian Physiotherapy Association: Protocol for premanipulative testing of the cervical spine. Austr J Physiother 34:97, 1988.

96. Olszewski J: Experimental ischaemia of the vertebral artery and its effect on brain stem auditory evoked responses in guinea pigs. Folia Morphol (Praha) 35:134, 1990.

97. Meadows J, Magee DJ: An overview of dizziness and vertigo for the orthopedic manual therapist, in JD Boyling, N Palastanga (eds). *Grieve's Modern Manual Therapy* 2d ed. Edinburgh, Churchill Livingstone, 1994.

CHAPTER 11

The Thoracic Region

Examination

Subjective

Thoracic pain can originate from the thoracic cage itself—the vertebras, ribs, sternum, manubrium, chondrium, intervertebral disks, zygapophyseal joints, costotransverse joints, and costovertebral joints—or from the structures enclosed by the cage—the heart, lungs, pericardium, pleura, bronchi, trachea, or diaphragm. The pain can be felt locally, or it can be referred to the shoulder area and even the arm. This is one area in which visceral causation must always be considered before musculoskeletal. Lung cancer and cardiac disease are among the leading causes of death in North America and cannot be discounted. Because of their linings, the heart and lungs are capable of causing pain that is musculoskeletal in type.

Heart attacks may not give the typical chest/neck pain or the classical ulnar hand and medial upper and lower arm pain, but may begin with aching in the deltoid and lateral upper arm area, and may even be on the right side occasionally. Ask about the onset and offset of whatever pains the patient is experiencing. If the pain is associated with general activity or emotional stress, refer the patient back to the physician. Pain of musculoskeletal origin should be associated with thoracic movements or postures. If pain is felt on deep respiration, it could of course be caused by movement of the ribs and the spine. However, if this is the case, you should be able to reproduce this pain with passive or active movements of the spine, and with careful questioning, the patient should be able to recall pain with activities other than simply breathing, however deeply. Pain felt only on respiration may be caused by cardiac ischemia;

the demand for deep breathing coincides with the need for more blood to the heart muscles. It may also be caused by pulmonary or pleural disorders. If respiratory pain is linked with changes in coughing or the product of coughing, the patient must be returned to the physician because this is just too much of a coincidence. Pleural pain can be very difficult to differentiate, even on the most tentative of bases. The attachment of the outer layer of the pleura means that as the ribs move, so does the pleura. Consequently, breathing and trunk movements can be very painful. Additionally confusing the issue is the type of pain produced by the parietal layer of the pleura: It is musculoskeletal. The diagnosis may have to be made retrospectively when treatment fails to improve the patient's condition.

Irritation of the diaphragm can cause shoulder pain. Diseases of the basal lung, stomach, spleen, liver, duodenum, and gall bladder may cause diaphragmatic irritation. Abdominal or low posterior thoracic pain and shoulder pain in the same patient is a red flag and may be caused by disease of one or more of the structures just discussed. This type of dissociated pain cannot be assumed to be musculoskeletal in origin and must be referred to the physician.

Upper thoracic pain associated with shoulder pain may well be pathomechanically linked with dysfunctional upper thoracic biomechanics causing the shoulder pain. In this case, look for the disturbed biomechanics in the thoracic spine and the shoulder. If this is found, a trial of treatment is in order, but if the treatment does not produce rapid improvement, the patient should undergo further medical assessment.

The thoracic pain leads the way in being affected by metastases (70% of spinal metastases affect the thoracic spine, 20% the lumbar, and 10% the cervical[1]) with possible subsequent cord compression. Direct invasion of the ribs does occur and can lead to reduction of shoulder movement if the muscles running from the ribs to the humerus or the scapula pull on the affected area. For the most part this may become apparent in the objective examination when passive movement away from the rib cage is painful and may have a spasm end feel, and isometric contraction of the adductor muscles is painful and weak. Palpation of the ribs may detect heat caused by the increased metabolism.[2]

Pain associated with diet or eating time is probably caused by visceral rather than musculoskeletal pathology. One patient gave a history of posterior thoracic pain when sitting to eat. The obvious thought is that compression of the spinal structures is causing the pain, possibly disk herniation. However, on further questioning, the patient said that he was able to sit for driving and watching TV but not for eating and had to eat standing at the sideboard. He was eventually diagnosed as having a hiatus hernia.

Rib fractures associated with trauma may also be associated with a sudden onset of severe pain, "cracking" sounds at the time of the injury, crepitus, pain, and strong respiration pain. Stress fractures may occur as a result of pathologies such as neoplastic invasion or because of strong and prolonged bouts of coughing in patients with the flu.

The spinal canal is relatively small compared with the cord in this region, and its blood supply is more fragile than that of other parts of the cord.[3] Posterior disk herniation or osteophytic encroachment may compress the cord or conus medullaris. Listen for complaints of bilateral lower limb paresthesia, urinary retention (which may be related as frequent urges but small volume), and lower limb incoordination or weakness.

Observation

Scoliosis is easily seen in this region as a rib hump on the convex side. Be careful about attributing the patient's pain to this condition, though, because it is frequently asymptomatic and only a coincidental finding.

Atrophy or hypertonicity of the paravertebral muscles (rotatores) can be seen more easily here than in the cervical or lumbar spines. Atrophy may be caused by spinal nerve compression from a disk prolapse, an osteophyte, or painful inhibition. Hypertonicity may suggest segmental facilitation arising from the spinal level where the hypertonicity is seen. With both hypertrophy and atrophy, the change may not be of sufficient magnitude to be seen but can be felt on palpation.

Watch rib excursion during quiet breathing. Later during the objective examination feel the excursion, and if it appears reduced, measure it. There should be at least a couple of inches of expansion in the base of the rib cage. Causes of reduced expansion are old age, ankylosing spondylitis, rib fractures or metastases, diaphragm paralysis, chronic asthma, and other chronic lung conditions.

Herpes zoster commonly affects the intercostal nerves between T5-10 (two thirds of all cases of herpes zoster),[4] so look for eruptions running along the dermatome. Remember that you may be seeing the patient early in the course of the condition, so the vesicles may not be apparent on the first or even second attendance but develop during subsequent examinations.

Active and Passive Movement Tests

The symmetrical capsular pattern of the thoracic spine is probably symmetrical limitation of rotation and side flexion extension loss and least loss of flexion, but traumatic arthritis may affect only the joints on one side if the traumatic force is asymmetrical. Presumably the capsular pattern is caused by irritation of the synovial joints, and in the spine, the most painful movement in cases of effusion is extension. Therefore, the loss is extension more than flexion, giving an asymmetrical loss of rotation and side flexion, a restriction of extension, and a lesser restriction of flexion. Because of the range of rotation, most "normal" musculoskeletal conditions of the thoracic spine will involve rotation and flexion or extension, with side flexion being minimally affected. Be careful of any patterns of restriction in which side flexion is more seriously affected than rotation. Neoplastic disease of the viscera or chest wall may present in such a manner.

The end feel of general rotation should be quite elastic in the nonelderly patient, presumably afforded by the chondral cartilage. Ankylosing spondylitis and osteoporosis change this end feel to a much stiffer end feel. In these patients, rib springing (be very careful in the patient suspected of being osteoporotic) affords the same end feel and there is a general loss of rib expansion with inspiration.

If flexion and extension are restricted to a greater extent than rotation and there are no other signs, a possibility is an anterior migration of the vertebra caused by instability through the disk and zygapophyseal joints. Essentially, both joints are jammed or subluxed into flexion. Posteroanterior pressure on the superior bone of the affected segment is usually extremely painful and produces a spasm end feel, whereas the same pressure on the inferior bone is less painful, with a springy or pathomechanical end feel. The clinical diagnosis is made from the biomechanical examination when the segmental restriction is identified.

Disk herniations are generally considered a rarity,[5] making up less than 1% of disk ruptures, and, unless they compress the spinal cord, can be more difficult to diagnose. In this study, 75% of thoracic disk herniations occurred below T8, with most (28%) occurring at T11-12. The majority occurred between ages 30 and 50, with the largest single age group being in the fourth decade (33%). Men were affected one and a half times more often than women were, and 67% of herniations were central or centrolateral.[6]

The pain of thoracic disk herniation is extremely variable, with Brown et al.[7] citing 13 different references on pain type and location. Their study on thoracic disks found that 67% had bandlike chest pain, 8% interscapular pain, 4% epigastric pain, and 16% lower limb pain. They also found that 20% of these patients had lower limb complaints, which included paresthesia (4%) and obvious weakness (16%). Of the 11 patients with lower limb symptoms, 9 had surgery. Certainly the pain can be intense and either runs around the chest wall or is felt in the dorsal and ventral aspects of the thorax. The diagnosis is more easily made if the pain is lancinating; otherwise, zygapophyseal or costal joint problems as well as dural irritation can cause somatic pain from a disk herniation. I have seen patients whose pain was so severe that the patient was admitted to the coronary care unit with a suspected myocardial infarction.

There is severe restriction of motion in a noncapsular pattern, usually with both flexion and extension being limited and very painful, together with one or both rotations. The end feel on at least one, and usually more, of these movements will be spasm.

Isometric Contractile Tissue Tests

Abdominal and intercostal muscle injuries do occur, often as a part of a rib fracture, and the appropriate tests will reproduce local pain. Posterior pain on isometric testing is much less likely to be caused by contractile lesions than is anterior or lateral pain. Usually, posterior pain produced by isometric testing is a result of compression or shearing of an acutely symptomatic spinal segment. Weakness with pain over the ribs may be caused by fracture when an intercostal muscle strain is not likely to produce weakness. Pain from an intercostal muscle injury is invariably local; its situation at the end of the dermatome and its superficiality do not facilitate its ability to refer pain.[2]

Neurological Tests

Neurological deficit is very difficult to pick up in the thorax. Sensation should be tested over the abdomen; the area just below the xiphoid process is innervated by T8, the umbilicus by T10, and the lower abdominal region level with the anterior superior iliac spines by T12. It is almost impossible to test above T8 because of overlap.

Similarly, testing muscle strength is difficult. In Beaver's test, the tester watches the umbilicus of the supine patient while the patient lifts the head. The abdominals are innervated by the lower six thoracic spinal nerves. If the umbilicus deviates diagonally, this suggests weakness in the diagonally opposite set of three abdominal muscles. For example, if the umbilicus shifts upward and right, the muscles in the lower left quadrant must be weak, and if this weakness is due to a spinal nerve palsy, the spinal nerve affected must be the tenth, eleventh, or twelfth thoracic nerve on the left.[8] Asking the patient to take a deep breath and hold it while the therapist presses a fingertip into the intercostal space can test the strength of the intercostal muscles. It should be equally difficult to penetrate the intercostal space with your finger on both sides.

A few reflexes are available to the examiners. Deep stroking with the end of the reflex hammer over the abdominal muscles tests the abdominal cutaneous reflex. Each quadrant is tested and compared to its opposite number. Skin rippling should occur or not occur equally in opposite quadrants. This test, when integrated with Beaver's test, can give the tester an idea of the strength of the abdominal muscles, at least a group of three abdominal muscles. Loss of two hemilateral segments occurs with central nervous system lesions. The cremasteric reflex can be carried out in males. The inner upper thigh is stroked, and the scrotum should elevate. If there is unilateral loss of the reflex and no central nervous system signs or symptoms, the loss of the reflex is probably from a first or second lumbar spinal nerve palsy. The reflex is not used very commonly among orthopedic physical therapists for two reasons: first, the obvious reluctance to look at the scrotal area, and second, because it can only be carried out in males. The spinal cord reflexes must be tested on patients with thoracic pain. Oppenheimer's clonus, and the extensor-plantar test looking for the Babinski reflex are all tested to evaluate the brain's ability to inhibit these reflexes and/or the reticulospinal tract's excessive contribution to the reflex.

Dural Tests

These are mostly central tests using neck flexion and the slump test. It is obvious that both of these dural tests also stress nondural tissues, and the pain may be coming from spinal nondural tissues. However, this is no different from the dural mobility tests used in other spinal regions, and their specificity as to tissue of origin is dependent on other tests. Inspiration moves the dura from the periphery by the moving ribs pulling on the intercostal nerves and moving the dura. Again, the results of this test must be compared to the active and passive movement tests.

1. History
- ❏ Age and sex
  - a. osteoporosis
  - b. neoplasm
  - c. cardiac conditions
- ❏ Spinal cord signs/symptoms
  - ❏ bilateral paresthesia, Babinski's reflex, clonus, spasticity
- ❏ Symptoms related to general exertion or emotional stress (cardiac problems)
- ❏ Symptoms related to eating (gastric ulcer, gall bladder disease)

2. Observation
- ❏ Rib hump (rotoscoliosis)
- ❏ Scars (surgery)
- ❏ Hyperkyphosis/lordosis (postural deficits)
- ❏ Rotatores atrophy (palsy)
- ❏ Rotatores hypertonicity (segmental facilitation)
- ❏ Reduced respiratory excursion (ankylosing spondylitis, old age, diaphragm weakness, pulmonary problems)

3. Articular Tests
- ❏ Active: flexion, extension, rotation, and side flexion
- ❏ Passive: flexion, extension, rotation, and side flexion
  - a. capsular or noncapsular patterns of restriction
  - b. onset of pain
  - c. end feel
- ❏ Resisted: flexion, extension, rotation, and side flexion
  - a. pain (minor contractile lesion)

    b. weakness (grade 3 tear or neurological)

    c. painful weakness (possible fracture or neoplasm)

4. Stress Tests

❑ Axial compression

    a. end-plate fracture

    b. disk herniation

    c. acute centrum fracture

    d. apophyseal joint inflammation

❑ Traction

    a. injury of the longitudinal ligaments

    b. acute apophyseal joint inflammation

❑ Anterior-posterior pressure

    a. anterior translation instability

    b. posterior instability

    c. acute zygapophyseal joint inflammation

    d. disk herniation

5. Dural Tests

❑ Neck flexion

❑ Slump test

❑ Bilateral straight leg raising

❑ Inspiration

    a. dural inflammation

    b. dural compression

    c. dural adhesions

    d. neural irritation

    e. nondural causes

6. Myotome (key muscles)

❑ Beevor's sign (lower six thoracic spinal nerves)

❑ Intercostal digital pressure while breathing (spinal nerve)

7. Dermatome

❑ T8 (xiphoid process)

❑ T10 (umbilicus)

❑ T12 (just below ribs to upper groin)

8. Reflexes

❑ Abdominal cutaneous reflex (central nervous system lesion or lower thoracic spinal nerve palsy)

❑ Cremasteric reflex (central nervous system lesion or lower thoracic spinal nerve palsy)

❑ Spinal cord reflexes (Babinski's reflex, clonus, deep tendon reflexes)

    a. corticospinal tract or cerebral lesion

Herpes Zoster[4]

This condition is being discussed in this section because the thorax is the most common region for it to make itself felt. It occurs much more commonly in the older person than the younger. Both sexes are equally affected, and no immunity is granted by an attack.

Herpes zoster is believed to be caused by a reactivation of the chicken pox infection and is infectious in those have not had chicken pox. Because of its low infection rate, it is nonepidemic in nature. Generally, reactivation occurs when the body is vulnerable. Old age, sickness, radiation therapy, lymphomas, and immunosuppressant drugs have all been known to permit its onset. About 5% if patients with shingles will be found to have a concurrent malignancy (about twice as many as for that age group). The condition affects the following structures:

- ❏ Inflammation of several unilateral adjacent spinal or cranial sensory ganglia
- ❏ Necrosis of all or part of the ganglia
- ❏ Inflammation of the spinal root and peripheral nerve ganglion
- ❏ A primarily posterior horn poliomyelitis
- ❏ A mild meningitis

Clinical features include:

- ❏ Itching
- ❏ Paresthesia
- ❏ Causalgia
- ❏ Radiculitis
- ❏ Sensory loss (uncommon)
- ❏ Motor palsy (uncommon)
- ❏ Malaise (occasional)
- ❏ Fever (occasional)

Within 72 to 96 hours of the pain onset, a rash erupts along the dermatome innervated by the affected ganglion. In the majority of cases (60%), the pain disappears within 4 weeks but in the remainder it can last for months. Usually one segment is involved, but in some cases, particularly when the cranial or limb nerve(s) is affected, two contiguous segments may be involved.

Any dermatome can be affected, but the condition most commonly affects T5-10, making up about 66% of cases, followed by the craniocervical region, where the condition tends to be more severe with greater pain and more frequent involvement of the meninges and mucus membranes.

Serious Disease Red Flags

Indication	Possible Condition
First episode of pain in the middle-aged to elderly patient	Neoplasm
Severe bilateral root pain in the older patient	Neoplasm
Wedging	Fracture (traumatic, osteoporotic, or neoplastic)
Onset/offset of pain related to general activity or stress levels	Cardiac
Onset/offset of pain unrelated to trunk movements	Ankylosing spondylitis, visceral disorder
Decreased and painful active contralateral side flexion with both rotations full-range	Neoplasm
Severe chest wall pain without articular pain	Visceral
Onset/offset of pain related to eating times or diet	Gastrointestinal or gall bladder disease
Bilateral paresthesia or central nervous system signs	Spinal cord compression

Notes

1. Roth P: Neurologic problems and emergencies, in RB Cameron (ed). *Practical Oncology.* Norwalk, CT, Appleton & Lange, 1994.

2. Cyriax J: *Textbook of Orthopedic Medicine,* vol. 1, 17(suppl):97 1992, 8th ed. London, Bailliere Tindall & Cassell, 1982.

3. Panjabi MM et al: Thoracic human vertebrae. Quantitative three dimensional anatomy. Spine 16:888, 1991.

4. Adams RD et al: *Principles of Neurology,* 6th ed, Part 4 (CD-ROM version). New York, McGraw-Hill, 1998.

5. Warren MJ: Modern imaging of the spine; the use of computed tomography and magnetic resonance, in JD Boyling, N Palastanga (eds). *Grieve's Modern Manual Therapy,* 2d ed. Edinburgh, Churchill Livingstone, 1994.

6. Arce KH, Dohrmann GJ: Protrusions of thoracic intervertebral discs. Neurol Clin 3:338, 1985.

7. Brown CW et al: The natural history of thoracic disc herniation. Spine 17:S97, 1992.

8. Hoppenfeld S: Orthopedic neurology: a diagnostic guide to neurological levels. Philadelphia, JB Lippincott, 1977.

CHAPTER 12

The Lumbar Spine

The lumbar spine and the neck are the two most common spinal regions treated by the generalist orthopedic therapist. Unlike neck pain, most low back pain is nontraumatically induced. As elsewhere in the spine, a multitude of tissues have the potential for being painful when provoked appropriately. In the lumbar spine, there is either experimental and/or clinical evidence for the disks, zygapophyseal joints, muscles, ligaments, and dural sleeve as pain sources.[1]

Disk herniations causing neurological deficits seem to be seen more commonly here than in the cervical spine, possibly in part because of the increased stress on the lumbar disk and also because of the different ways in which the two disks degenerate.[2] The lumbar disk retaining its, albeit drier, nucleus into old age whereas the cervical disk's nucleus disappears at all but the lowest level by the middle twenties.

Anatomically, the areas are distinct: The spinal cord inhabits the cervical spine canal whereas the cauda equina, the cord terminating at about the first lumbar level, inhabits the lumbar spine. This means that a cervical posterior disk herniation compressing the contents of the spinal canal may cause an upper motor lesion, whereas in the lumbar spine the result will most frequently be a lower motor lesion. This compression of the cauda equina is the most frequent pathology in the lumbar spine. There are no uncovertebral or costovertebral joints to protect the intervertebral canal and its contents from disk compression as there are in the cervical and thoracic regions. Certainly the cervical disk and possibly the thoracic disk are radically different from their lumbar counterparts in makeup.

However, with all of this concentration on the lumbar disk as a source of disability, it should be realized that symptomatic externalization of the disk is considered by most authorities to be a rare occurrence, possibly being responsible for only about 5% of cases of low back pain.[3]

Serious Pathology

Given the possibility of cancer in younger and older populations, age must be considered from the perspective of disk degradation. The older patient is also less likely to have a disk herniation because the disk has been successfully tested without previous failure over its lifetime and the person is generally putting less adverse stress on the disk because activity levels tend to drop with age. In addition, degenerative changes have made the spine and the disk stiffer, with changes in the zygapophyseal joints and in the disk itself. The possibility of metastatic disease must always be considered because 20% of spinal metastases occur in the lumbar spine.[4] It is very unusual for the young patient, say up to about the middle twenties, to suffer from symptoms of a disk herniation because it usually takes some time for nontraumatic degradative processes to superimpose themselves on the degenerative changes. However, exceptions do occur. Recent literature gives the age of 9 years as the youngest patient age with established lumbar disk herniation.[5]

In the younger patient with acute low back pain, neoplastic disease should be considered first. One study looked at the clinical differences between children suffering from disk herniations and those with spinal tumors of all types. Spinal neoplastic disease in children tends to affect both legs, whereas disk herniations in the same group mainly affect one leg. Abdominal pain may be present in the neoplastic disorder and is usually absent in disk lesions. Neurological deficits are more commonly caused by neoplasms than by disk herniations in this age group. The study also found that the younger the child, the greater the likelihood that neoplastic disease is the cause of the symptoms. Most of the children in the neoplastic group were under 10 years of age.[6]

As far as an upper age limit is concerned, I have seen a 65-year-old woman with acute articular signs, radicular pain, segmental sensory loss, and weakness that imaging studies subsequently confirmed as a fifth lumbar disk herniation with first sacral nerve compression. The literature offers examples of patients over 70 years of age with disk herniation. However, the pathology seems to differ from that found in patients less than 60 years old. In the patient over 60, the nucleus does not appear to be a major factor in the condition. The main pathology is anular sequestration or avulsion of the cartilaginous end-plate, which then herniates posteriorly with the anulus. It must be remembered that disk herniation in both the young and older populations is an oddity, and other causes of disklike signs and symptoms must be considered and excluded before accepting the diagnosis of disk herniation.

Intervertebral Disk Pathologies

There are various ways of classifying disk lesions, based on the size, the location, or the composition of the herniated material. The classical method of quantifying disk lesions is based on the size of the externalization and the material that has herniated as follows[7]:

1. *Protrusion.*   This is a relatively small bulge on the disk with no migration of nuclear material. It may be caused by a weakness in the anulus, possibly the result of the alignment of circumferential fissures or a radial tear. There are biomechanical effects but often no dural or neural compromise.

2. *Prolapse.*   There is migration of the nucleus, but it is constrained by the anulus and is not externalized. The bulge is much larger, and if it is a clinical rather than an imaging entity, dural and neural signs can be expected. Of the movements, flexion tends to provoke pain more than extension, and the patient has trouble sitting and bending.

3. *Extrusion.*   The nuclear material has become externalized, and the pressure effect is much larger than the prolapse. Neurological deficit can be expected. All movements tend to reproduce the pain, and the patient is uncomfortable with both flexion and extension activities and postures. There is often deformity in the form of kyphosis combined with straight deviation or with scoliosis.

4. *Sequestration.*   The extruded nuclear material has fragmented and lies in the spinal canal. The effects of this condition depend on the sizes of the fragments and their locations.

This classical categorization based mainly on nuclear migration has recently been challenged. The concept of disk degeneration being a pathological process that is of itself painful has been questioned for quite some time. Certainly, common sense would dictate that if degeneration of the spinal segment were painful then almost everybody would be painful all of the time, as this is an almost universal and nonreversible process.

Age changes (degeneration) in the disk are initially biochemical, with a reduction in number and alteration in composition of proteoglycans and a decreasing level of chondoitin sulfate. The other major changes include increases in nuclear collagen and in collagen-proteoglycan binding. The nucleus becomes less elastic, that is, stiffer and less hydrophilic. The now less than optimally handled compression stresses start to randomly separate the anular lamellae, causing small fissures and cracks termed *circumferential tears,* which may become larger. Because of selective resorption of the horizontal trabeculae in the vertebral body and subsequent collapse of the vertical trabeculae, the intervertebral disk height actually increases by about 10% over adult life. Degradation occurs from disruption of the nucleus (presumed to be caused by end-plate fracture) and resorption of nuclear material, with subsequent disk height loss, and possibly becomes symptomatic because of compression of sensitive structures. Alternatively, there may be radial tearing of the anulus and migration of liquefied nuclear material through the tear, resulting in prolapse or extrusion. For an excellent review of disk degeneration and degradation read Brogduk and Twomey.[1,8]

Another method of classification is to consider disk lesions as contained or uncontained herniations. In the contained herniation, the nucleus is disturbed but its migration remains within the anulus. This would have effects similar to those of a protrusion or a small prolapse. The uncontained herniation would essentially be the equivalent of a large prolapse or extrusion. Contained disk lesions tend to have minimal or no neurological deficit, minor dural signs, and moderate articular signs. Uncontained disk herniations were more severe in their articular, dural, and neural signs and symptoms, resembling extrusions.[9]

Another concept is that of metaplastic proliferation of fibrocartilage, the formation of a lump of immature collagen on the anulus fibrosis, possibly caused by granulation of an anular tear. In his study of 21 surgical cases for low back and leg pain, Lipson[10] biopsied the discal material found to be protruding. He found that this material was not nuclear but newly formed fibrocartilage. He concluded that "proliferative metaplastic fibrocartilage, synthesized by the annular fibroblasts, is the source of herniated disc, and replaces the traditional concept of herniation of pre-existing disc tissue."

Whichever classification method or terminology is used, the clinical signs and symptoms remain paramount for treatment and prognosis. The finding of neurological deficit does not indicate a good prognosis, and treatment will not be very aggressive, with intermittent traction and pain-free exercise predominating. Manual therapy in these cases is not likely to afford much relief and may worsen things. At the other end of the spectrum, the diagnosis of small protrusion is very presumptive but much more easily treated. Exercises and/or manual therapy may well correct the problem very quickly.

It appears that the pathology and clinical presentation of the elderly patient with a disk prolapse tend to differ from those of the younger. The herniated material is a mixture of anulus fibrosis and avulsed cartilaginous end-plate material.[11] Disk herniation in the elderly patient tends to resemble central spinal stenosis, with less severely affected straight leg raise and more severely affected walking ability.[9]

Among the more reliable signs and symptoms for disk herniations are

❏ Radicular (lancinating) pain
❏ Radiculopathy

❑ Severely restricted straight leg raise (the more restricted, the more reliable)[12]

❑ Crossed straight leg raise

❑ Limited walking ability (more common with extrusions and sequestrations)

❑ Severely restricted lumbar range

Another diagnostic consideration in the elderly patient is spinal stenosis.[13,14] Although stenosis may be caused by disk herniation, postfracture callus formation, or spondylolisthesis at any age, developmental stenosis is mainly the scourge of the older patient. Frequently there are structural predispositions in the form of a trefoil spinal canal or an abnormally narrow canal that lend themselves to narrowing from arthrotic changes in the zygapophyseal joints. In both central and lateral stenosis, the pain is exacerbated by extension postures or activities such as prolonged standing and walking respectively. Central stenosis generally causes low back and bilateral or unilateral leg pain, whereas lateral stenosis is frequently unisegmental and unilateral. The leg pain is usually not of the severe variety experienced with disk herniation and is only uncommonly lancinating. The patient with central stenosis usually complains of mild to moderate aching in the backs of the legs. This is evoked or exacerbated by walking or standing and relieved by flexing the spine either by sitting or squatting. Simply stopping walking does not alleviate the symptoms; the spine has to be flexed.

The articular and dural signs of stenosis are much milder than are those accompanying a disk herniation. Neurological signs are unusual and if present tend to be mild, often confined to hypoesthesia and mild reduction in the deep tendon reflexes. The major pathology in this condition is thought to be caused by the obstruction diminishing the blood flow to the dural sleeve and/or the nerve, causing ischemia of these structures.

Intermittent claudication syndromes can be spinal or peripheral.[15] Peripheral claudication usually affects the gluteal or calf muscles and can be confused with referred pain from the lumbar spine. The condition is a demand ischemia caused by stenosis of the arteries to the spine, the nerve roots, or the peripheral muscles. The patient tends to be middle-aged or elderly, with the usual risk factors for atherosclerosis.[16] Spinal claudication is linked with spinal stenosis,[17] and it, rather than compression-induced conduction problems, may be the main cause of the patient's symptoms. If the spinal cord is affected either from cervical, thoracic, or high lumbar stenosis, the symptoms are weakness, tightness, numbness, and/or a strangulated feeling in the lower limb and trunk.[18]

Initially, before the condition becomes severe, the patient complains of buttock or calf pain on walking a set distance on the level or decreased distance on hills. The pain is relieved when the patient simply stops walking for a set period. The flexion required for the relief of pain from spinal stenosis is not need to relieve this pain. Later as the condition progresses, the amount of effort needed to provoke the pain lessens and the amount of rest time required to relieve it increases until the pain becomes almost continuous. Other vascular signs, such as the loss of peripheral pulses and color changes, become obvious as the disease progresses.

Obviously the clinical diagnosis becomes easier to make as the condition worsens, but these patients will not reach your facility. The early atheroscelorotic patient presents the diagnostic problem. The diagnosis will be made more difficult if the patient also has coincidental low back pain.

Repeated or sustained contractions of the affected muscles will eventually reproduce the patient's symptoms. The condition is usually a systemic one affecting both legs. However, one side is usually worse than the other, and as a consequence, the symptoms normally experienced by the patient are unilateral because when the pain starts, the patient stops. However, continued exercising of the asymptomatic leg after the symptoms occur in the leg complained of will usually cause this leg to become symptomatic.

Spinal cord intermittent claudication is usually caused by cervical or thoracic conditions such as atherosclerosis or compression of spinal arteries that impair blood flow to the cord. In thoracic claudication, the patient commonly complains of weakness, paresthesia, and numbness in the legs, and a choked-off feeling in the legs and trunk, mainly on walking. When the symptoms are present, there is evidence of spinal tract compromise, particularly of the spinothalamic tracts.[18] Sustained or repeated exercises may reproduce the symptoms, but spinal compression may be needed.

The need to accurately diagnose the disease is obviously important, because this patient needs to be on appropriate medication and a walking program[19] rather than having his or her back treated.

Spondylolisthesis may have its first onset in childhood or in adulthood, or it may be delayed into middle age and develop as a result of segmental degenerative/degradation and a narrow facet angle[20] or as a result of trauma or pathology.[21] The condition really affects those under 40 years old and is more common in females. The signs and symptoms are usually far from clear-cut in these patients. There is usually mild to moderate back and/or leg pain that is made worse with extension activities and postures, and more typically is stenotic, in that there is neurogenic claudication of the fifth lumbar spinal nerves. Only about 50% of these cases show evidence of overt neurological involvement.[22] Anular splitting has been found to accompany degenerative spondylolisthesis[23] and may complicate both the treatment and the diagnosis.

Degenerative spondylolisthesis will generally present with a stenotic type of history, with pain being worse with prolonged standing or other extension activities or postures. The pain tends to be neurogenic in nature, only uncommonly becoming acute or causing overt neurological signs or symptoms. A step deformity might be palpable in standing and if present denotes the lower vertebra of the affected segment.

In comparison, isthmic spondylolisthesis in the young patient usually has its onset under the age of 18 and may be related to some relatively minor trauma. The causation of isthmic spondylolisthesis is not well understood; the roles of genetics, family, and chance have all been debated. The pars articularis is deficient, and the signs and symptoms are variable but can be much worse and more evident than in degenerative spondylolisthesis, usually coming on in the early half of the second decade. Typically moderate symptoms are low back pain with radiation into the buttock and posterior thighs. Only rarely is there neurological involvement.[24] If isthmic spondylolisthesis is severe, the patient will be kyphotic, with guarding and spasm of the hamstrings to limit the anterior slippage. There is bilateral sciatica, often of the radicular pain variety, with limitation of both straight leg raises. Neurological signs may be present depending on the severity of the migration and the length of time the patient has had the condition. If a step deformity is present, it will denote the bone of the segment superior to the affected one because the spinous process of the deficient vertebra is left behind as the centrum slides forward. The major effect of a significant spondylolisthesis of either type is central stenosis, so expect similar provocative factors.

Urinary bladder dysfunction is a key finding in the history. Prostate cancer may be associated with nocturia, hematuria, urinary hesitancy, or acute retention. Back pain may be referred directly from the prostate or bladder but may also be caused by metastatic invasion.[25]

Low back pain, urinary sphincter dysfunction, saddle anesthesia, bilateral sciatica, and multisegmental sensory and motor deficits characterize cauda equina lesions, whereas lesions of the spinal cord or the conus medullaris may cause a neurogenic bladder.[25] In these cases, spasticity of the internal sphincter results in frequent urges with little to show for them. The pressure rises in the bladder until it and muscular contraction force the sphincter open, but only for a very short period until the pressure drops and it can close again. Mild compression of the cauda equina, possibly caused by hypertonicity of the external sphincter, may cause similar effects, but as the pressure on the neurological tissue increases, incontinence intervenes.

Almost invariably, compression of the cauda equina from a disk herniation will involve severe low back pain and bilateral sciatica with seriously reduced ranges of movement of the trunk. However, it is worth noting that although the position of the conus medullaris tip (that is the spinal cord) is given as L1, it is variable and follows a normal distribution around the lower third of L1, ranging from the middle of T12 to the upper third of L3.[27] Consequently, it is perfectly possible for an L2-3 lesion, disk, or neoplasm to compress the spinal cord (conus). The pain may be of various types and in various locales, depending on the source.

The pain can be local, referred, or radicular, depending on the structures irritated. Funicular or central pain is caused by compression of the descending spinal cord tracts (spinothalamic) and tends to be diffuse and deeply aching or burning. Its presence denotes involvement of the conus medullaris.

Increasing pressure on the cauda equina may also result in genital dysfunction in the form of genital sensory loss,[28] with impotence in males and frigidity in females.[29,30] Penile deviation may also occur. The same compression may also result in a lack of expulsive power during defecation.

Patients complaining of only back pain and urinary problems must be cleared for prostate cancer in men and gynecologic problems in women. Incontinence in women without back pain is may be stress incontinence. However, if the incontinence is not related to physical stress or, if the patient is a man, bladder infections or prostate cancer are possibilities. The orthopedic physical therapist should rarely encounter these presentations; the lack of back pain makes it very unlikely that the patient will seek out our services.

Segmental Instability

In addition to obvious spondylolisthesis, another type of instability might exist that is more subtle. Grieve described this patient in 1982.[31] Stating that removal of the posterior elements of the mobile segment (neural arch and ligaments) made no difference to the range of movement in the sagittal plane, he concluded that the limiting tissue to these movements must be the disk. Farfan[32] demonstrated that segments with "degenerated" disks had appreciable lateral shear that was not present if the disk was intact. Consequently, the stability of the segment appears to rely on both the anterior and posterior components, and if one or both are intact, instability is neither perceptible nor significant; essentially, the segment is stable.

Grieve[31] felt that typical patients who might be suffering from segmental instability were

- ❏ The young nurse or housewife
- ❏ The tall young man
- ❏ The young man in his late twenties or early thirties with undetected osteochondrosis
- ❏ The women of around 40 years old with mild degenerative spondylolisthesis

❏   The post–surgical fusion patient
❏   The man in his late fifties or sixties

As is apparent, this is quite a spectrum, and if it does nothing else, it suggests that almost anybody is vulnerable to this type of instability. This is quite different from Schneider's opinion that the age group is almost invariably young (discussed later).

In the same article, Grieve felt that the following criteria typified segmental instability.

❏   Long-term nonacute low back pain and early morning stiffness
❏   A history of ineffective conservative treatment
❏   Bilateral posterior creases in the flanks
❏   Full-range pain-free movements in the early stages
❏   Abnormal quality of movement, with hinging or angulation, wiggling, or using the thighs to "walk" on returning to the erect position after flexion
❏   Cautious active movements in the later stages (the patient knows what is likely to happen)
❏   Tenderness at one segment
❏   A slight "boggy" end feel on testing the accessory movement of the affected level
❏   Excessive physiological movements on segmental testing
❏   Spondylolisthesis on palpation
❏   Increased sagittal movements on x-rays

Schneider[33] gives the following as criteria, all of which he feels must be present, for diagnosing segmental instability:

❏   Age group twenties to thirties
❏   Recurring episodes of pain and loss of mobility
❏   Simple onset
❏   Relatively rapid resolution
❏   Lumbar pain without or without radiation into one or both buttocks and/or posterior thighs
❏   Abnormal spinal movements in the sagittal plane, with or without painful arc
❏   Abnormal compliance detected on accessory movement palpation, indicating loss of stiffness or increased neutral zone at one segment

Schneider's list is a good, general guide, but it does not allow for exceptional patients. Instability can and does occur before age 20; isthmic spondylolisthesis is a case in point. Because we do not know how precisely how sensitive our manual techniques are, we cannot exclude a patient from this diagnosis based on our palpation. Other possible indicators are

- ❏ Trauma
- ❏ Repeated unprovoked episodes or episodes following minor provocation
- ❏ A feeling of instability
- ❏ Giving way
- ❏ Inconsistent symptomatology
- ❏ Minor aching for a few days after a sensation of giving way
- ❏ Consistent clicking or clunking noises
- ❏ Protracted pain (with full-range motion)
- ❏ Posterior or abdominal creases (lumbar spondylolithesis)
- ❏ Spinal ledging (step deformity)
- ❏ Spinal angulation on full-range motion
- ❏ Inability to recover normally from a full-range motion
- ❏ Excessive active range of motion
- ❏ Hypermobility in the spine
- ❏ Recurrent subluxations (articular locking)
- ❏ Subluxation (needs to be tested after reduction)
- ❏ Constant clicking, slipping, or clunking
- ❏ No constant pattern of dysfunction
- ❏ Positive stability tests

It can be seen from my list that I tend toward the greater inclusivity of Grieve, but to keep this simple, here are what I think of as minimums in the diagnosis of functional segmental instability:

- ❏ Frequent episodic back pain
- ❏ Unpredictable onset of the pain relative to the function of the back
- ❏ Minor or no provocation for pain onset
- ❏ Abnormal quality of movement during testing
- ❏ Full range of motion when nonsymptomatic
- ❏ Any treatments have failed or have afforded only temporary relief.

In addition, there are screening tests that can be carried out in the spine (lumbar H and I and the cervical figure of eight or half-circumduction tests) and in the peripheral joints (quadrants tests).

If passive motion testing demonstrates a hypermobility, the presence of an underlying instability should be suspected and its possibility investigated. For a segment to be unstable, all of the important segmental structures that control the effect of the stress must be inadequate. For example, there may be degradation or degeneration of the disk, but if the zygapophysial joints are stable, they will prevent abnormal anterior migration of the vertebra.

Relatively minor intervertebral instability is probably common in the over-30 age group, but how many of these instabilities are pertinent to the patient's presentng problem is arguable. This of course raises a very real dilemma for the therapist: Does the discovered instability require treatment, or can it safely be ignored as an asymptomatic consequence of the patient's age or activities? The determination of the relevance of the instability is based on the judgment of the therapist, who must appraise the instability's importance in the context of the entire musculoskeletal examination.

The division of segmental instability into functional and clinical types is useful. *Functional instability* suggests that it interferes with the patient's function and is relevant and significant. A *clinical instability* is one that is found on clinical testing but does not affect the patient's life. Presumably, the patient has learned to control the segment automatically. The former requires treatment; because the latter does not, it has already been stabilized. Only the history can differentiate the two.

Examination

History

The history has already been discussed in general terms in Chapter 1; the following will discuss the subjective examination as it relates to the lumbar spine.

Age is a factor. As already discussed, the very young and very old do not usually present with severe back pain. In the young, nontraumatic ongoing pain without a history of the patient being heavily involved in sports may indicate serious disease or isthmic spondylolisthesis. In either case, it would be prudent to get whatever objective testing you can before initiating treatment. In the older patient, any pain that is not obviously stenotic must be suspect, especially if it is the first episode.

A family history of low back pain is believed to be a predictor for degenerative (degradative) disk disease,[34] but of course this information can only be used in combination with other data generated by the total examination. Among coincidental medical conditions, diabetes may be significant. A recent study has found that diabetes alters the biochemistry of the disk in such a way that it may predispose these patients to low back pain from disk degradation.[35]

Be alert for evidence of serious disease. Paresthesia without pain or with minimal pain may suggest neurological disease. Constant pain, especially when the patient is not disabled by the inability to move, may suggest cancer. Rapidly progressing, unprovoked, severe pain may also suggest cancer or an infection. Be careful of anterior or perineal pain, especially when they are isolated from any back pain, because they may be caused by visceral conditions. Complaints of urinary dysfunction that have not been previously diagnosed need to be. Even if you believe that the diagnosis is something as benign as stress incontinence, it is worthwhile informing the physician of your finding and ascertaining if he or she wants you to go ahead with treatment or wait until this problem has been clarified. Bilateral leg pain, especially with extensive spread, is only rarely caused by a simple disk herniation and almost never by zygapophyseal joint dysfunction. Be alert for cauda equina compression problems and other serious diseases. Cyriax described forbidden area pain as follows:

> First and second lumbar disc lesions are extremely rare; third lumbar lesions contribute five percent of the total. There thus exists an upper lumbar region about five inches wide—"the forbidden area"—where pain is very seldom the result of a disc lesion. Pain in the forbidden area suggests ankylosing spondylitis, neoplasm, caries, aortic thrombosis or reference from a viscus.[15]

Cyriax was not a believer in the zygapophyseal joint as a source of pain and so did not include dysfunctions of this joint in the possible causes of forbidden area pain, but even with this limitation, it is still worth being cautious with patients who complain of pain in this region; most lumbar dysfunctions from all sources will cause mid- or low lumbar pain.

On the less serious side, consider from the history whether the problem mainly affects the patient's function in flexion or extension. Disk herniations will generally be made worse by flexion activities or postures such as sitting, bending, slouching, and lifting, whereas stenotic conditions, including spondylolisthesis, will be exacerbated by extension activities and postures. Such things as prolonged standing, walking (slow walking such as browsing in a shopping mall is really a flexion activity), and overhead work cause extension. However, be aware of extension activities and postures that, although they exacerbate the pain, have little to do with spinal dysfunctions. Early peripheral intermittent claudication is a prime example of this. The patient will relate pain provoked by walking and eased by resting. However, in this case, the resting position can be any position, as long as the patient stops walking. The stenotic patient relating the history will tell you that simply stopping walking is not enough to eliminate the pain (this just swaps one extension activity for another) but adopting a flexion posture (squatting, bending, or sitting) is necessary.

Remember also that there are causes of low back and lower limb pain other than disk herniation, spondylolisthesis, and central stenosis. Zygapophyseal joint dysfunction may affect flexion or extension, and only be during the differential and biomechanical objective examinations can these conditions be diagnosed even provisionally.

Patients with segmental instability will generally complain of episodic pains that are provoked with minimal stress or no predictable stress at all. They may tell you that they can do a certain activity ten times in a row without problems but the eleventh time they get into trouble. They may complain of a sharp twinge type of pain followed by mild to moderate aching that is independent of movement. They may describe episodic locking in the form of sudden, short, sharp pain followed by moderate to severe pain on various movements. Usually the time spent suffering during these episodes is short, but occasionally they last longer. Patients will often tell you of a long history of treatment. They typically get good relief from chiropractic initially, requiring only two or three treatments, but as the condition progresses, the treatments become less effective and the recovery time longer while the time between episodes becomes progressively shorter, so what was once a short-term nuisance is now a disability.

Observation

Here are some points to bear in mind when observing the patient.

1. *Good posture* and *bad posture* are subjective and judgmental terms that are usually based on one clinician's ideas. There is no evidence that the concept of vertebral vertical stacking is the best posture or that it reduces symptoms or disability, nor is there any evidence to the contrary. Do not be too much of a rush to correct what may be an innocuous posture.

2. Generally, you have no idea of what the patient's posture was like before seeing him or her during the examination; consequently, you have no idea if the current posture is habitual or results from the condition bringing the patient in to see you. Do not jump to conclusions about cause and effect.

3. Variations from what you consider normal (including scars, muscle atrophy, etc.) may have nothing whatsoever to do with the patient's current problem.

4. Posture is not necessarily an accurate reflection of function in that patients do not function in the position in which we observe them. Do not place undue importance on observation of the static patient. Integrate it with other examination techniques.

Observe the patient's freely adopted standing posture from the front, back, and both sides. Do not spend long minutes pondering the patient's posture. If you cannot tell fairly immediately that there is something abnormal in the patient's stance, then whatever may be there will probably be insignificant. At this stage, we are looking for the obvious; if nothing can be seen within 2 or 3 seconds, move on. The use of a gown, although politically correct, is definitely an obstruction to effective and efficient observation. However, I suspect that we are stuck with this obfuscating garment, especially as it has now reached the point where even men are being offered them.

This is not the time to make a judgment about the patient's habitual posture. As has already been discussed, the adopted posture is probably not habitual at all, but a response to the pain that brought the patient in. Consequently, any thoughts that you may have regarding cause and effect from a postural perspective should wait until you have more information about the patient's condition. By all means make a note of the presenting posture so that you can assess what if any changes occur with treatment, but do not immediately consider postural therapy, you do not yet have enough information.

Look at the patient's general stance. Is he or she standing with one leg flexed at the knee and hip? This is often seen in acutely painful patients, who adopt this posture to relieve tension on the neuromeninges. Is there an obvious deformity? This usually takes the form of a lateral deviation, which may be a straight shift or a rotoscoliosis. Depending on the extent of the articular and neuromeningeal signs, the rotoscoliosis may be a consequence of a disk herniation. The straight lateral deviation may be the result of remote influences such as leg length discrepancy, or it may be more local, such as a transverse instability through the segment. However, other, less common causes such as acute zygapophyseal joint dysfunctions cannot be excluded as yet.

Imagine a plumb line dropped down from the nose to the floor. Does it fall equally between the feet, or does it fall to one side? When you are looking from the side, does the plumb line fall in front of or behind the patient's feet when it should fall between them? If the patient appears to be leaning to one side, this might indicate a shorter leg on that side, which, might or might not be relevant. If the patient is leaning forward or backward, this may indicate a balance problem, in which case it is usually very easy to push the patient off balance in the direction of the lean. If this occurs, a clinical assessment of the patient's balance will not be a waste of time.

Take note of the spinal curvatures. Is there a scoliosis, and if so, to what extent? Most, if not all, of your patients will have some degree of scoliosis, probably as a normal result of life. However, in some it will be significant. Is it much larger than your experience allows you to believe is normal? Is it a smooth curve, does it angulate, or is it more linear than curvilinear? This last is almost never developmental and will probably turn out to be a result of lumbar dysfunction. Angulation may indicate a hypermobility, especially if movement worsens it.

If a scoliosis or lateral shift is found, try to correct it manually. Does it correct easily and painlessly? If it does, it is probably compensatory for a remote problem. Is there severe pain and spasm? The cause is more likely to be significant lumbar pathology such as a disk herniation. Deviations that partially correct with or without some discomfort but with some degree of difficulty respond well to the McKenzie shift correction technique and extension protocol.

The association of a lateral list and back pain goes back more than a hundred years,[36] but its association with lumbar disk herniation is a little more recently described.[37] Cyriax stated that patients demonstrating a gross lateral deviation with sciatica and minimal back pain almost always required surgical intervention.[15] It is also a point of common wisdom that because of the influence of the iliolumbar ligaments, a lateral deviation of any size cannot occur at the lumbosacral junction.

The reason for the list is generally held to be irritation of the spinal nerve and/or its dural sleeve, and the direction of the list is throught to be a function of the position of the disk herniation and the spinal nerve. According to this theory, if the spinal nerve/dural sleeve is compressed on its lateral aspect, the list will be contralateral to relieve the pressure. If the compression is medial (axillary), the list will be ipsilateral for the same reason.[38] This last observation based on the anatomic construct has largely been accepted by the physical therapy community and is used to differentiate a lateral protrusion from a medial one. However, a surgical study has thrown serious doubt on this concept. Based on the list, the researcher predicted the level and site of the disk lesion and compared these with what was found on surgery. In the event of those patients who underwent surgery, there was no correlation between the side of the list and the site of the disk pressure on the spinal nerve or between the presence of a list and the level of the disk lesion.[39] It seems reasonable that what Porter found would be the case. Too many variables are associated with back pain in general and disk herniations in particular for us to be able to take one feature of the patient's clinical presentation, such as a list, and make such definitive statements. One point that Porter made in his article was that lateral lists associated with disk herniation were almost invariably gravity induced, disappearing on lying down or hanging, whereas those accompanying osteoid osteoma and infections remained constant regardless of the position of the patient. If this is true—and in my experience, most if not all lateral lists do correct with lying down—it would suggest that the examining therapist be especially cautious if a non-gravity-dependent list is encountered.

Does the lordosis seem excessive or reduced? A flat back may indicate systemic disease or may be the result of spasm in acute back problems. It is also seen in symptomatic isthmic spondylolisthesis in children because the hamstrings contract to limit anterior migration. Does the lordosis fall within *your* acceptable parameters (there does not seem to be an accepted range of normal), but the patient sways backward at the hips in a swayback posture?

Is there atrophy, and if so in which muscles? Does it fall into a segmental distribution? If so, you may be looking at a spinal nerve palsy. However, because of myotomal overlap, atrophy is not very likely to be observed as a result of this lesion unless it is extremely long-lasting. Profound atrophy is more likely to be caused by peripheral nerve disease or compression, or by muscle-wasting diseases.

Scars are from old injuries or surgeries and should prompt further questioning about previous medical conditions and surgeries.

Look for creases in the posterior trunk, which if present may indicate areas of hypermobility and/or instability. If creases are found, look to see if they worsen with movement. If they do not, the patient may have a clinical but not functional instability, an important point when considering stability therapy. A very low abdominal crease is strongly suggestive of spondylolisthesis.

Birthmarks, deformities, fat pads, and hair tufts are congenital deficits in the integumentary system and probably indicate underlying anomalies in the systems derived from the same embryological segments.[40]

Repeat your observations with the patient sitting and look for changes. Major changes indicate involvement of the leg in the patient's posture. If posture worsens in sitting, the legs are probably compensating, and if it improves, there is a good chance that the legs are part of the problem.

Active and Passive Movements

The six cardinal movements—flexion, extension, both side flexions, and both rotations—are tested by having the patient move through these ranges and applying careful overpressure at the end of the range as the passive test. The examination assesses the following:

- ❏ Range of motion
- ❏ Quality of motion and mode of recovery from end-position
- ❏ Symptoms produced (type and location)
- ❏ Variations in symptom reproduction and range between passive and active tests
- ❏ End feel
- ❏ Patient anxiety (willingness)

Range of Motion

Flexion and extension ranges can be hard to gauge as far as normality is concerned, because there is nothing objective to compare them with. Certainly, look to see if the lumbar spine is moving throughout its length or if all or most of the movement is coming from the hips and thoracic spine. A modification of Schober's test may help. Put one finger on the sacrum and a finger of the other hand on an upper lumbar or lower thoracic spinous process. During flexion, the distance between the fingers should increase by about 50%, and during extension, it should decrease by about the same amount. If you find that there is little or no separation or approximation of your fingers, the spine is failing to flex or extend regardless of how far forward or backward the patient can bend. If you are satisfied that the spine is moving into flexion, you must ask the patient, How far can you normally bend? Compare the current range with what the patient is telling you. For extension, you do not have this convenience, because no normal patient knows how far he or she can bend backwards. As an aside, a positive Schober's test may indicate the presence of ankylosing spondylitis, especially if it does not improve with warmup.[41]

Look at the formed curve in flexion and extension to ensure that it is smooth. A fairly common finding in extension is an angulation, which usually denotes an area of instability. In flexion, look especially at the lumbosacral angle. This should remain flattened or even convex. The junction is not designed to flex very much, and if this area is convex, there is again the possibility of hypermobility and/or instability. During extension, watch for posterior creases: If these are unilateral, they may indicate an area of rotational instability or hypermobility, and if they are bilateral and symmetrical, an extension hypermobility and anterior instability.

During side flexion, look at the spinal curve and see if it is smooth, if there is an area or areas where no motion is occurring, or if there is an angulation present. Do not make the mistake of thinking that the point at which the side flexion curves is the problem segment. Rather, this is the first segment that is capable of side flexing. Even if it is hypermobile, the chances are that it is the result of a hypomobility in the non-moving segment or segments.

Rotation should produce a C curve in the lumbar and thoracic spines. Look for this and be sure to check out those segments that do not join the party.

Quality of Motion

During flexion, the patient may deviate at the end of the motion, during the motion, or in the middle of the motion (arc). Just as standing deviation is believed by many to be caused by irritation of the dura and/or spinal nerve (root), trunk deviation during flexion is thought to be associated with a disk herniation. Again, the direction of the deviation is supposed to determine if the pressure is applied to the lateral or medial side of the nerve root. However, there is no direct evidence for this, and the same objections that were made to static deviation being a predictor of level and site obtain here. Other causes of deviation through or near the end of the flexion range are

❏ Neuromeningeal adhesions
❏ Flexion hypomobility of one or more segments on the contralateral side
❏ Flexion hypermobility of one or more segments on the ipsilateral side
❏ A structural scoliosis or hemivertebras
❏ A flexion hypomobility of the contralateral hip
❏ A short leg on the ipsilateral side

Deviations in the middle part of the range that correct before the end of the range is reached may be caused by a small disk protrusion contacting the dural sleeve. A painful arc on straight leg raising should accompany this, although the addition of weight bearing may make only the flexion arc.[16]

A failure to recover from the end range of a movement in the same manner as the movement occurred may indicate instability. This usually occurs at the end range of flexion, when the patient is momentarily incapable of extending except by walking up his or her legs, pulling to one side or the other, and extending, or extending the hips first and then the spine in a sort of a jerk movement.

Symptoms

Is the end of range symptomatic? If so, what are the symptoms? Are they those that the patient was complaining of, or new and possibly irrelevant? Are they neurological or somatic symptoms? How far down the leg does the pain go? Most studies on pain referral from nonneurological sources in the lumbar spine find that its spread is generally confined to above the knee or, in more severe cases, as far as the ankle, with the degree of distal referral being directly proportional to the intensity of the stimulus.[42] The location of the pain may afford a rough estimation of the location of the lesion, but because of the degree of overlap in innervation of somatic tissue, no definite level can ascribed. The location of paresthesia or neurological pain may be of more use in helping to determine the level of the problem, but radicular pain tends to be so fast that the patient can usually only remember its intensity.

Cyriax noted that leg pain on any movement other than trunk flexion was not a sign for a good prognosis.[15] The reproduction of somatic posterior thigh pain may be caused by referral from local tissues or may be dural referral in the same manner as the straight leg raise, and although it may suggest a disk herniation, it may be minor and treatable. If the latter is the case, you should expect the straight leg raise or the sitting straight leg raise to produce similar pain. If it does not, the leg pain is probably coming from a nondural tissue and the lesion is probably not an externalized disk herniation, although it could be a contained herniation. In either case, the outlook is better than it would be if a herniation were compressing sensitive structures.

On the other hand, posterior leg pain coming on with extension, rotation, or side flexion is not a good sign. The lumbosacral dura is either unaffected or being relaxed with these movements, so stretching it cannot be the cause of the symptoms. If the dura is the source of the pain, the disk herniation is large enough to compress the dura, and/or in a position where it can, and a poorer result can be expected. Possibly the worst-case scenario is the patient with bilateral sciatica who is fixed in flexion such that any attempt to straighten results in bilateral radicular pain in the posterior legs. This would suggest a fairly massive prolapse or extrusion that could possibly rupture the posterior longitudinal ligament and compress the cauda equina.

Variations in Symptom Reproduction and Range Between Passive and Active Tests

Some increase in range is to be expected during the passive test over that found in the active movement. However, a very large increase would suggest that either the patient is trying to put one over on you or, more commonly, the patient is very anxious. In the latter case, the pain is usually very acute and the patient has learned from hard experience that bending in a particular direction will cause severe pain. Respect what you find, and carry on the examination with more care than you might normally.

End Feel

For me this is more important than measuring the range. The end feel will afford information about the restrictor to the movement. First, whether it is a normal or abnormal restrictor, and if it is abnormal, what it is. I know that it is thought that one should not overpress into the painful range, but if we follow that particular tenet, we will never feel spasm, an empty end feel, or most of the others that are significant, because nearly all significant end feels will be associated with pain. The overpressure must be done carefully, especially into painful ranges, but it must be done. The exception to this in the lumbar spine is when radicular pain is reproduced. Here the patient moves out of the range so quickly that it is impossible to apply overpressure, and it is cruel to try. In addition, we can have a pretty good idea that the end feel will be spasm.

Patient Anxiety (Willingness)

The patient's anxiety can be gauged from both the subjective and the objective examinations. We have looked at one aspect of this with the large increase in passive over active movement, but also watch patients and see how reluctant they are to move. Reluctance to move is generally an indication of very acute pain.

Neurological Tests

These are simply the local application of the principles discussed previously. A slowly increasing resistance to breaking the contraction so as to ensure that maximal effort has been given tests muscle strength. With practice, it is easy to tell when a patient is not giving maximal effort because the break in the contraction is completely different from what occurs because of inhibition or your overcoming the patient's maximal contraction. If there is weakness, repeat the tests to determine if there is abnormal fatigability. As stated earlier, no studies support the common observation that abnormal fatigability occurs with nerve root palsy, but many clinicians believe it does. Look at the distribution of the weakness. Is it segmental, isolated to one muscle, or in a nonsegmental group of muscles? If a nonsegmental group is weak, is there another pattern of distribution, such as a peripheral nerve or around a joint (possible articular inhibition)? If a group of muscles that do not fall into an articular or peripheral or nerve root palsy pattern is affected, you must be concerned that the weakness is caused by an upper motor neuron lesion. If this is the case, be very careful when observing the results of deep tendon reflex testing, the extensor-plantar response, and the clonus tests.

A segmentally distributed weakness associated with normal or even brisk reflexes and a normal sensation of hyperesthesia may be caused by a neurophysiological response phenomenon termed *segmental facilitation.*[43] Paralysis is evidence of either peripheral nerve lesions or neurological disease.

Sensation should be tested initially with a pinprick to map out the hypoesthetic region. Does this region fall within the confines of a dermatome? There is overlap between the areas of skin innervated from different segments, but an area of exclusivity can be sought that will be considerably less sensitive than the surrounding hypoesthetic area. If a peripheral nerve is affected, anesthesia can be expected in the skin supplied by that nerve and the edges between the hypo or anesthesia and the normal sensation are sharp as opposed to the diffuse boundaries seen with nerve root palsies.

With peripheral nerve palsies, you can expect areflexia in the area of the nerve's innervation. Spinal nerve palsies will usually be hyporeflexic rather than areflexic, and central nervous system conditions that result in decreased inhibition will lead to hyperreflexia.

Neuromeningeal Tests

The Straight Leg Raise Test For a review of the straight leg raise, read Urban's article.[44] The straight leg raise in the form of Lasegue's test was described by Lasegue over a hundred years ago.[45] When it is severely restricted or crossed, the straight leg raise is considered one of the more reliable signs of disk herniation.[11] However, small degrees of restriction have many causes. Vucetic and Svensson investigated to see if physical signs could determine the degree of disk herniation against surgical findings. They found that only lumbar range of motion and the crossed Lasegue sign were of any real value.[11]

It is generally accepted that the first 30 degrees or so of straight leg raising, when it is not painful, does not move the dural sleeve or the spinal nerve and its roots but takes up the slack (crimp) in the sciatic nerve and its continuations. Between 30 and 70 degrees, the spinal nerves, their dural sleeve, and the roots of the fourth and fifth lumbar segments and the first and second sacral segments move. After 70 degrees, all movement has been taken up, and now these structures undergo increasing tension.[40] It must be remembered, however, that structures other than the neuromeninges of the lumbosacral plexus are being stressed as the test is being carried out. These other tissues include the hamstrings and gluteus maximus muscles, the hip joint, the sacroiliac joint, and the lumbar spine.[46] In addition, in the symptomatic patient the initial 30 degrees may not be crimp being taken up, as it is in the nonpainful subject. The spinal nerve and/or its dura may be tractioned upward by the disk herniation, or if the dura is inflamed, it may be so irritable that any tension put upon it provokes an extreme reaction.

For the straight leg raise to be positive for reduced dural mobility, the range should be limited by spasm to less than 70 degrees. Flexing the knee must alleviate the pain and allow a greater range of hip flexion. If the spinal nerve or root is inflamed, the pain reproduced should be neurological in nature. It is worth noting that one study using cinematography of marked pelvises in healthy young adults found that the ipsilateral hemipelvis started moving before 9 degrees of straight leg raise had been obtained and continued throughout the hip movement.[47]

Even when the straight leg raise is limited below 70 degrees by spasm, the cause may still not be the neuromeninges. Hamstring injuries and acute lumbar joint or sacroiliac joint lesions may restrict the range. The adjunctive tests (neck flexion, ankle dorsiflexion, medial hip rotation, Lasegue's test, bow-stringing, etc.) may or may not alter the pain, but if they do, they add to the evidence supporting dural compromise as part of the diagnosis. If neck flexion carried out at the point where the straight leg raise is positive increases or decreases the pain, then almost certainly the problem lies somewhere in the neuromeningeal system. A decrease in pain could indicate that neck flexion is pulling the dural sleeve and/or spinal nerve off of the medially located disk herniation (axillary herniation); increased pain with neck flexion could suggest a laterally placed herniation. If the hamstrings are suspected as the cause of the limitation, test them directly by isometric contraction testing.

In the cross straight leg raise, lifting the asymptomatic leg causes pain in the symptomatic side because it pulls the neuromeninges caudally. This caudal displacement has been speculated to result in compression of the dural sleeve against a large or medially placed disk herniation if one is present, causing pain in the resting symptomatic side. Apart from its use as an adjunctive confirmatory test for the straight leg raise, it may be more important than the straight leg raise test as it appears from the studies of Vucetic, Svensson, and Supic[12] (cited earlier) to be more valid for lumbar disk herniation.

The straight leg raise in sitting looks at factors other than just the stretch on the neuromeninges of L5-S2. The most common interpretation of the patient who complains of pain during the straight leg raise test when lying but not when sitting is either hysterical or malingering.[48] More interesting is the patient who has more pain in the seated straight leg raise test than in the supine. It is difficult to argue the increased pain from an increased tension perspective, and perhaps a more realistic suggestion might be that the pain increase might be caused by increased bulging of a disk protrusion or herniation. If so, the patient's outlook for recovery is presumably poorer, because the disk is less stable.

The addition of other tests, including neck flexion, medial hip rotation, ankle dorsiflexion, and so on are all designed to move or stretch the neuromeninges in ways other than that brought about by the straight leg raise and thereby confirm the positive test. However, an observation that I have made is that if neck flexion is applied while the straight leg raise is maintained in the painful position, it can sometimes reduce or eliminate the pain. In these patients traction applied from the thorax seems to be more effective than when it is applied from the pelvis. A possible interpretation of this is that the lesion is a medial prolapse and neck flexion lifts the dura and spinal nerve off of the disk.

A retrospective study[49] on the straight leg test as a predictor of disk herniation on postsurgical patients found the following:

❑ 77% of cases with positive straight leg raise had disk prolapse.
❑ In 85% of herniations, the straight leg raise was positive below 30 degrees.
❑ In 76% of herniations, it was positive between 30 and 60 degrees.
❑ In 63% of herniations, the straight leg raise was positive between 60 and 90 degrees.

This demonstrates that the more restricted the straight leg raise is, the more likely it is to be a disk herniation causing that limitation.

False positive results were as follows:

- ❏ 7% of nonherniations had a positive straight leg raise below 30 degrees.
- ❏ 16% of nonherniations had a positive straight leg raise between 30 and 60 degrees.
- ❏ 19% of nonherniations had a positive straight leg raise between 60 and 90 degrees.

This shows that the more restricted the straight leg raise is, the less likely it is to be something other than a disk herniation. Finally, 87% of patients operated on had a cross straight leg raise.

The slump test described and popularized by Maitland[50,51] combines the seated straight leg raise, neck flexion, and lumbar slumping to assess the mobility of the neuromeninges and their continuation into the posterior legs. This gives very little, if any, extra information on the lumbar spine over that provided by the straight leg raise while sitting together with the accompanying adjunct tests in the acute or subacute patient. Either the straight leg raise and its various adjunctive tests, including the seated test and neck flexion, should be done or the slump test should be used. It seems to me that doing both tests is simply redundant. Because almost all of the investigations validating neuromeningeal tests have been carried out on the straight leg raise, this is the one that I will stick with. However, the lumbar slump test will increase the compression forces through the disk, may sensitize the test to increased disk bulging, and is more likely to demonstrate the presence of dural adhesions than the straight leg raise.

Maitland also described the use of the straight leg raise as a treatment when there are no musculoskeletal restrictions and when the therapist is certain of what he or she is trying to achieve, that is, stretching the structures within the spinal canal. Here, the technique is more useful than simply using the straight leg raise because it allows a stronger stretch to be imparted to the tissues within the canal.[47]

The Prone Knee Flexion Test This test, which was first described by Wasserman in 1918, is the femoral nerve's neuromeningeal equivalent of the straight leg raise, using the hip extension and knee flexion to move and stretch the femoral nerve termination in the quadriceps muscle to move the L2, L3, and part of the L4 neuromeninges.[15] However, this test has not been researched as fully as the straight leg raise. It has been inculpated in upper lumbar disk herniations,[52,53] especially when hip extension is added.[54] Dyck advocated neck flexion as an adjunct to the test, and its effects were further investigated in normal subjects by Davidson.[55] Christodoulides considered the reproduction of sciatica with this test pathognomonic of an ipsilateral lateral disk protrusion at

L4-5.[56] In one 73-year-old woman with back and left anterolateral thigh pain and a crossed "femoral nerve stretch test," a far lateral disk herniation was found at L3-4. The author[57] considered the cross femoral nerve stretch test to be a valid test for symptomatic disk herniations above L4, although the sample size of one is a little small to talk of pathognomy. Another view is that the test actually compresses the nerve roots via the extending lumbar spine,[58] although there is little evidence for this concept and it is generally not the accepted view.

The relative lack of investigation about its specificity and sensitivity makes the prone knee flexion test a problematic test for hypomobile or irritable neuromeninges. The patient lies prone, and the ischium is fixed so that the pelvis cannot rotate anteriorly as the test progresses. The knee is then flexed, and if necessary (that is, no pain is reproduced) the hip is extended while knee flexion is maintained. We do not have enough information about where in the range this test is positive or for what, so it can only be considered to be strongly positive for the neuromeninges if movement is limited and painful in the anterior thigh prior to reaching 90 degrees and weakly positive for these tissues if movement is limited or painful after 90 degrees.

The same limitations as to specificity are present for this test as were present for the straight leg raise. The quadriceps and the sacroiliac and lumbar joints may all cause pain and limitation of prone knee flexion. However, the better fixation that can be effected at this joint reduces the ability of the spinal and sacroiliac joints to affect the test. The quadriceps muscles should be tested directly and isometric contractions if they are suspected of being the cause of the limitation.

A modification of this test incorrectly called the *slump prone knee flexion test* (it is spinal flexion, not slumping, and the patient is in a side lying position, not prone) has been described[51] and does possess some advantages over the prone test. The extension factor is abolished with contralateral hip and knee flexion, but a flexion complication replaces it. However, this is stable throughout the test. On the other hand, fixing the ischium rather than the innominate during the prone test can stabilize lumbar extension. In the end, it probably comes down to which test you are most comfortable with.

Compression Test The supine patient's hips and knees are flexed until there is obvious pelvic backward rotation; this will be somewhere around 100 degrees of hip flexion. Cranially directed pressure is then applied against the patient's feet or buttocks as if to push the patient up the bed. This provides an axial compression force on the lumbar spine. Putatively this tests vertical stability and integrity. Pain reproduced on this test supposedly arises from end-plate fractures, centrum fractures, or disk herniations. Although there is no objective evidence for these assertions, it seems likely that these lesions would be sensitive to compression forces. Whether the test can produce enough compression to detect all degrees of these lesions is something else. There is also little information on how often these tests are positive for conditions other than those listed here. My experience has been that the majority of these tests found to be positive on acute low back pain patients are found to be negative within 2 or 3 weeks, suggesting that many conditions causing a positive compression test are less profound than end-plate or body fractures or disk herniations. However, a couple of useful things do come from this test. First, if the test reproduces radicular pain in the posterior leg, the very strong possibility is that a disk herniation is present. Second, the test is useful as an indicator as to when the patient can return to a sedentary job.

Torsion Test The patient lies supine, and the therapist fixes the twelfth thoracic spinous process. He or she then reaches over the patient, grasps the anterior superior iliac spine, and pulls it directly backward, imparting a torsion force to the lumbar spine. This produces pure (axial) rotation, of which there should only be a very minimal amount. Classically, a positive test for torsional (rotational) instability is the reproduction of the patient's pain. However, there are other potential reasons for this pain, inflamed zygapophyseal joints being the most likely candidates. To claim that there is instability present, either there must be an increase in the neutral zone or there must be more axial rotation present than there should be. Again, this test has not been validated (or invalidated) but is useful when it is integrated with the history and other examination findings that might suggest segmental instability (discussed earlier).

H and I Test A common characteristic of directional instabilities is inconsistent hypomobility. That is, if the joint is moved in one direction, the movement may be hypermobile but does not sublux into the instability and become hypomobile. However, when the joint is moved in the opposite direction, it subluxes into the instability and becomes hypomobile. An example of this is an anterior instability in the lumbar spine. When asked to bend forward, the patient can do so with little if any trouble. However, after reaching full range, he or she cannot extend without walking up the legs. This characteristic is exploited in the H and I test.

The patient is asked to actively flex forward as far as possible and then side flex, say to the left. The range of motion and the end feel are compared with that found on left side flexion followed by flexion. If there is a hypomobility into extension and left side flexion present, the patient will not be able to get into that posterior quadrant regardless of how he or she tries. However, suppose that left lateral instability is present at one segment. The first part of the test would not demonstrate any hypomobility because the patient would sublux laterally only after flexing, so the motion would not be reduced. However, if the quadrant position were initiated with side flexion, the resulting subluxation would jam the joint, prevent any further motion from occurring, and so limit the quadrant.

The H and I test is quite useful as a quick test once its limitations are understood and allowed for. However, this test has the same problems as other screening tests, including

1. False negatives

2. Nondiscriminatory (picks up irrelevant instabilities)

4. Does not differentiate between a rotational and a lateral instability

5. Has not been validated (or invalidated)

To assist in the evaluation of the instability's relevance, a history denoting instability must be present. If the instability does not cause symptoms either directly or indirectly, its treatment is almost certainly not required because the patient has already managed to do what we would teach him or her, that is, stabilize. In the case of the spine, the instability should be associated with a clinically detectable hypermobility. If the instability is not sufficiently gross to produce a discernible hypermobility, it is unlikely to be a cause of symptoms or dysfunction and so does not require treatment.

Lumbar Differential Diagnostic Examination

History

1. Age
- ❏ Young
  - a. neoplasms
  - b. atypically disk lesions
  - c. infections
  - d. spondylolisthesis
- ❏ Old
  - a. vertebral metastases
  - b. prostate cancer
  - c. stenosis
- ❏ 30 to 50
  - a disk herniation
  - b. degenerative spondylolisthesis
  - c. zygapophyseal joint dysfunction

2. *Pain*
- ❏ Radicular (lancinating)
  - a. Neurological tissue irritation from
    - disk compression
    - adhesions
    - spondylolisthetic traction effects
    - dorsal root ganglion compression
- ❏ Somatic
  - a. anulosis fibrosis injury
  - b. contained herniation
  - c. zygapophyseal joint inflammation or dysfunction
  - d. ligament injury
  - e. muscular injury
  - f. bone disease or fracture
  - g. diskitis
  - h. visceral disease
  - i. metastatic invasion
- ❏ Causalgia
  - a. neurological tissue irritation
  - b. central nervous system disorder
  - c. spinal nerve root irritation
  - d. peripheral nerve irritation

3. *Paresthesia*

4. *Neurological Compromise*
- ❏ Segmental
  - a. disk herniation
  - b. lateral stenosis
  - c. low-level central stenosis
- ❏ Multisegmental
  - a. disk herniation (no more than two levels)
  - b. higher-level or multilevel central stenosis
  - c. multilevel lateral stenosis
  - d. cauda equina compression or tumor
- ❏ Nonsegmental
  - a. spinal cord lesions
  - b. brainstem lesions
  - c. multiple sclerosis or other neurological disease

5. *Bladder, Genital, and Bowel Complaints*
- ❏ Incontinence with back pain
  - a. cauda equina syndrome
  - b. bladder infection with coincidental back pain
  - c. bladder cancer

❏ Retention with back pain
  a. cauda equina syndrome
  b. spinal cord compression
❏ Hesitancy with back pain
  a. prostate cancer
  b. gynecologic disorders
❏ Impotency, frigidity, penile deviation with back pain
  a. cauda equina syndrome

Sequencing the Objective Examination
Standing

1. *Observation*

Gross deformities such as
❏ lateral lists
  a. leg length discrepancies
  b. disk herniation
  c. transverse instability
❏ hyperkyphoses
  a. disk herniation
  b. spondylolisthesis
  c. ankylosing spondylitis
  d. sacroiliitis
❏ hyperlordoses
  a. fixed postural deficit
❏ step and wedge deformities
  a. spondylolisthesis (step)
  b. compression fracture (wedge)
❏ skin creases
  a. extension hypermobility (posterior and bilateral)
  b. torsional instability (posterior and unilateral)
  c. spondylolisthesis (low abdominal)
❏ scars
  a. postsurgical
  b. traumatic
❏ birthmarks (not moles)
  a. underlying vertebral deformity

2. *Articular*
❏ active movements (flexion, extension, and side flexions)
  a. capsular (arthritis or arthrosis)
  b. noncapsular (disk herniation, zygapophyseal joint dysfunction, fracture)
  c. full range (hypermobility, instability, visceral)

> d. deviations (disk protrusion or herniation, zygapophyseal joint dysfunctions, instabilities)
> e. painful arcs (disk protrusion or herniation)
> ❏ passive movements (flexion, extension, and side flexions)
> a. arthritis or arthrosis
> b. noncapsular (disk herniation, zygapophyseal joint dysfunction, fracture)
> c. full range (hypermobility, instability, visceral)
> d. end feel (spasm, normal capsular, abnormal capsular)

3. Muscular
> ❏ isometric tests (flexion, extension, and side flexions in stretched condition)
> a. muscle tear (unlikely)
> b. disk herniation
> c. fracture
> d. acute zygapophyseal joint inflammation
> ❏ palpation along the suspect muscle-tendon unit
> a. tenderness (tear or tendonitis)

4. Neurological
> ❏ plantaflexion (S1 palsy)

Sitting

1. Observation
> ❏ changes in posture
> a. improvement (leg length discrepancy, lower limb pain)
> b. worsening (legs were compensating for spinal problem)

2. Articular
> ❏ active and passive ranges of trunk rotation
> a. thoracic spine
> b. lumbar spine
> c. sacroiliitis

3. Muscular
> ❏ isometric rotation
> ❏ palpation along the suspect muscle-tendon unit

4. Neurological
> ❏ motor reflexes can be tested in this position but prone is better for L3 (quadriceps)
> ❏ deep tendon reflexes
> a. L3 (quadriceps)
> b. S1 (plantaflexors)

5. Dural
> ❏ slump test (nonspecific)

❏ weight-bearing straight leg raise (L4-S2)
❏ neck flexion (nonspecific)
❏ cough (nonspecific)

Supine

1. Articular
❏ sacroiliac anterior primary stress test
  a. sacoiliitis
  b. fracture
❏ compression
  a. vertebral body fracture
  b. end-plate fracture
  c. disk herniation
  d. acute zygapophyseal joint inflammation
❏ traction
  a. anulus fibrosis tear
  b. longitudinal ligament tear
  c. disk herniation (if traction reduces pain)

2. Dural
❏ neck flexion (nonspecific)
❏ straight leg raise and adjunctive tests (L4-S2)
❏ cough (nonspecific)

3. Neurological
❏ motor
  a. L2 (hip flexion)
  b. L3 (knee extension)
  c. L4 (ankle dorsiflexion)
  d. L5 (extensor hallucis or * peronei)
  e. S1 (* peronei)
❏ sensory hypo- and hyperesthesia and pattern of distribution
❏ reflexes
  a. deep tendon reflexes
      L3 (quadriceps)
      L4 (tibialis anterior)
      L5 (extensor digiti minimi and peroneus longus)
      L5 (* medial hamstring)
      S1 (peroneus longus and Achilles tendon)
      S2 (* lateral hamstring)
  b. spinal cord reflexes
      extensor-plantar

---

*There are more questions concerning the principle segmental innervation of these muscles.

clonus

deep tendon hyperreflexia

4. *Arterial patency tests (special tests)*
- ❏ femoral popliteal, dorsalis pedis, and posterior tibial arteries' pulses
- ❏ repeated or sustained exercise for the suspected ischemic muscle group

Side Lying

1. *Articular*
- ❏ sacroiliac posterior primary stress test
  - a. sacroiliitis
  - b. fracture

2. *Neurological*
- ❏ motor
  - a. L5 (hip abductor)
- ❏ sensory
  - a. hypo- and hyperesthesia and pattern of distribution

Prone

1. *Articular*
- ❏ posteroanterior pressure
  - a. pain
  - b. reactivity of mobile segment
  - c. end feel
- ❏ lumbar torsion
  - a. pain
  - b. end feel

2. *Palpation*
- ❏ hypertonicity
  - a. segmental facilitation
- ❏ atrophy
  - b. disk herniation
  - c. inhibition (pain, instability)
- ❏ skin changes
  - a. orange peel (segmental facilitation)
  - b. trophedema (segmental facilitation)
  - c. papery (sympathetic dystrophy)
- ❏ tenderness
- ❏ reactive (myotactile response)
  - a. segmental facilitation

3. *Dural*
- ❏ prone knee flexion with adjunctive tests (L2, L3)

4. Neurological
- ❏ motor
  - a. L5-S1, 2 (knee flexion)
  - b. S1-S2 (gluteus maximus)
  - c. L3 (knee extension)
- ❏ sensory
  - a. hypo- and hyperesthesia and pattern of distribution

Summary of Disk Lesions

Type	Typical Features
Protrusion (no migration of nuclear material)	Backache Perhaps minor dural signs No neurological signs
Prolapse (migration of nuclear material within the anulus)	Backache Obvious articular signs with severe flexion limitation Dural signs Probable minor to moderate neurological signs
Extrusion (externalized nuclear material)	Backache Obvious articular signs with severe flexion and extension limitation Dural signs Probable minor to moderate neurological signs Probable radicular pain
Sequestration (fragmentation of externalized nuclear material)	Highly variable, depending on the positioning and size of the disk fragments Probable signs of an extrusion or prolapse
Contained (herniation contained within the anulus)	Similar to a protrusion or small prolapse
Uncontained (herniated material escaped the anulus)	Similar to a prolapse or an extrusion
Posterolateral herniation	The bulge or nuclear material is potentially compromising the posterolateral corner of the segment.
Posterior	The bulge or nuclear material is potentially compromising the posterior aspect of the segment, specifically the cauda equina.
Vertical	Rupture of the end-plate
Anterior	Mechanical block to movement; no direct involvement of neuromeningeal tissues
Far lateral or foraminal	Usually the upper levels are affected. There may be no back pain and little in the way of articular signs. There are usually strong neurological signs.

Medial or axillary compression	The disk is compressing the medial aspect of the nerve root.
Lateral compression	Compression of superolateral aspect of the spinal nerve/root/dural complex
Anular tear	Established in the elderly patient, in whom it presents as spinal stenosis; not as well established in younger patients because a cause of pressure effects but does exist and may be painful in itself
Metaplastic proliferation	The formation of collagen on the outside of the disk; effects depend on its size

The following table gives the various neurological findings that may be found with disc herniations compressing a specific spinal nerve or nerve root. The same provisos that applied to the table on neurological deficits in the cervical spine apply here. Because of the oblique orientation of the lumbar spinal nerve roots, a moderate-sized disk herniation can compress its own nerve root level if the herniation is posterolateral or the one below if it is a little more posterior. A large herniation will be able to compress two levels, but three-level involvement will not be caused by a single disk prolapse unless it is very central and compromising the cauda equina. At the upper lumbar levels, the orientation is more horizontal, so there is less chance of the herniated disk compressing two roots. However, an upper lumbar disk may compress the spinal cord/conus medullaris and give upper motor neuron signs. Also remember that L1 and 2 disk herniations are uncommon, and palsy signs may be caused by neoplastic disease. If a disk herniation is present, it may present as a far lateral herniation with dural and neural signs but little articular restriction.

Level	Myotome Test	Dermatome	Reflex
T12	Beevor's test (abdominal lower quadrants)	Lower abdomen	Abdominal cutaneous
L1	Hip flexion	Inguinal area Anterior scrotum	Cremasteric
L2	Hip flexion Hip adduction	Outer groin across the anterior thigh to the medial thigh above the knee	Cremasteric

(continued)

L3	Hip adduction Knee extension	Lateral hip across the anterior thigh to the medial aspect of the knee and the upper medial lower leg	Knee jerk
L4	Knee extension Foot inversion	Lateral lower thigh across the anterior thigh to the lower medial lower leg and the dorsum of the foot and big toe	Knee jerk Tibialis anterior and posterior
L5	Distal great toe extension Foot eversion Hip abduction	Lateral thigh Lateral lower leg Dorsum of the foot and medial toes Middle plantar aspect of the foot	Extensor digitorum brevis Perone
S1	Foot eversion Plantaflexion Hip extension or gluteal squeeze	Lateral border of the foot and fifth toe Lateral border of the lower leg and thigh	Achilles' tendon Perone
S2	Knee flexion	Medial heel, posterior calf and thigh	Lateral hamstring
S3	None	Medial thigh and saddle area	Anal wink
S4	None	Saddle area Posterior scrotum	Anal wink

Serious Disease Red Flags

Indication	Possible Serious Condition
Unrelenting nocturnal pain	Neoplasm, severe inflammation, infection
Bladder, bowel, or genital dysfunction associated with back and leg pain	Cauda equina syndrome
Bladder, bowel, or genital dysfunction not associated with back and leg pain	Prostatitis, bladder infection, stress incontinence
Saddle paresthesia/hypoesthesia	S4 palsy (cauda equina syndrome)
Vertebral wedging	Fracture
Bilateral sciatica with negative straight leg raise	Cauda equina syndrome
Bilateral multisegment signs with bilateral leg pain	Cauda equina syndrome
Bilateral multisegment signs with unilateral leg pain	Multiple sclerosis
Bilateral multisegment signs without leg pain	Neurological disease
Paralysis in nonperipheral nerve distribution	Neurological disease

Severe low back pain with relatively normal flexion but severely decreased side flexion	Ankylosing spondylitis
Flat back without severe pain	Ankylosing spondylitis
Three or more nerve roots involved unilaterally	Neoplasm
Nonadjacent roots involved	Neoplasm
Forbidden area pain	Neoplasm, ankylosing spondylitis, kidney pathology, aortic aneurysm
L1 or L2 palsy	Neoplasm, ankylosing spondylitis
Nontraumatic bilateral capsular pattern	Ankylosing spondylitis, neoplasm
Step deformity	Spondylolisthesis
Sign of the buttock	Various severe diseases of the hip or buttock
Weak and painful hip flexion	Neoplasm, fracture transverse process, spondylolisthesis

Notes

1. Bogduck N, Twomey LT: *Clinical Anatomy of the Lumbar Spine,* 2d ed., pp 107–120, 145–159. Edinburgh, Churchill Livingstone, 1991.

2. Twomey LT, Taylor JR: Joints of the middle and lower cervical spine: age changes and pathology. Man Ther Assoc Austr Conf, Adelaide, 1989.

3. Mooney V: Where is the pain coming from? Spine 12:754, 1987.

4. Roth P: Neurologic problems and emergencies, in RB Cameron (ed). *Practical Oncology.* Norwalk, CT, Appleton & Lange, 1994.

5. Jankowski R et al: Lumbar intervertebral disk herniation in children. Neurol Neurochir Pol 30:435, 1996.

6. Martinez-Lage JF et al: Disc protrusion in the child. Particular features and comparison with neoplasms. Childs Nerv Syst 13:201, 1997.

7. DePalma AF, Rothman RH: *The Intervertebral Disc.* Philadelphia, WB Saunders, 1970.

8. Bogduck N, Twomey LT: *Clinical Anatomy of the Lumbar Spine,* 2d ed., pp 161–173. Edinburgh, Churchill Livingstone, 1991.

9. Jönsson B, Strömqvist B: Clinical appearance of contained and noncontained lumbar disc herniation. J Spinal Disord 9:32, 1996.

10. Lipson S: Metaplastic proliferative fibrocartilage as an alternative concept to herniated intervertebral disc. Spine 13:1055, 1988.

11. Harada Y, Nakahara S: A pathologic study of lumbar disc herniation in the elderly. Spine 14:1020, 1989.

11A. Vucetic N, Svensson, O: Physical signs in lumbar disc herniation. Clin Orthop (333):192–201, 1996.

12. Supic LF, Broom MJ: Sciatic tension signs and lumbar disc herniation. Spine 19:1066, 1994.

13. Arnoldi JR et al: Lumbar spinal stenosis. Clin Orthop 115:4, 1976.

14. Verbiest J: Pathomorphological aspects of developmental lumbar stenosis. Orthop Clin North Am 6:177, 1973.

15. Cyriax J: *Textbook of Orthopedic Medicine,* vol. 1, 8th ed. London, Balliere Tindall & Cassell, 1982.

16. Murabito JM et al: Intermittent claudication: a risk profile from the Framingham Heart Study. Circulation 96:44, 1997.

17. Takahashi K et al: Changes in epidural pressure during walking in patients with lumbar spinal stenosis. Spine 20:2746, 1995.

18. Kikuchi S et al: Spinal intermittent claudication due to cervical and thoracic degenerative spine disease. Spine 21:313, 1996.

19. Regensteiner JG et al: Exercise testing and exercise rehabilitation for patients with peripheral arterial disease: status in 1997. Vasc Med 2:147, 1997.

20. Kim NH, Lee JW: The relationship between isthmic and degenerative spondylolisthesis and the configuration of the lamina and facet joints. Eur Spine J 4:139, 1995.

21. Wiltse LL: Classification of spondylolysis and spondy-lolisthesis. Clin Orthop Rel Res 117:23, 1976.

22. Bolesta MJ, Bohlman HH: Degenerative spondylolisthe-sis. Instr Course Lect 38:157, 1989.

23. Ito S et al: Specific pattern of ruptured annulus fibrosis in lumbar degenerative spondylolisthesis. Neuroradiology 32:460, 1990.

24. Hensinger RN: Spondylosis and spondylolisthesis in chil-dren. Instr Course Lect 32:132, 1983.

25. Gomella L, Stephanelli J: Malignancies of the prostate, in RB Cameron (ed). *Practical Oncology.* Norwalk, CT, Ap-pleton & Lange, 1994.

26. Jaradeh S: Cauda equina syndrome: a neurologist's per-spective. Reg Anesth 18:474, 1993.

27. Saifuddin A: The variation of position of the conus medullaris in an adult population. A resonance imaging study. Spine 23:1452, 1998.

28. Haldeman S, Rubenstein SM: Cauda equina syndrome in patients undergoing manipulation of the lumbar spine. Spine 17:1469, 1992.

29. Tay EC, Chacha PB: Midline prolapse of a lumbar inter-vertebral disc with compression of the cauda equina. J Bone Surg Br 61:43, 1979.

30. Khan SA et al: Neurologica erectile dysfunction second-ary to intradural paraganglioma of the cauda equina. Urol Int 46:119, 1991.

31. Grieve GP: Lumbar instability. Physiotherapy 68:2, 1982.

32. Farfan HF et al: Mechanical disorders of the low back. Philadelphia, Lea & Febiger, 1972.

33. Schneider G: Lumbar instability, in JD Boyling, N Palas-tanga (eds). *Grieve's Modern Manual Therapy,* 2d ed. Edinburgh, Churchill Livingstone, 1994.

34. Kanamori MH: Familial predisposition for lumbar degen-erative disease. A case control study. Spine 23:1029, 1998.

35. Robinson D et al: Changes in proteoglycans of interverte-bral disc in diabetic patients. A possible cause of in-creased back pain. Spine 15:849, 1998.

36. Remak E: Dtsch Med Wochenscher 257, 1881. (From Porter, RW: Back pain and trunk list. Spine 2:596, 1986.)

37. Bianco AJ: Low back pain and sciatica. Diagnosis and indications for treatment. J Bone Joint Surg Am 50:170, 1968.

38. DePalma AF, Rothman RH: *The Intervertebral Disc.* Philadelphia, WB Saunders, 1970.

39. Porter RW: Back pain and trunk list. Spine 2:596, 1986.

40. Beals RK et al: Anomalies associated with vertebral mal-formations. Spine 18:1329, 1993.

41. Roberts WN: Effects of warming up on reliability of an-thropometric techniques in ankylosing spondylitis. Arthri-tis Rheum 31:549, 1988.

42. Bogduk N, Twomey LT: *Clinical Anatomy of the Lumbar Spine,* 2d ed. pp 151–159, 1991.

43. Patterson MM: A model mechanism for segmental facili-ation. J Am Osteopath Assoc 76:62, 1976.

44. Urban LM: The straight leg raising test: a review. J Or-thop Sports Phys Ther 2:117,

45. Lasegue C: Considérations sur la sciatique. Arch Gen Med Paris 2:258, 1864.

46. Mooney V, Robertson J: The facet syndrome. Clin Orthop 115:149, 1976.

47. Bohannion R et al: Contribution of pelvic and lower limb motion to increases in the angle of passive straight leg raising. Phys Ther 65:474, 1985.

48. Nehmkis AM et al: The predictive utility of the orthope-dic examination in identifying the low back pain patient with hysterical personality features. Clin Orthop 145:158, 1979.

49. Hakelius A, Hindmarsh J: The comparative reliability of preoperative diagnostic methods in lumbar disc surgery. Acta Orthop Scand 43:234, 1972.

50. Maitland GDM: Negative disc exploration: positive canal signs. Austr J Physiother 25:125, 1979.

51. Maitland GE: The slump test: examination and treatment. Austr J Physiother 31:215, 1985.

52. Estridge MN et al: The femoral nerve stretching test. J Neurosurg 57:813, 1982.

53. Dyck P: The femoral nerve traction test with lumbar disc protrusions. Surg Neurol 6:136, 1976.

54. O'Connell JEA: Protrusions of the lumbar intervertebral discs. J Bone Joint Surg Br 33:8, 1954.

55. Davidson S: Prone knee bend: an investigation into the effect of cervical flexion and extension. Proc Manip Ther Assoc Austr 5th Biennial Conf, Melbourne, 235, 1987.

56. Christodoulide AN: Ipsilateral sciatica on femoral nerve stretch test is pathognomic of an L4/5 disc protrusion. J Bone Joint Surg Br 71:88, 1989.

57. Kreitza BG: Crossed femoral nerve stretching: A case re-port. Spine 21:1584, 1996.

58. Herron LD, Pheasant HC: Prone knee flexion provocative testing for lumbar disc protrusion. Spine 5:65, 1980.

CHAPTER 13

The Pelvis

We have three joints to consider here, the two sacroiliac joints and the pubic symphysis. Depending on which school of thought you follow, the sacroiliac joints are almost never a problem or the scourges of mankind. Occasionally a middle ground is discussed in which the joints can produce problems on occasion, but this middle ground is usually dismissed by most therapists as being nonsensical. Recent research has indicated that the sacroiliac joint might be inculpated in up to 30% of cases of very low back or buttock pain.[1] My opinion is that the sacroiliac joints need to be treated in about 10 to 15% of all low back pain patients; that is, I subscribe to the middle-of-the-road theory when it comes to these joints. Fortunately, when you are making a differential diagnosis, the various theories on minor pathologies and biomechanics of the sacroiliac joints are not particularly important.

The musculoskeletal conditions affecting the pelvis include those of the sacroiliac joint and those of the pubic the symphysis. The sacroiliac lesions fall into two main groups; (1) those that are demonstrable from the selective tissue tension examination, more precisely the primary stress tests, that is, pain provocation tests, (major lesions); and (2) those that can only be diagnosed from the biomechanical examination (minor lesions). This discussion will concern the major lesions of these joints.

The sacroiliac joints are vulnerable to severe diseases in the form of metastatic invasion and pyogenic arthritis. Secondary deposits in the sacrum usually present clinically as deep local aching pain that is increased by sitting and lying and lessened by walking. There may be radicular symptoms if the tumor compresses the sciatic nerve, and there may be tenderness over the greater sciatic notch, possibly with radicular pain.[2]

Sacroiliac Joint Examination

Pain from the inflamed sacroiliac joint tends to be over the posterior aspect of the joint and into the buttock, with occasional radiation down the posterior thigh to the knee. The pain rarely goes below the knee. If the ventral ligament is injured, the pain can be felt in the lower groin. The patient usually complains of pain on walking, either on heel strike or just before heel off. Almost pathognomonic is a sharp pain that wakes the patient as he or she turns in bed. Tuberculosis, pneumococcus, salmonella, and a host of other organisms can cause pyogenic sacroiliitis.[3] These conditions should be positive on pain provocation tests, including the primary stress tests; the pain in most cases will be deep and constant and disturb sleep. Cyriax maintains that septic bursitis and tumors affecting the sacrum or ilium will cause the sign of the buttock.[4]

Primary Stress Tests

The principle differential diagnostic tests for sacroiliitis are the anterior and posterior primary stress tests.[4] The anterior stress test, also called the *gapping test,* is carried out with patient supine. The examiner stands to one side of the patient, crosses the patient's arms over the pelvis, and places the palms of the therapist's hands on the anterior superior iliac spine. Keeping the elbows straight, the therapist leans on his or her hands. Crossing the arms ensures that the applied force is lateral, tending to push the ilia away from the sacrum. This tends to gap the anterior aspect of the sacroiliac joint, stressing the ventral ligament and compressing the posterior aspect of the joint. A positive test is one that reproduces the patient's pain, which must be centered over the sacroiliac joint(s) either anteriorly or posteriorly, unilaterally or bilaterally.[4,5]

The posterior stress test also called the *compression test,* is carried out with the patient lying on the side. The therapist applies downward pressure on the side of the uppermost innominate with his or her hands or forearm. This generates a medial force that tends to gap the posterior aspect of the joint and compress its anterior aspect. Again, the reproduction of pain over one or both sacroiliac joints is considered positive.[4,5] The dorsal long ligament is accessible just below the posterior inferior iliac spine[6] and should be palpated for tenderness, which would tend to confirm the test.

For the most part, it is believed that these tests are sensitive for arthritis or, if groin pain is reproduced, for ventral ligament injury. They are not believed to be positive for any other sacroiliac ligament tears because these are thought to be too massive to be injured and the bone would fail before the ligament.

The Fortin finger test for the sacroiliac joint has been validated as being sensitive for sacroiliitis.[7] This is not so much a test as an observation. It is considered positive if the patient puts a finger on an area a little inferior and medial to the posterior superior iliac spine. Though it is sensitive for pain arising from the sacroiliac joint, it is not specific.

Secondary Stress Tests

Three secondary tests will be discussed. The dorsal shear test is done with the patient supine. The hip ipsilateral to the joint to be tested is flexed to about 90 degrees and semiadducted until it feels stable. The therapist slides his or her cranial (to the patient) hand under the near-side innominate and palpates the posterior superior iliac spine with the middle finger and the first or second sacral tuberosity with the index finger. A downward force is applied along the long axis of the femur. This tends to push the innominate posteriorly on the sacrum. Of course, this movement should not occur, and if it is felt to occur between the palpating fingers, instability is considered to exist.

Cranial and caudal stress testing is carried out with the patient prone. The therapist applies strong pressure with the heel of the caudal (to the patient) hand to the apex of the sacrum and the heel of the other hand to the superior aspect of the posterior superior iliac spine. A shearing force is then applied to the bones that tends to displace the innominate inferiorly. No movement should occur. Superior nominate stress testing is carried out by switching the hands so that the hand on the apex of the sacrum moves to the inferior aspect of the posterior superior iliac spine. The other hand moves to the base of the sacrum, and again the two bones are sheared on each other, the force tending to push the innominate cranially. Any movement between the two bones is considered to be evidence of instability.

The primary stress tests are considered to be evidence of the presence of a sacroiliitis unless there is isolated groin pain, in which case, the pain could be arising from an injury to the much smaller ventral sacroiliac ligament. If the tests are painful after trauma, especially in the elderly patient, consider fracture as a diagnosis, especially if the posterior primary stress test is as painful as the anterior (which is caused by the decreased leverage with the posterior test), because it should be less painful in sacroiliitis. The primary stress tests do not differentiate the cause of the arthritis. This could be

- ❏ Systemic arthritis (ankylosing spondylitis)
- ❏ Traumatic arthritis
- ❏ Microtraumatic arthritis (cumulative stress)

Sacroiliac Arthritis

Clinical Presentation

1. Pain
- ❏ posterior aspect or groin pain alone (uncommon)
- ❏ radiation usually confined to the posterior thigh

❏ walking, either at heel strike or at midstance
❏ frequently wakes the patient when turning in bed

2. Motion
❏ extension most painful
❏ ipsilateral side flexion and rotation less so
❏ flexion least of all

3. Single leg hopping
❏ hopping on the affected side leg reproduces the patient's pain
❏ usually reduced if a SI (sacroiliac) belt is applied

4. The anterior and possibly the posterior primary stress tests are positive.

Integration of the results of the primary and secondary stress tests will help determine which type of arthritis is present. If there is a history of major trauma with an onset of pain soon thereafter, the chances are that it is a simple post-traumatic arthritis. In this case, the secondary stress tests should be negative (for instability, the test will probably be painful) because trauma will fracture bone before tearing the sacroiliac ligaments (except the ventral, and one study failed to find nerve receptors in this ligament[8]).

If the secondary stress tests are positive post-traumatically, the likelihood is that there was an underlying instability present prior to the injury. If there is no history of trauma associated with the positive primary stress tests and the secondary stress tests are negative, systemic arthritis must be investigated with blood tests and x-rays. If the secondary stress tests are positive, the chances are that this is a microtraumatic arthritis.

From a management perspective, the type of arthritis must be determined. If it is a simple post-traumatic arthritis, anti-inflammatory modalities and rest should resolve the problem. If it is microtraumatic arthritis, the source of the ongoing stress needs to be determined and addressed. This force often originates from an extension hypomobility of the hip, in which case mobilizing this joint will reduce the continuing stress on the sacroiliac joint. If it is believed that a systemic arthritis is present, the patient should be referred back to the physician for the appropriate imaging and laboratory tests.

Ankylosing Spondylitis[9] This is a systemic chronic spondyloarthropathy. It may be associated with Reiter's disease and psoriatic arthritis. Involvement of the sacroiliac and peripheral joints and the absence of the rheumatoid factor characterize all of these arthropathies. Other similarities include involvement around the ligament attachment rather than the synovium and involvement of the eyes, skin, lungs, and bowel.

The disease is distributed almost equally between both sexes, with men generally having the more severe form affecting the spine whereas women tend to have the peripheral joints more affected. There is a 10 to 20% risk that the offspring of patients with the disease will later develop it.

Typically, at least in established cases, mobility loss tends to be bilateral and symmetrical. There is loss of spinal movement on flexion, which shows up on Schober's test. There is often a history of lower limb peripheral involvement (20 to 30% of patients) such as arthritis, plantafasciitis, or Achilles' tendonitis. The patient may relate a history of costochondritis, and on examination, rib springing may give a hard end feel. There is often decreased basal rib expansion, and the glides of the costotransverse joints and distraction of the sternoclavicular joint are decreased.

Four features may appear in the history:

❑ Insidious onset
❑ Age less than 40 years
❑ Persistence for more than 3 months
❑ Morning stiffness and improvement with moderate exercise

If you are considering a systemic arthritis as a possible diagnosis, inquire about

❑ Other joint problems
❑ Morning pain and stiffness
❑ General health

Examine for

❑ Other joint involvement from the history and from the objective examination
❑ Cervical and thoracolumbar rotation and flexion, Schober's test, occiput-wall and occiput-chin distance, trunk flexion, finger-floor distance, and chest expansion.[10]

Radiographic Findings In early cases, there may be squaring of the superior and inferior margins of the vertebral bodies and later the bamboo spine in severe cases.

Laboratory Findings The mainstay of lab tests is the HLA B27 (human leukocyte antigen B27). It is present in 90 to 95% of caucasian patients and 6 to 8% of the nonankylosing population. The erythrocyte sedimentation rate is elevated in about three quarters of these patients.

The synovium fluid tests are negative in contradistinction to most other inflammatory arthropathies.

Minor Conditions of the Sacroiliac Joint   These are biomechanical lesions of the joint and may be painful in themselves, or they may be asymptomatic but, because of the stress they apply to other joints, cause pain elsewhere in the lumbar spine. This is not a book on the biomechanical aspects of orthopedic therapy, but it does seem worthwhile bringing the subject up, at least for a short discussion. It has only been relatively recently that the sacroiliac joint was unequivocally found to move.[11-13]

There are numerous ways of testing the sacroiliac joint biomechanically, including (position testing, my personal all-time unfavorite), checking the glides, assessing the end feels for innominate rotation, abduction, adduction, assessing the sacral unilateral flexion and extension, and so on. The number of different tests should give you some idea of how unsatisfactory the state of the art is in evaluating the sacroiliac joint.

Before embarking on the biomechanical examination of the sacroiliac joint, my suggestion is that you clear the lumbar spine as much as possible. This will save time (after all, the sacroiliac joint is responsible for only a minority of low back pain) and will reduce the number of false positives generated by lumbar conditions.

Pubic Instability   In some cases of trauma and sometimes with childbearing, the pubis can be destabilized. This results in a very severe and painful lesion, one that is not easily missed. The pain is local to the pubic area, with the patient quite disabled and with all movements and weight-bearing postures very painful. The lesion generally shows up on one-legged weight-bearing x-rays and often requires surgical intervention to stabilize the symphysis.

A clinical test has been designed in which one pubis is sheared cranially or caudally on the other, but given the usual severity of the condition the test is usually redundant.[14]

Sign of the Buttock   This syndrome is described here because of its location, not because it is necessarily pathology at the sacroiliac joint. The sign of the buttock is actually seven signs that indicate the presence of serious pathology posterior to the axis of flexion and extension of the hip (although I once saw a patient who had all of the signs except buttock swelling for over 2 years and had never been diagnosed). The sign of the buttock includes almost all of the following (with the occasional exception of buttock swelling):

- ❏ Limited straight leg raising
- ❏ Limited trunk flexion

❏ Limited hip flexion
❏ Noncapsular pattern of restriction of the hip
❏ Painful weakness of hip extension
❏ Swelling of the buttock with some pathologies
❏ Empty end feel on hip flexion

The limited straight leg raise, trunk flexion, and hip flexion are all aspects of hip flexion loss and not a result of the constant-length phenomenon, so when you carry out the straight leg raise and find it limited to, say, 40 degrees, flexing the knee does not greatly increase the range.

Among the pathologies that may cause the sign of the buttock are

❏ Upper femoral osteomyelitis
❏ Upper femoral neoplasm
❏ Infective sacroiliitis
❏ Ischiorectal abscess
❏ Infective trochanteric/gluteal bursitis
❏ Rheumatic fever with bursitis
❏ Ilial neoplasm
❏ Fractured sacrum

The sign of the buttock is rare, but you cannot afford to miss it because it is usually caused by some serious pathology.[4]

Notes

1. Schwarzer AC et al: The sacroiliac joint in low back pain. Spine 20:31, 1995.

2. Foley KM: Diagnosis and treatment of cancer pain, in AI Holleb (ed). *Textbook of Clinical Oncology.* Atlanta, American Cancer Society, 1991.

3. Le Dantec L et al: Peripheral pyogenic arthritis. A study of one hundred seventy-nine cases. Rev Rhum Engl Ed 63:103, 1996.

4. Cyriax J: *Textbook of Orthopedic Medicine,* vol. 1, 8th ed. London, Balliere Tindall & Cassell, 1982.

5. Lee D: *The Pelvic Girdle.* Edinburgh, Churchill Livingstone, 1989.

6. Vleeming A et al: The function of the long dorsal sacroiliac ligament: its implication for understanding low back pain. Spine 21:556, 1996.

7. Fortin JD, Falco FJ: The Fortin finger test: an indicator of sacroiliac pain. Am J Orthop 26:477, 1997.

8. Grob KR et al: Innervation of the sacroiliac joint of the human. Z Rheumatol 54:117, 1995.

9. Schumacher JR (ed): *Primer on the Rheumatic Diseases,* 10th ed. Atlanta, Arthritis Foundation, 1993.

10. Viitanen JV et al: Correlation between mobility restrictions and radiologic changes in ankylosing spondylitis. Spine 29:492, 1995.

11. Smidt GL et al: Sacroiliac motion for extreme hip positions. A fresh cadaver study. Spine 22:2073, 1997.

12. Kissling RO, Jacob HA: The mobility of the sacroiliac joint in healthy subjects. Bull Hosp Joint Dis 54:158, 1996.

13. Lund PJ et al: Ultrasound evaluation of sacroiliac motion in normal volunteers. Acad Radiol 3:192, 1996.

14. Lee D: *The Pelvic Girdle.* Edinburgh, Churchill Livingstone, 1989.

PART II

Case Studies

Post-MVA Chronic Dizziness

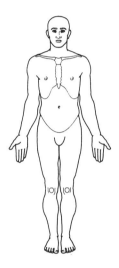

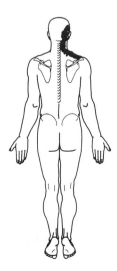

Subjective Examination

An otherwise healthy 33-year-old woman complains of ongoing neck pain since a hyperextension injury in a car accident 6 months earlier. There was no direct impact in the accident, no loss of consciousness, and no memory loss. Initial pain onset was the day following the accident. The initial pain was felt in the right neck and upper trapezius with occipital headache along with nausea, lightheadedness, and unsteadiness. This nonvertiginous dizziness was initially present on every neck movement, but after a week or so it was felt only on right rotation combined with extension. She was put into a soft cervical collar for a week by her GP and given analgesics. She continued to work as a medical secretary. The pain eased off somewhat during the next 3 weeks, and by 6 weeks she was almost painfree, except for some mild soreness in the right upper cervical spine. The dizziness was gone by 3 weeks post-accident.

She continued to have mild discomfort in the right suboccipital area intermittently but nothing that interfered with function, and she did not feel it was of sufficient intensity to warrant treatment other than aspirin as required. This condition continued until 3 months ago when the suboccipital pain increased in intensity and was accompanied by type 2 dizziness (giddiness and nausea). The first episode of recurrent pain lasted 2 weeks and the second 6 weeks. She had no previous physical treatment, each time being treated by her physician employer with analgesics, muscle relaxants, and anti-inflammatories.

This, the third episode, started 4 days earlier. She complains of right-sided upper cervical and occipital pain and type 2 dizziness for the last 3 days.

What are you thinking at this point? How will you proceed with the examination? ☞

Cervical Case 1 Continuation

The important aspect of this case is to make sure that the dizziness has a benign etiology. After this has been established, then it is reasonable to look at the musculoskeletal dysfunction.

Among the possible causes of this lady's dizziness are cerebral or brainstem concussion, medication, labyrinthine concussion, brainstem damage, cervical joint damage, and vertebrobasilar ischemia. Cerebral or brainstem concussion as a cause of her dizziness is very unlikely because there was no history of being knocked unconscious or of amnesia. Also, the dizziness is intermittent with long periods between episodes. Medication is a possible cause, and questions about the association between the ingestion of her medication and her dizziness are necessary. However, while she was taking analgesics and anti-inflammatories during the acute stage, the dizziness improved, so this is an unlikely etiology.

Her history indicated no previous ear pain, pops, or clicks and no immediate dizziness, and her dizziness was not of the vertigo type. These facts tend to move the diagnosis away from benign paroxysmal positional dizziness from labyrinthine concussion. However, the periods between episodes of pain are free from dizziness. The dizziness seems to be associated with her cervical pain. If labyrinthine concussion was the source, then dizziness should be present at times other than when the neck is painful. The fact that the dizziness is related to her neck pain getting worse and better as her neck pain does would suggest cervical joint causes.

Vertebrobasilar insufficiency as a cause is unlikely. There is no good reason for the episodic nature of the symptoms if the artery was the cause. No symptoms other than the type 2 dizziness would suggest other cranial nerve involvement, but this consideration is marginal because many cranial nerves when injured do not cause symptoms that are obvious to the patient. But because cervical rotation combined with extension reproduces her dizziness and these movements are also the most stressful movements for a single vertebral artery, this diagnosis cannot be excluded on the history alone. The most likely cause of the dizziness is cervical joint dysfunction, but the main concern is with the condition of the vertebral artery.

Objective Examination

Investigate the most serious symptoms first—the dizziness. Assume that it is neurovascular in origin and go from there.

1. Cranial nerve and long tract tests (the latter if the cranial nerves are positive)
2. Craniovertebral ligamentous stress tests (transverse anterior shear and Sharp-Purser, and alar)

3. Dizziness reproduction tests (leave right rotation/extension until last)

4. Differentiation tests (body rotation under the right rotated/extended head and Hautard's test)

If everything is clear with above examination, proceed to the remainder of the musculoskeletal examination, the upper quadrant scan, and then the biomechanical examination. The cranial nerve examination was negative except that during ocular tracking, the patient experienced mild vertigo when looking to the right and upward. The ligament stress tests were negative. The results of the dizziness tests were: reproduction test for right rotation/extension produced mild lightheadedness; body rotation test with left rotation under the extended head produced mild lightheadedness; and Hautard's test was negative.

Extension and right rotation were painful and slightly limited. The other movements were full range and painfree. There were no signs of neurological deficits. There were no dural signs and the upper limb tension tests were painfree.

No working diagnosis was possible from these results, so a biomechanical examination was carried out. The passive and accessory intervertebral movement tests for combined extension and left-side flexion were positive at the right C2/3 zygopophyseal joint with a pathomechanical (jammed) end feel. Do these results strengthen or weaken the postulate that the dizziness is caused by the cervical joints? What is your treatment plan?

Please turn to page 395 for solutions.

A First Instance of Headaches and Neck Pain

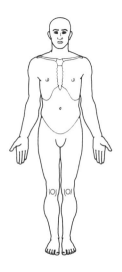

Subjective Examination

A 35-year-old woman woke with pain 3 days earlier. The pain was felt over the right suboccipital region and the right neck on an intermittent basis. She related that the pain was worse with prolonged sitting especially if reading or watching TV and was much more severe for about an hour upon waking. She described no neurological pain or paresthesia. The pain sites and intensity were unchanged since the onset. She could find no reason for the pain and had no history of anything similar or any medical problems of note. The patient worked as an office cleaner.

Objective Examination

Right rotation and extension were about 30% limited with jammed end feels and pain. The other ranges were full range and painfree. Posteroanterior pressures over C2/3 were painful. Neurological testing was negative and there were no dural signs.

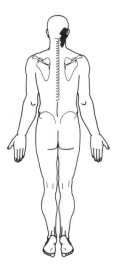

What are you thinking at this point? How will you proceed with the examination? ☞

Cervical Case 2 Continuation

There is no real cause for concern. This is the first episode. The pain is typically cervical in its distribution. Although the differential diagnostic examination affords no positive information, we can be fairly certain that the symptoms are not due to a disk herniation.

A question that should be asked about the pain increase in the morning concerns sleeping. In what position does she sleep? How many and of what types of pillow does she use? She stated that she slept on her right side with one foam pillow.

A biomechanical examination was carried out, which demonstrated restricted physiological and accessory intervertebral movements at C2/3 into extension on the right with a pathomechanical or jammed end feel.

The diagnosis is the right C2/3 zygopophyseal joint flexion pathomechanical hypomobility (extension subluxation).

She was treated with active exercises after manipulation of C2/3 or nonrhythmical jerky mobilizations. The patient responded well to the first treatment with the patient painfree until she slept that night. The next morning the pain had returned and was as intense as ever. What do you do next?

Please turn to page 395 for solutions.

A Sudden Onset of Neck and Arm Pain While Lifting

lancinating
Tearing, darting,
sharp cutting
Pain

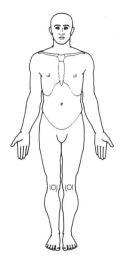

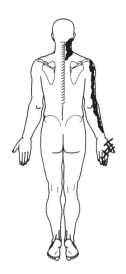

Subjective Examination

A 28-year-old nurse, while lifting a patient with a partner, experienced a sudden onset of severe right neck pain with referred nonlancinating pain in the right deltoid when her partner slipped and let go of the patient. The nurse was forced to take the full weight of the patient for a few seconds. When asked if her head was twisted into flexion, extension, or rotation at the time of the accident, she said no.

The accident occurred 6 days ago. She was initially treated by the physician with analgesics and with time off work. Since the accident, the pain has progressed with the referred pain now felt down the posterolateral upper and lower arm with mild aching in the index finger and thumb. Paresthesia had been present for the last 2 days in the index finger and thumb, and lancinating pain on extending and/or turning the head to the right was felt in the posterolateral upper and lower arm. X-rays were taken at the time of the injury and were read as negative. At this time, the physician's diagnosis was changed to cervical disk herniation and an anti-inflammatory was prescribed in addition to the analgesic. The physician also referred the patient for physical therapy.

The patient had no history of neck or arm pain and no medical history of relevance.

What are you thinking at this point? How will you proceed with the examination? ☞

Cervical Case 3 Continuation

Disk prolapses are not overly common in the cervical spine, but this does seem to be the case with this patient. The immediacy of the pain argues for fairly substantial tissue damage. The mechanism of injury is likely to be compression. Because the patient did not relate that any excessive movements occurred, torque and shear are less likely to be the underlying causative forces. Compression in the absence of rotation or angular displacement is unlikely to damage the joints, ligaments, or muscles because these are nowhere near the ends of their ranges, but are more likely to cause compression fractures or disk failure. The lancinating pain and the paresthesia are pathognomonic of neural tissue involvement. Again, it is difficult to see what else might be causing these conditions other than compression by a disk. Because no head or neck displacement of any great degree occurred, overstretching of the spinal nerve roots or brachial plexus is unlikely. Given her age, lateral stenosis is also not a strong candidate especially because the X-ray was negative.

The delayed onset of the lancinating pain would suggest an inflammatory component to the condition, whereas the delayed onset of the more distal referred pain and paresthesia could be indicative of a worsening condition. The distribution of the paresthesia into the index finger and thumb indicates involvement of the C6 root.

The provisional diagnosis from the history is worsening C5/6 herniation with compression of the C6 spinal nerve or root. If the objective examination does not demonstrate considerable painful limitation of the cervical spine, the diagnosis will have to be reviewed. In addition, you can expect to find motor signs in the form of paresis in the C6 distribution.

Objective Examination

On observation, the patient was a healthy looking female without any obvious deformity or atrophy.

There was severe limitation of motion in the neck. Flexion was about 30° and produced neck pain; extension was 20° limited by spasm and caused lancinating arm pain with overpressure. Left rotation was almost full range and reproduced mild neck pain. Right rotation was 30° and caused lancinating pain into the right arm and was limited by spasm. Left-side flexion was limited to about 50% of the expected range and reproduced the nonradicular radiating pain in the right arm. Right-side flexion was limited to about 75% of the expected range and produced neck pain.

Compression produced neck pain, and traction did not affect the patient. Posteroanterior pressures caused local pain and spasm when applied over C5/6.

Sensation testing demonstrated loss of pinprick and light touch sensation over the radial aspect of the right index finger and over the dorsal aspect of the thumb. Pinprick was reduced in the same areas but also

distinctly specific to a condition

over the dorsolateral aspect of the forearm. There was moderate weakness of the elbow flexors and wrist extensors. Deep tendon reflexes were normal throughout the arms.

There is no need of the upper limb neural tension (provocation) tests because these will not clarify the diagnosis nor help determine treatment. What is your diagnosis and treatment?

Please turn to page 395 for solutions.

4

A Good or Bad Prognosis in This Post-MVA Patient

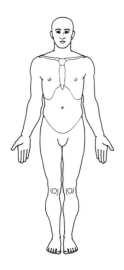

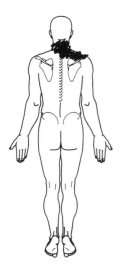

Subjective Examination

A 42-year-old woman was attended 4 days after suffering from a rear-end collision. She was driving the car that was rear-ended and her car had been moving forward at the time of the accident. Her car was hit directly in the rear. The woman's head was facing forward. Because she was aware of the impending impact, she braced herself against the wheel with her arms. She did not hit her head nor did she loose consciousness nor did she suffer from any amnesia.

At the time of the accident she felt some mild neck pain, which was worse the next day upon waking. The pain was felt in mid to lower cervical spine with radiation to the right upper trapezius. She did not complain of headaches, dizziness, or paresthesia. The pain was felt to level off that same day and was described by the patient as moderate reaching a level of 5 on a scale of 1 to 10. In addition to the posterior cervical pain there was very mild pain in the left anterior mid-cervical area. There had been no change in the pain since this time. She was still working as a high school teacher. The pain tended to be a little worse at the end of the day and better in the morning. She had no trouble sleeping.

The patient had no history of neck or arm pain and no medical history of relevance. From her history, what is her likely prognosis? Discuss how you would continue her examination and what results you expect.

What are you thinking at this point? How will you proceed with the examination? ☞

Cervical Case 4 Continuation

There are number of indicators that this patient should have a good prognosis.

1. The extension force was symmetrical in that her head was facing directly forward and the force was straight on to the rear of the car. One study found that a critical prognostic point was inclination of the head at the time of impact (poor prognosis).

2. There was no direct head trauma, no loss of consciousness, and no amnesia, thereby minimizing the possibility of concussion and traumatic brain injury.

3. She was aware of the impending impact, another factor that appears to offer a good prognosis.

4. The peak of the pain was delayed. Immediate onset of severe pain suggests profound tissue damage, such as a fracture or ligamentous tearing, and offers a poor prognosis.

5. The peak of the pain was moderate. The more severe the pain, the poorer the prognosis.

6. There were no neurological symptoms.

Despite the good prognosis, it is best to approach cervical trauma carefully. Vertebral artery damage is still a possibility. One study using magnetic resonance angiography demonstrated that 1 in 10 whiplash victims may have one damaged artery and be either asymptomatic or have minimal symptoms. The sequence outlined on page 177 should be followed for all traumatic necks regardless of how minor the damage appears to be. The examination is not overly long and goes a little further to ensure the safety of this higher risk patient.

Objective Examination

There was nothing of note on observation. The fracture and cranial nerve tests were negative, and there were no signs of spinal nerve or nerve root involvement. Craniovertebral ligament stress testing was negative, and the dizziness tests (vertebral artery tests) were unremarkable. Cervical range of motion was as follows. Extension was about 80 percent of the expected range and reproduced posterior neck pain. Flexion was full range and painless. Both rotations were about 80° with pain felt on the opposite side of the posterior neck. Both side flexions reached about 30° and produced mild pain ipsilaterally. In addition, left rotation caused some very mild left anterior neck pain. Compression and traction were negative even though isometric right rotation caused mild left anterior neck pain. Posteroanterior pressures over C5/6 produced mild central discomfort.

Biomechanical assessment found that extension at both C5/6 zygopophyseal joints was restricted with a <u>minor spasm</u> end feel.

What is your diagnosis and treatment? Have you changed your prognosis?

Please turn to page 396 for solutions. ☞

Facial Impact in a Post-MVA Patient

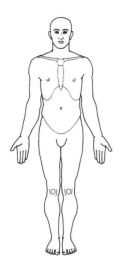

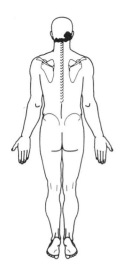

Subjective Examination

A 38-year-old man was rear-ended 9 weeks earlier. His head was turned upward and to the right while he looked in the rearview mirror on hearing the brakes of the car behind. He was not wearing a seat belt and was thrown forward, hitting his face on the steering wheel. He denied being knocked unconscious but he could not remember anything that happened for about half an hour following the accident. After the accident he was taken to the emergency room where his neck was X-rayed and proved to be negative. He also had X-rays taken of his face because he complained of severe pain in the left side of his face. The X-rays demonstrated an undisplaced fracture of the zygoma, an area that had not been painful for the last week or so.

At the time of the accident he could not remember what pains he experienced but at the hospital 30 minutes later he had severe pain in the right suboccipital area and both sides of the posterior upper neck. The patient was treated with narcotic analgesics for the facial pain and a soft collar for the neck. He was advised to see his own physician. He also experienced vertigo continuously at first and then intermittently after the first day. The emergency room physician said that this was just a reaction to the accident and that it would disappear. After 3 days, the vertigo was felt only while lying on his right side.

He saw his family doctor the next day. The physician replaced the narcotics with Tylenol and told him to remove the collar. He took a couple of days off work. When he returned to work as a welder he was unable to tolerate the weight of the welding mask and had to stop work.

Objective Examination

The upper posterior neck pain improved only very slowly and at 4 weeks he was still off work but was moving better. The suboccipital pain was unchanged. The vertigo was felt more frequently now, especially when he extended and right rotated his head. He also complained of nonvertiginous dizziness in the form of nausea and giddiness when turning his head to the left. This had been noticed over the previous few days as his range of motion increased. At 4 weeks, his physician referred him to an orthopedic surgeon who ordered an MRI that showed a posterior disk prolapse at C5/6. The surgeon referred him to physical therapy with a diagnosis of post-whiplash C5/6 disk prolapse for traction and ultrasound.

What are you thinking at this point? How will you proceed with the examination?   ☞

Cervical Case 5 Continuation

This man is in trouble. He suffered a concussion as evidenced by his postaccident amnesia. The facial impact is a poor prognostic indicator. He may have occult cervical fractures such as subchondral or pedicular fractures or rim lesions. Severe pain only 30 minutes after the accident is not a good sign. The probability is that this pain was immediate but unremembered. Another problem the patient faces is his work. Welding is a problem for the posttraumatic neck patient due to the weight of the mask and the positions the welder has to adopt.

The vertigo may have been the result of a vertebral artery injury, labyrinthine concussion, or cervical joint receptor dysfunction. However, vertebral artery damage sufficient to cause immediate vertigo lasting continuously for a day would probably have manifested more obvious central nervous signs and symptoms, sooner rather than later. Cervical joint receptor dizziness is also unlikely because the vertigo was a function of head position and motion not cervical movement as demonstrated by its onset in lying down on the right side. The most likely explanation for the vertigo is labyrinthine concussion. Given the consistency of the provoking position otoconia displacement is the likely cause of the benign positional paroxysmal vertigo.

The MRI diagnosis of a C5/6 disk prolapse is probably not relevant to the patient because there is no low cervical or upper limb pain.

Objective tests need to be carried out carefully and progressively with the assumption that the vertebral artery has been damaged. The sequence outlined on page 177 is as complete and as safe as any other sequence of testing.

Objective Examination

Gentle compression through the head did not reproduce pain. Although there was some minor discomfort with isometric testing of both rotations and flexion, the discomfort was not severe nor was it associated with inhibited weakness. There were no cranial nerve signs, although the body-tilting test (minimized Hallpike-Dix) produced some very mild vertigo on backward and forward tilting. No neurological deficits were noted when the long tracts or the spinal nerves were tested. The Sharp-Purser and other craniovertebral stability tests were negative.

On testing the dizziness with reproduction tests (so-called vertebral artery tests), left head and neck rotation produced mild type 2 dizziness, whereas combined rotation and extension reproduced his vertigo. Cranial nerve testing while the patient was dizzy was negative. Body rotation to the right produced the same mild type 2 dizziness that left neck rotation caused, whereas extension and left rotation of the body under the head did not reproduce the patient's vertigo that was felt with head right rotation and extension.

The patient was markedly limited into right rotation (45°) and reproduced mild suboccipital pain. Left rotation (about 60°) was moderately painful in the occipital region and produced dizziness. Extension was limited by about 50% and produced somewhat stronger right suboccipital pain than did the other movements. Flexion was just short of full range and painfree. Both side flexions were limited, right-side flexion to about 50% of the expected range and left by about 25%, and neither produced pain. Posteroanterior pressures over C2/3 produced pain and a jammed end feel, whereas over the other levels these pressures were negative.

Because no working diagnosis could be reached concerning the musculoskeletal system, a biomechanical examination was carried out. There was restriction of both side flexions combined extension at the atlantooccipital segment, although full range could be obtained if hold-relax techniques were employed carefully. Both rotations were limited at the atlantoaxial segment, although they could be increased to near normal with hold-relax techniques. Extension and right side flexion and left translation was limited at C2/3. There was also a restriction of inferior gliding of the right zygopophyseal joint. No movement dysfunctions could be felt at any other cervical level.

What are your thoughts concerning the diagnosis and treatment of this complex patient.

Please turn to page 397 for solutions.

Neck Pain and Vertigo During Lifting

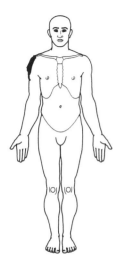

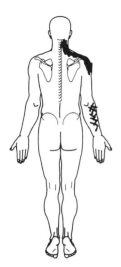

Subjective Examination

A 36-year-old woman attends your clinic. Two days earlier while lifting a heavy suitcase from the trunk of her car, she experienced a sudden onset of acute nonradicular (somatic) pain in the right neck, upper trapezius, and deltoid areas plus paresthesia in the dorsolateral forearm. She also experienced immediate vertigo that lasted an hour but has not been present since. The next day, in addition to her previous symptoms, she experienced radicular (lancinating) pain in the dorsolateral aspect of the upper and lower arm.

The patient had no history of neck or arm pain or vertigo. X-rays were negative. The physician diagnosed her as a C5 radiculopathy from a cervical disk herniation.

Objective Examination

On observation there was no torticollis or any other unusual signs.

Right rotation, right-side flexion and extension were both severely limited and caused lancinating pain and paresthesia reproduced into the right posterolateral upper and lower arm.

There was hypoesthesia to pinprick in the right posterolateral forearm. Profound weakness was felt when right elbow flexion strength was tested, whereas wrist extension was only slightly weak. The biceps deep tendon reflex was reduced when compared with the left arm. All other reflexes were normal.

Are there any other tests you would like to do? Can you make a diagnosis and begin management of this patient?

What are you thinking at this point? How will you proceed with the examination? ☞

Cervical Case 6 Continuation

The lancinating pain and paresthesia would suggest either a C5 or C6 dermatome involvement. However, there are no symptoms into the hand, specifically in the thumb or index finger, so it is probably the C5 spinal nerve that is being compromised. The delay in the onset of the lancinating pain would indicate an inflammatory process rather than preexisting adhesions at the spinal nerve or nerve root level. The C5 involvement is further demonstrated by elbow flexor weakness, biceps tendon hyporeflexia, and hypoesthesia along the C5 dermatome. It is less likely to be a C6 radiculopathy because there is no involvement of the brachioradialis reflex or the sensation of the thumb and index finger and the wrist extensor weakness is mild. Most of us would have probably used mechanical traction and a hard collar on this patient because we have very little else to offer a frank disk herniation with neurological deficit.

However, the patient's vertigo has not been considered and is the atypical factor in this case. There is really no good explanation for it. Vertigo is not likely to arise from the neck problem because it came on very suddenly and then disappeared even though the cervical pain remained. There was no direct or indirect trauma to the head. Consequently, cerebral and brainstem concussion or contusion can be essentially ruled out as can labyrinthine concussion. However, if the patient produced a strong Valsalva maneuver, a dramatic change in middle ear pressure might have ruptured the tympanic or vestibular membrane. However, there was no ear pain or noises associated with the vertigo, as is frequently the case with middle ear damage, and the vertigo abated rapidly.

Another possibility is that the vertebral artery is being compressed or has been damaged by the presumed herniating disk. In this case, there may have been reactive vasospasm that lasted for a short while and did not recur. The patient's pain is preventing her from moving into the compromising position.

The objective examination must investigate the vertigo.

In fact, this patient was very lucky. During the movement tests, she complained of blurred vision when she turned her head to the right. Initially the therapist ignored this and carried on with the testing. However, at the end of the examination, the patient asked what the therapist thought might have caused the dizziness, which made the therapist rethink. Right rotation was again tested with the therapist facing the patient who noticed very mild left lateral nystagmus.

What are you going to do now and what do you think is happening?

Please turn to page 399 for solutions.   ☞

Acute Torticollis in a 10-Year-Old Boy

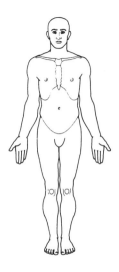

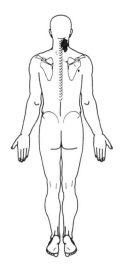

Subjective Examination

A 10-year-old boy in obvious distress is referred with a diagnosis of acute torticollis and a prescription of "assess and treat." He is complaining of severe right posterior neck pain of less than a day's duration, the pain starting upon waking this morning (4 hours ago). The previous day he had been roughhousing with his friends but cannot remember any particular incident that might have caused the problem. His mother did not send him to school, and he spent the morning lying down waiting to see the physician. He has no history of neck pain or any medical history of significance. The physician gave him Tylenol and referred him to physical therapy.

Objective Examination

On observation, this was a normal healthy boy with a left torticollis that was side flexed right and rotated right and slightly extended so that the patient's head twists a little upward and to the left.

He had painfree full range into left rotation and flexion but attempts to right rotate or left-side flex produced acute neck pain. Right-side flexion had almost full range but produced moderate pain, and extension was full range provided it was carried out in the line of the deformity. The end feel on right rotation and left-side flexion was spasm, which was palpated in the sternomastoid.

Diagnose, prognose, and treat.

What are you thinking at this point? How will you proceed with the examination? 🖝

Cervical Case 7 Continuation

Diagnosis This is a typical case of adolescent torticollis. The etiology is not well understood but the spasm of the sternomastoid appears to be a fairly consistent component. However, as always, the spasm is an effect rather than a cause. The problem seems to lay in the articulations of the upper neck.

Prognosis If you treat patients with this condition, they tend to recover in about 7 days. If you do not treat them, they recover in a week. However, although treatment does not shorten the recovery overall, it reduces the acute pain and restores full function within a day, leaving the patient with some mild soreness to contend with over the next 6 days or so.

Treatment One advocated treatment is to manipulate the dysfunctional segment, usually the atlantoaxial or C2/3. But if you are not keen on manipulating children, which I would rather avoid, another effective treatment is available.

Manual traction repeated many times during the initial treatment session and applied through the line of the deformity is extremely and almost uniformly effective and reduces at least 80% of the patient's pain within a few hours. Hot packs applied prior to the traction helps the patient relax and a soft collar appears to help prevent relapse. At the very least, a soft collar is comforting to the patient. The child is instructed to lie down in a comfortable position for that day and night. Usually by the next morning, the patient is ready to get rid of the collar and return to school. Usually further treatment is unnecessary.

If this patient does not recover quickly and easily, what would you be thinking and what would you do?

Please turn to page 400 for solutions.

Head Forward Posture and Arm Symptoms

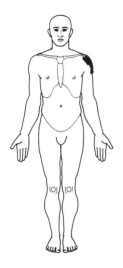

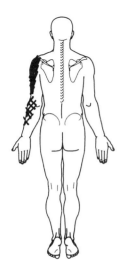

A 53-year-old man complaining of mild neck and left deltoid and lateral upper arm ache is referred. The aching had been present in the neck on and off for about 5 years with the initial onset unremembered but unassociated with any specific incident. The deltoid and lateral arm ache had come on about 3 years ago, again from no apparent cause. Recently, he had felt pins and needles around the lateral aspect of the elbow. The pain and paresthesia was made worse by prolonged sitting, especially driving, and also if he stood for too long. Sleeping eased the symptoms.

The patient had received chiropractic and physical therapy in the past, initially with good results but recently with no improvement. A recent X-ray showed degeneration in the lower cervical levels.

Objective Examination

The patient had a head forward posture with a deep crease running horizontally across the base of the neck. There was generalized stiffness in the neck with all movements being somewhat limited with a capsular end feel and with none of the movements reproducing the patient's pain. There were no neurological deficits and the upper limb tension tests were negative. Posteroanterior pressures did not produce pain but were stiff from C5 to T1. A biomechanical examination disclosed equal flexion and extension stiffness bilaterally at C5–C7 except for an extension hypermobility at C5/6 beneath the crease in the neck.

Diagnose, prognose, and treat.

What are you thinking at this point? How will you proceed with the examination? ☞

Cervical Case 8 Continuation

The paresthesia is a neurological symptom, so we need to try to figure out what is causing it. It seems mechanically provoked as evidenced by the increase in symptoms with standing and driving. However, a disk lesion is not the cause because his range of motion is not acutely disturbed nor do any of the movements provoke pain. The stiffness in the neck is generalized and seems local to the lower levels (as seen from the posteroanterior pressures). Radiographic evidence of degeneration is not a clinical diagnosis. Many individuals function quite well without knowing if there is degeneration present. However, in this case, it has probably caused the stenosis. Biomechanically there is an extension hypermobility at C5/6 but otherwise generalized flexion and extension hypomobility throughout the rest of the lower cervical spine.

Diagnosis is left C5 degenerative lateral stenosis with compromise of the C5 spinal nerve or root. Typically lateral stenosis in the neck produces more paresthesia than pain. Having identified it, what now?

Please turn to page 400 for solutions.

Acute Torticollis in a 5-Year-Old Girl

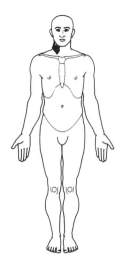

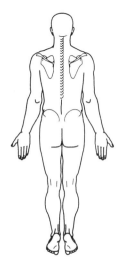

Subjective Examination

A 5-year-old girl is referred with a diagnosis of torticollis. She complained of pain in the right anterolateral neck that had been present for 2 days. Although there was no apparent cause, the pain had been present continuously since the onset. Any movement increased her pain. She woke frequently during the night with acute pain.

She had no history of similar pain and no medical history of relevance.

Objective Examination

On observation her neck was rotated to the left and side flexed to the right. Any attempt to correct the torticollis caused severe pain. All movements except right rotation and right-side flexion were impossible without acute pain.

There were no neurological deficits. The upper limb neural tension (provocation) tests, as far as they could be tested given the torticollis, were not painful.

Please turn to page 401 for solutions.

263

Headaches and Neck Pain After a Fall

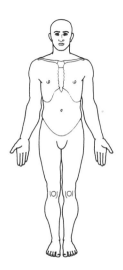

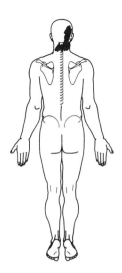

Subjective Examination

A 41-year-old woman complaining of posterior upper neck pain and right suboccipital and occipital headache attends for treatment. The onset of the pain was 3 months earlier after a fall when she hit her head. She denied being knocked unconscious and could remember everything about the injury except for a few minutes after the fall. Mild upper neck pain, worse on the right, was felt immediately, but the pain was much worse the next morning upon waking. In addition to the occipital headache, the patient was also experiencing a mild deep diffuse ache throughout the head that was worse when she was tired or when she exerted herself. This ache had been present since the accident but had been never severe.

She complained of difficulty concentrating, sleeping, and staying motivated and felt tired and run down most of the time. She also complained of intermittent type 2 dizziness during which she would become unsteady and lightheaded occasionally on rapid position changes from sitting to standing or the reverse or on sudden turns. She denied vertigo, and there was no predictable pattern of provocation to these episodes of dizziness.

The neck and occipital pain was worse with prolonged sitting, especially if she was reading. It flared up with strong exertion. The three or four times she had tried to go back to work as a practical nurse, the exacerbation had been so acute that she only managed a day or two. When the pain flared up, it spread into both upper trapezia and from the occipital region over the head to the right eye. Essentially she had been off work since the accident and was covered by Worker's Compensation. Previous treatments included chiropractic treatments that relieved her neck and head pain for a few hours relief and physical therapy in the form of ultrasound, stretching, and cranial sacral therapy. This provided no relief at all and the stretching, if overly vigorous, increased her headaches.

She had a history of episodic low-back pain over the previous 4 years that was associated with an on-the-job injury. She had taken some time off work for this. Her medical history included treatment for depression 10 years earlier, which improved with Elavil. She had not been troubled with it since then, but she did seem depressed during the interview.

What are you thinking at this point? How will you proceed with the examination?   ☞

Cervical Case 10 Continuation

It would be easy to label this patient as having chronic pain syndrome based on her past injury and work record, her lack of motivation and vague symptoms, and her previous history of depression. However, such labeling would be unfair until all exhaustive tests had been carried out both by the therapist and by other, more appropriately trained health care practitioners.

Although most of her complaints are part of the clinical picture of the depressed patient with chronic pain syndrome and/or secondary gain issues, they are also part of the presentation of the patient with post-concussion (posttraumatic head injury) syndrome. In addition, the pain and other symptoms started almost immediately after the accident, did not progress, and are local without involvement of other body areas, a usual accompaniment to chronic pain syndrome. Her apparent depression may be real, and given her disability and ongoing pain, she would be entitled to be somewhat depressed. Or it may only be apparent because the therapist was sensitized to it by her previous history of depression. In any case, it is something for her physician to decide upon but she does need some guidance in order to bring up the subject with her doctor.

It is safer and fairer to assume chronic pain syndrome and prove or disprove it than to assume that there is a physical basis for her disability. It is likely that she was concussed, even though she denies being unconscious. The history of amnesia after the injury is almost pathognomonic of concussion or worse. On the bright side, the symptoms are not progressing and the condition is 3 months old, so more serious considerations such as a slow intracranial bleed can be excluded.

The two distinct types of headache with this lady are the typical cervical headache in the occiput with occasional spread occipitofrontally and orbitally when exacerbated and the diffuse deeper headache. The former is related to head and neck movements and postures, while the latter is associated with tiredness and physical fatigue, which is probably part of the head injury syndrome. The presence of dizziness may also be part of the head injury or it may be associated with chronic pain syndrome. But because it came on very quickly after the injury, the former is the more likely possibility.

Her cervical pain and occipital headache are typical and should normally respond to appropriate physical therapy. The fact that it did not suggests that either inappropriate therapy or complicating factors that prevent effective therapy from working.

Whatever else may be said of this patient, she has had a head injury. In addition to the musculoskeletal examination she requires a cranial nerve examination and perhaps a recommendation to her physician that a neuropsychiatric evaluation be carried out to try to determine if traumatic brain injury has occurred. There is no evidence from the history that any damage to the vertebral artery occurred but examination should exclude the possibility as far as the tests are able so that the source of her dizziness can be found. The remainder of the examination is routine.

Objective Examination

The patient looked tired but otherwise had no obvious postural deficits or deformities.

Cranial nerve testing was negative except that during the tracking tests for the third, fourth, and sixth nerves, she experienced mild short duration vertigo and longer lasting nausea. Body-tilting tests did not reproduce her dizziness. Craniovertebral ligament stress testing, including Sharp-Purser, were negative for both instability and symptomatology.

Dizziness was not reproduced on any of the so-called vertebral artery tests and Hautard's test was negative. As the vertebral artery appeared to be normal (given the lack of cranial nerve signs and the negative tests), the Hallpike-Dix test was carried out. This reproduced her dizziness when her head was in both left and right rotation and extension. The dizziness came on almost immediately and disappeared within a minute. No cranial nerve signs were discovered on testing while she was dizzy.

She had full range cervical movements with extension and left rotation reproducing her neck and head pain. Both movements had a jammed (subluxed) end feel, whereas all other movements of the neck were painfree and had normal end feels.

There were no signs of neurological deficit. All neuromeningeal (dural and neural tension) tests were negative.

Compression and traction were negative. Posteroanterior pressure over the spinous process of C2 and over the back of C1 neural arch reproduced her headache and local tenderness. The posterior suboccipital muscles were hypertonic and tender to moderate palpation.

It seems probable that the occipital headache is due to a dysfunction in the craniovertebral joints, but exactly where cannot be ascertained from the examination. A biomechanical examination is required.

Passive physiological and accessory (arthrokinematic) movement testing determined that there was an extension pathomechanical hypomobility (subluxation) at the left atlantooccipital joint and a flexion pathomechanical hypomobility at the left C5/6 zygopophyseal joint.

Diagnose, treat, and prognose.

Please turn to page 401 for solutions. ☞

Post-Manipulation Vertigo

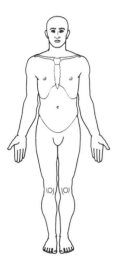

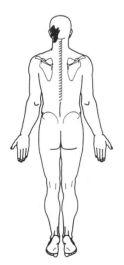

Subjective Examination

A 42-year-old woman had been treated by another therapist for cervical pain with manipulative therapy (high-velocity, low-amplitude thrust techniques) for left occipital headaches. Her response to treatment had been to suffer vertigo for about an hour after each treatment. Although the headaches had improved slightly, the therapist had been unwilling to discontinue the treatment, telling her that the vertigo was caused by cervical joint dysfunction and would eventually disappear. After 4 sessions she discontinued treatment herself and went back to her doctor, who then referred her to you.

Her neck pain had been present intermittently for 6 months but she could relate no cause. She had no history of neck pain or of vertigo.

What are you thinking at this point? How will you proceed with the examination?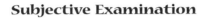

Cervical Case 11 Continuation

This case points out the requirement for adequate training in manipulative therapy. The actual techniques can be very simple; unfortunately, so can some of the practitioners. One of the documented causes of severe adverse complications in manipulative therapy is the failure to recognize potential or actual neurological signs or symptoms. The previous therapist's contention that the post-manipulative vertigo was arthrogenic in origin could possibly be true, but it should not be the first assumption. The possibility that it was caused by vertebrobasilar ischemia had to be the foremost consideration and should have been excluded. Compression of the artery during the manipulation could also have resulted in vasospasm either as a result of simple compression or possibly of intramural damage. The other possible cause of the vertigo is a labyrinthine condition. If the amount of head displacement was excessive during the manipulation and if the stupidity of the therapist in pursing manipulation in the face causes vertigo, anything is possible. Although it is possible that the vertigo was due to the cervical joint, cervical dizziness usually comes in the form of type 2 (nonvertiginous) dizziness, and when it does produce vertigo, it is relatively mild and of short duration.

This patient, at least potentially, is an accident waiting to happen, and every care must be taken. The less-experienced therapist should probably refer this patient to another therapist with more experience.

Objective Examination

The examination should be progressive and gradual so it can be halted at the earliest sign or symptom of neurological involvement. The examination of the cranial nerves was negative. There were no long tract signs of motor paresis, spasticity, pain or light touch, vibration or proprioception sensation or vibration loss. There were no signs of segmental palsy, and all neuromeningeal tests were negative. The craniovertebral ligament stress tests were negative. The dizziness (vertebral) tests were negative. She had full range movement in the neck with pain on flexion and left rotation. The biomechanical examination disclosed a flexion pathomechanical hypomobility (extension subluxation) at the left atlantooccipital joint.

Where do you go to here from here?

Please turn to page 403 for solutions.

Retro-Orbital Headaches

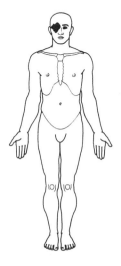

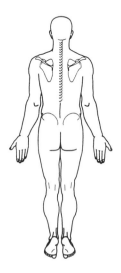

Subjective Examination

A 44-year-old woman was attended for treatment for right orbital headaches that had been present for 2 days and that were diagnosed as being caused by "cervical migraine." She could not relate any cause and stated that the headaches had started suddenly with mild aching that built up to a severe pain within hours of the onset. The pain was present all the time but, since the initial build up, was no more or less severe. She complained of photophobia and wore sunglasses whenever out in the sunlight or in a bright room. She did not associate the headache with neck movements or posture.

She had no history of similar pains, although she did suffer from neck pain and headaches running from the right occiput over the head to the right eye episodically. The last episode of this was a year earlier and had been treated successfully with manipulative therapy.

She had no medical history of relevance. She works as a legal secretary and does not smoke or drink alcohol.

Objective Examination

She had full range painfree movements in her neck. The temporomandibular joints opened equally, normally, and painlessly. She has some loss of atlantooccipital flexion bilaterally and atlantoaxial flexion and both rotations.

Develop a diagnosis and treatment plan.

Please turn to page 404 for solutions.

Headaches and Low Cervical Pain

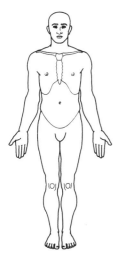

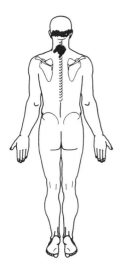

Subjective Examination

A 24-year-old man was involved in a front-end collision as a driver. He suffered mild pain in the lower cervical region immediately after the accident, but the pain was much worse the next morning (15 hours later). He saw his physician the following morning with moderate pain (about a 6 on a 1 to 10 scale) in the lower neck and a moderate occipital headache (a 4 on the same scale), which he had first felt upon waking. The neck pain and the headache were fairly constant. Due to the short duration of the problem, he had not had an opportunity to discover what activities and postures increased the pain. He had not experienced any numbness, paresthesia, or dizziness.

He denied any history of neck pain or ongoing headaches nor did he have any medical history of significance. He works as an auto mechanic.

His physician referred him to a physical therapist, who attended him 2 days later or 4 days after the accident. At this time, the lower cervical pain had leveled off but was made worse with prolonged flexion when reading or if watching TV for more than an hour. The headache was a little worse and was especially strong in the morning and after reading. He had not returned to work at his point.

X-rays of his cervical region were negative.

Objective Examination

His range of motion was reduced in flexion to about 75% of the expected range and in extension to about 50% of the expected range. Flexion and extension produced lower cervical pain. Both rotations were slightly limited to about 90% of their normal range, and both were uncomfortable in the lower neck at the ends of range.

There was no neurological deficit in the form weakness, sensory loss, or reflex changes. His cranial nerves were not tested.

What are you thinking at this point? How will you proceed with the examination? ☞

Cervical Case 13 Continuation

The occipital headaches are spatially and functionally dissociated from the lower cervical pain. From a spatial perspective, this can happen, but it is not common. Usually there are times when the pain runs between the painful areas. The headache was worse with prolonged neck flexion, but none of the tests were able to reproduce the headache. Again, this is not rare or even uncommon. One reassuring aspect is that the headaches were linked to neck flexion.

At this point, there is not enough information to make a diagnosis or to develop a specific treatment plan. A biomechanical examination was carried out.

The craniovertebral joints were normally mobile. Testing did not provoke the headache or any other pain either at the time of testing or later. There was a bilateral extension hypomobility at C7/T1 with a pathomechanical end feel. Flexion had a normal end feel (that is normal range) but was painful at the end of range. All other segments appeared to be moving normally.

Diagnose, prognose, and treat.

Please turn to page 404 for solutions.

CERVICAL CASE 14

Pins and Needles After an MVA

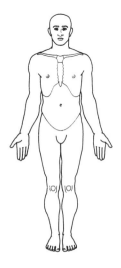

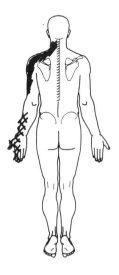

Subjective Examination

A 32-year-old female was involved in an automobile accident when the car she was driving was rear-ended while stopped at an intersection. She complained of immediate moderate pain in the left posterolateral neck, which was worse that evening, 5 or 6 hours later. The next morning, the pain in the neck was a little worse and had extended to include the left deltoid region to the middle of the humerus. She also complained of paresthesia in the left index finger and thumb and up the posterolateral aspect of the forearm to the lower third of the radius. She had first felt paresthesia while washing her hair in the shower that morning.

She works as a computer technician and decided to take the day off work to see her doctor. He prescribed anti-inflammatory medication and told her to go back to work after the weekend (this was Thursday). At this time she had problems moving her neck, especially backward and to the left. Both movements were very painful and restricted. She rested over the next few days and was feeling better by the time she returned to work on Monday. The shoulder pain had disappeared and the posterolateral neck pain was much easier. She still felt the paresthesia mildly when washing her hair.

She worked for the next 2 days. During this time, the neck pain gradually worsened and the deltoid pain resumed and spread to the elbow. The paresthesia was much stronger but remained in the same location. The range of motion in the neck decreased and flexion now caused her paresthesia.

She saw her physician again on Thursday. He advised her to continue working, to increase her medication, and to work through the pain. By the middle of the following week, the symptoms had increased to the point where she simply could not continue to work. She returned to her physician, who took her off work and referred her to physical therapy.

On attendance, she stated that the neck pain was present mainly on movement and on prolonged flexion. The pain woke her occasionally while sleeping, although she could not say what provoked it—sleeping position or movement. The lateral upper arm pain was present to some extent all of the time but was worse when the neck was worse. The paresthesia was intermittent, being felt whenever the neck was flexed or when washing her hair and more recently whenever she lifted her arm more than 90° from her side.

She did not complain of dizziness or paresthesia anywhere other than in the left hand. She denied any history of cervical problems and had no medical history of relevance. X-rays were negative and her physician did not feel that an MRI or CT scan was necessary.

Objective Examination

Cranial nerve, long tract, and fracture tests were negative. Progressive dizziness testing through Hautard's test was negative. Craniovertebral ligament testing was negative.

Flexion was about 50% of the expected range and reproduced neck and lateral upper arm pain and her paresthesia. Extension was about 75% of the expected range and caused local posterolateral neck pain. Right-side flexion was full range but reproduced her paresthesia. Left-side flexion was about 50% of right-side flexion and produced posterolateral neck pain and her paresthesia. Right rotation was full range and painfree. Left rotation was about 50% of right and produced posterolateral neck pain, left lateral upper arm pain, and the paresthesia.

Muscle testing found mild fatigable weakness of the lateral rotators of the left shoulder and moderate fatigable weakness of the left elbow flexors and wrist extensors. There was slight loss of pinprick sensation over the paresthetic area but no loss of light touch in this or any other area. Her reflexes were equal and normal on both sides. Moderate to strong compression of the cervical spine produced left neck pain. Traction did not have any effect.

Do you have a diagnosis, treatment plan, and prognosis for this lady?

What are you thinking at this point? How will you proceed with the examination? ☞

Cervical Case 14 Continuation

Diagnosis From the patient's symptoms it seems likely that she has a disk herniation compressing the sixth nerve root. The amount of compression seems moderate because the sensation loss and weakness are not profound and there is no change in the deep tendon reflexes. Possibly she damaged her disk in the accident and this caused some compression of the sixth nerve root. Continuing to work may have caused more herniation and increased nerve compromise.

Neither the subjective examination or the objective examination indicate any central neurological or neurovascular involvement.

Traction did not make her symptoms worse (although it did not relieve them either), so it is not contraindicated as a treatment. The lack of lancinating pain would suggest that the nerve root is not inflamed, so she should be able tolerate traction.

As a point of interest, I did not use the upper limb neuromeningeal tension or provocation tests because there did not seem to be any point. The clinical signs were very clear—distinctly affected range of motion with some of the movements reproducing her paresthesia. The paresthesia and hypoesthesia appear in a clearly delineated C6 zone, and her weakness is distributed in the C6 myotome.

Treatment She should remain off work until the continuous pain subsides and changes to intermittent pain. A hard collar should be considered for this patient because physiological movements are causing arm pain and paresthesia. Mechanical traction is also a possibility after a trial manual traction treatment or two to ensure that it will not exacerbate her condition.

Prognosis Some factors suggest a good prognosis and some factors indicate a bad one. On the plus side, the pain was delayed and there was no immediate severe loss of motion. On the down side is the overriding presence of neurological symptoms. This presence is one of the worse prognostic factors in post-whiplash patients.

The patient was treated with a hard collar, manual and then mechanical traction, and painfree exercises every day. She was also advised on sleeping positions—her pillows were reduced from two to one and in order to keep her off of her stomach, a golf ball was placed in her pajama pocket.

This treatment scheme was continued, with modifications and additions, for 3 weeks. The patient noted no improvement in the last two treatment sessions. The collar was removed at this point. The lateral arm pain was no longer present. The posterolateral neck pain was very local to left mid neck. The paresthesia was still present, but less noticeable, and was felt on overhead arm movements away from the side such as hair washing.

On examination, the range of motion had increased. Extension was limited to about 10% of the expected range and caused local soreness. Flexion was full range and painfree. Right-side flexion was slightly limited, while all other movements were full range and painfree.

The muscle weakness was observed only on testing the wrist extensors and was very mild starting at a grade 4+ and reducing to a grade 3+ over six repetitions. Pinprick sensation was normal and the tendon reflexes remained normal.

This lady had made substantial improvement but her pain had not leveled off. Where do you go from here? Does she need any other clinical examinations? Do you continue with her current treatment or change it? Does she go back to work?

Please turn to page 406 for solutions.

Lateral Elbow Pain

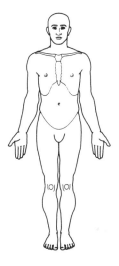

Subjective Examination

A 53-year-old man complaining of right lateral elbow pain was referred by his physician with a diagnosis of tennis elbow. The pain had been present for 4 weeks and was felt during and after staining his sundeck. For the first few days, the pain was present all of the time but was worse whenever he used his hand. On attendance, the pain was felt only on use but it was disabling. He had not been able to work as a plumber since the injury.

The patient had no history of elbow pain but said that he suffered the occasional neck ache for no apparent reason. This pain was felt in the posterior neck and was not referred to his arms. He had no medical history of relevance.

Objective Examination

The elbow had full range and painfree movements. Isometric wrist extension and radial deviation were painful at the lateral aspect of the elbow. There was tenderness to palpation over the lateral epicondyle. The pain on isometric testing was less when the test was carried out with the patient wearing a tennis elbow support.

Do you have a diagnosis and what are the potential causes?

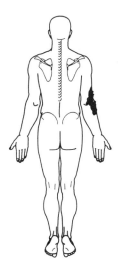

What are you thinking at this point? How will you proceed with the examination? ☞

Cervical Case 15 Continuation

This man is suffering from an epicondylar tennis elbow as demonstrated by the isometric tests and the location of the tenderness. However, there are numerous causes of tennis elbow, including: cervical biomechanical dysfunction, direct trauma, wrist hypomobility, elbow hypomobility, and true overuse.

Repeating the isometric tests in various head and neck positions can quickly screen the neck. If the patient's pain is significantly reduced, then the neck is playing a role. If the pain is completely relieved, there is no pathology at the elbow. However, only biomechanical testing can definitively exclude the neck clinically. A positive examination only demonstrates the presence of a biomechanical dysfunction. It is up to the therapist to judge the dysfunction's association with the tennis elbow. Cervical dysfunction may be contributing or causing this man's elbow problem.

Direct trauma would be obvious in the patient's history, which is not a factor in this case.

If the wrist cannot extend, then the wrist extensors may become overactive in an attempt to fully extend the wrist. Biomechanical testing will demonstrate the hypomobility.

The common elbow dysfunction that underlies tennis elbow is the abducted ulna. Here the ulna is unable to fully flex or supinate and shifts the wrist into ulna deviation. This limits radial deviation and the radial deviators overwork trying to attain full range. In this case, the biomechanical examination of the wrist did not show any dysfunction.

True overuse is, in my opinion, an unusual cause of tennis elbow. A history of significant overuse that is unfamiliar for that patient is necessary in order to make this diagnosis.

In this case, the screening tests for the neck are negative. Biomechanical testing of the neck found hypomobility at the atlantooccipital joints into extension bilaterally and hypomobility at the left C3/4 zygopophyseal joint.

Diagnose and treat.

Please turn to page 407 for solutions.

Is Her Post-MVA Headache Arising From Her Neck?

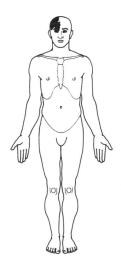

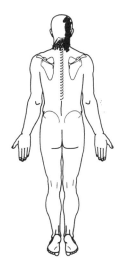

Subjective Examination

A 34-year-old woman complaining of neck pain and headaches is referred for treatment. She gave a history of being involved in a motor vehicle accident, when the car she was driving was struck from the rear 2 weeks earlier. She experienced a mild posterior, right neck ache almost immediately. By the next morning, the cervical pain was much worse and accompanied by a right occipitotemporal headache. The cervical pain and headache were initially present continuously and relieved only by analgesics. But over the last week, the headache became intermittent and was felt upon waking and at the end of the day. The cervical pain was also present at the end of the work day, on various movements, and on prolonged flexion positions such as reading. She experienced no other pains or paresthesia.

She did not hit her head during the accident, denies being knocked unconscious, and was able to remember everything about the accident. She had no medical history of relevance or any previous neck pain. She had not experienced any dizziness, nausea, or visual symptoms.

In general she thought that her pain was improving. She was able to do more, especially over the previous few days. Initially she took a couple of days off work as a taxi dispatcher, but then returned to work. Although working aggravated her neck, the pain was less the last few days.

From this information can you determine if the headache is referred from the cervical spine; if the prognosis is good, bad, or indifferent; or if the patient needs to wear a cervical collar?

What are you thinking at this point? How will you proceed with the examination? 🖝

Cervical Case 16 Continuation

The headache is probably referred from the neck. The onset of the more severe cervical pain and the onset of the headache occurred simultaneously. The distribution of her headache is typical of a cervicogenic headache because its onset and provocative factors coincide.

Her prognosis is good. The onset of pain was delayed. There were no neurological signs or symptoms and she was making a steady recovery. Additionally she was fully functional.

This patient should not need to be put into a collar because she not only functioned without a collar but also improved without a collar.

Objective Examination

Extension was about 50% of the expected range and reproduced her right cervical pain. Flexion was almost full range and pulled on the posterior neck. Right rotation and right-side flexion were about 60% and 30%, respectively, of the expected range with both reproducing her neck pain. Left-side flexion and left rotation were full range and painfree. None of the limited ranges produced spasm, but all had a harder than usual end feel, which in the case of right rotation felt pathomechanical.

Compression and traction were painless. The cranjovertebral stress tests were negative.

All neurological tests including those for the cranial nerves and spinal nerve roots were negative. Biomechanical testing indicated a loss of extension with a pathomechanical or subluxed end feel of the right C2/3 zygopophyseal joint, which was also painful during the test. Although none of the tests reproduced her headache, she did complain of its onset after the examination was finished.

Do any of these objective findings alter the likelihood of the headache being referred from the neck, or her prognosis, or her need for a collar? What treatment would you initiate?

Please turn to page 407 for solutions.

Medial Arm Paresthesia

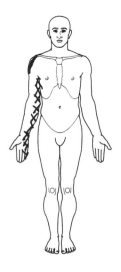

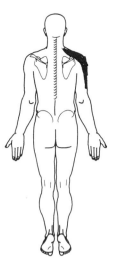

Subjective Examination

A 56-year-old man is seen complaining of pain in the left upper trapezius with radiating pain into the lateral upper arm with paresthesia in the left medial upper arm and forearm and ulna border of the hand and the little finger. The upper arm pain had been present for 6 weeks, gradually increasing in severity over that time until it had become a constant ache. The paresthesia had been felt for the last week and was becoming more intense.

He had been receiving treatment at another clinic with no improvement, and when the paresthesia started, he switched clinics. The treatment consisted of manual therapy and exercises, and when this failed to provide relief, mechanical traction was substituted.

The patient could relate no apparent cause and had no history of cervical or arm pain. The patient had no medical history of relevance. He had quit smoking a year earlier but retained his smoker's cough. He works as a millwright in a paper mill.

Objective Examination

Flexion was full range and painfree. Extension was full range and produced mild pain in the upper left trapezius. Left-side flexion was full range and painfree. Right-side flexion was about 30% of that seen with left-side flexion and had a strong spasm end feel. Right-side flexion also reproduced the upper trapezius and lateral arm pain and the paresthesia in the ulna border of the lower arm and hand. Both rotations were full range and painfree. Isometric left-side flexion was painful but all other isometric tests were negative. Compression, traction, and posteroanterior pressures were all negative. Severe pinprick sensation decreased over the ulna border of the hand and the entire fifth finger. There was weakness of finger flexion and finger abduction and adduction. No reflex changes were noted. The upper limb tension test for the ulna and median nerve components were both positive in that they reproduced the paresthesia as well as the lateral arm pain.

Offer a diagnosis and treatment.

What are you thinking at this point? How will you proceed with the examination?   ☞

Cervical Case 17 Continuation

The absence of a cause is a yellow flag and the condition is worsening as evidenced by the onset of paresthesia in the eighth cervical and first and second thoracic dermatomal areas. However, the pattern of motion restriction is unusual in that flexion and extension and the rotations are largely unaffected. Because the posteroanterior pressures were painless (as were compression and traction), the spinal segments are less likely to be involved. These findings (or their lack) would tend to exclude a disk herniation as a cause. The patient's age would allow spinal stenosis as a potential cause; however, the pain does not seem to be related to neck positions. The failure of mechanical treatment is another cause for concern.

Weakness of the intrinsic hand muscles has been recognized as an uncommon result of disk herniation, but may be present in thoracic outlet syndrome and various other brachial plexus lesions, including Pancoast syndrome. In general, this is not typical of the cervical problems normally seen by orthopedic therapists and requires great care on the part of the therapist. If this is Pancoast's syndrome, what do you expect to find on further examination? What are the common causes?

Please turn to page 408 for solutions.

Hand Paresthesia

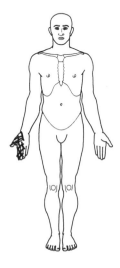

Subjective Examination

A 45-year-old man complaining of paresthesia in the right hand is referred by his family doctor with a diagnosis of carpal tunnel syndrome. The paresthesia was felt in the palmar aspect of the right hand covering the middle and index fingers and thumb. The symptoms had been present for a week and had no apparent cause.

The patient had no history of wrist or neck pain. He is a controlled insulin-dependent diabetic but has no other medical history of relevance. He is a nonsmoker and works as a management consultant.

Velocity conduction studies were negative.

Objective Examination

The wrist and fingers had full range painfree movements. Isometric tests were negative. Phalen's and Tinnel's tests reproduced his symptoms as did sustained extension. Venous obstruction tests (circumferential pressure just above the wrist) were negative. Sensation over the hand was normal.

The scanning examination of the neck was negative.

Is the above information sufficient to make a diagnosis and initiate treatment?

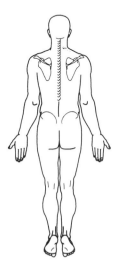

What are you thinking at this point? How will you proceed with the examination? ☞

Cervical Case 18 Continuation

The differential diagnoses with these symptoms are thoracic outlet syndrome, ulnar nerve entrapment at the elbow or wrist, cervical radiculopathy, and carpal tunnel syndrome. Cervical radiculopathies produce segmental symptoms. The closest distribution of paresthesia that would typically come from the neck would be due to pressure on the sixth nerve root. This could give paresthesia in the thumb, index finger, and the radial part of the middle finger but it is felt on the dorsal rather than the palmar aspect of the hand. Ulnar nerve entrapment would give paresthesia along the ulna border of the hand and two fingers. Thoracic outlet syndrome tends to affect the entire hand and frequently has a vascular component. All in all, carpal tunnel syndrome does seem the likeliest diagnosis. The negative nerve conduction velocity studies do not exclude the diagnosis but may simply not be sufficiently sensitive.

There is no obvious cause for the paresthesia, although the patient is an insulin-dependent diabetic and the paresthesia could be an early manifestation of diabetic neuropathy. However, the absence of cause could possibly indicate a double crush syndrome,[1] which could explain the negative nerve conduction studies. The upper limb neural tension tests can be useful in determining if a double crush syndrome exists. In this case, the tests for the median nerve components reproduced the symptoms when the neck was side flexed away from the symptomatic side.

This finding required a biomechanical examination, which demonstrated hypomobility with a pathomechanical (jammed) end feel of the right zygopophyseal joint of C5/6. A biomechanical examination of the wrist and elbow failed to find any dysfunction.

What are your thoughts on etiology and treatment?

---

1. A double crush syndrome occurs when neural tissue is compromised at two or more points, neither of which is sufficient alone to cause symptoms but, when taken together, become clinically significant because their combined contribution decreases axoplasmic flow.

Please turn to page 408 for solutions.

"Frozen Shoulder?"

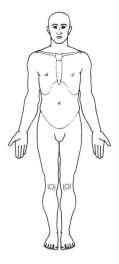

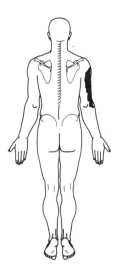

Subjective Examination

A 34-year-old woman complaining of right lateral arm pain is referred by her family doctor with a diagnosis of "frozen shoulder." The pain is felt over the lower part of the right deltoid and extends to the right lateral elbow. It had been present for 3 weeks initially as a mild ache but built up over 2 weeks to its present level. She could relate no obvious cause and had not undertaken any unusual activities with her upper limbs.

She had no history of similar pains and no medical history of note.

The pain was intermittent, being felt only on certain movements of the arm, which included lifting the arm from her side and putting it behind her back.

Objective Examination

Her cervical spine had full range motion. Apart from slight pain on extension and right rotation, she was painfree. There were no neurological deficits. The upper limb tension tests could not be carried out due to the limitation in her range of movement at the shoulder. Compression, traction, and posteroanterior pressures were negative.

Her shoulder was limited to 130° of elevation and 120° of abduction. Medial rotation was almost full range, but when combined with extension (as if you were putting your hand into your back pocket) was very limited and painful. Lateral rotation was almost full range and painfree with the arm by the side but limited if tested in abduction.

Isometric lateral rotation was painful and there was tenderness along the infraspinatus tendon.

The patient is exhibiting a noncapsular pattern of restriction,[2] excluding the diagnosis of frozen shoulder (capsulitis, adhesive capsulitis, or any of its other synonyms). However, to confirm this, an evaluation of the glenohumeral joint's glide needs to be undertaken.

The presence of pain on isometric testing of lateral rotation coupled with limitation of medial rotation/extension and tenderness along the tendon would argue strongly for a diagnosis of infraspinatus tendonitis.

289

Biomechanical testing of the shoulder demonstrated that all glides and lateral traction were normal. This effectively eliminates articular restrictions as a cause of her range limitation.

2. According to Cyriax, this is most often a limitation of lateral rotation, then abduction, and least of all limitation of medial rotation.

What are you thinking at this point? How will you proceed with the examination?   ☞

Cervical Case 19 Continuation

If the joint is not limiting her cervical movement, the muscles must be causing the restriction. Given the time frames the muscle's inextensibility can only be due to hypertonia and not to structural shortening. One cause of hypertonicity of this type is cervical joint dysfunction. To include the neck as contributory, oscillatory general cervical traction was applied for a minute or so and the shoulder re-examined. Elevation increased to 160° and abduction to 150°. Medial rotation/extension was still limited and painful.

A biomechanical examination revealed hypomobility into extension at the right T1/2 and an extension hypermobility at C6/7 and C7/T, both of which were slightly painful.

Diagnose and treat!

Please turn to page 408 for solutions.

A Third Case of Torticollis

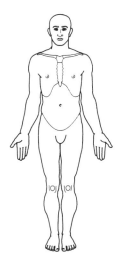

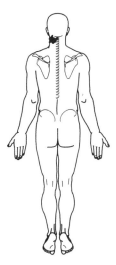

Subjective Examination

A 15-year-old girl is referred with a diagnosis of torticollis. She complains of left suboccipital pain that has been present on and off for 10 months. The onset had no apparent cause and started as severe suboccipital pain and the torticollis. This pain was relieved with physical therapy in about 4 weeks. It recurred about a month later, again for no apparent cause. On this occasion, physical therapy did not help. She tried chiropractic treatments with very limited relief. An X-ray taken at this time was negative.

Within a month from the onset of this episode, the torticollis disappeared but the patient continued to feel a mild to moderate level of pain. The next episode of acute pain and torticollis occurred 3 weeks later and lasted for 4 weeks. When the acute pain and torticollis abated again, she continued to feel constant aching in the suboccipital region that was more severe than the previous pain. The constant pain between episodes was rapidly and profoundly relieved by one tablet of aspirin taken 4 times a day and the patient was managing this pain well with this medication.

Two more episodes of acute pain and torticollis followed with the period between each episode being filled with an increasingly intense suboccipital ache. She saw an orthopedic surgeon during this episode. His diagnosis was "torticollis due to mechanical strain." He told her that this condition would clear up and was probably just growing pains. (She had grown an inch in the previous 4 months.) The most recent episode started one week ago and her physician decided to try physical therapy again.

She was very active before this problem started. She played volleyball and baseball, and she skied and skated during the winter. She had no history of this type of condition nor any medical history of note.

What are you thinking at this point? How will you proceed with the examination? ☞

Cervical Case 20 Continuation

A few things must be considered. First, she is at the upper age limit for adolescent torticollis, plus this condition more commonly affects boys than girls. Second, the torticollis did not clear quickly as it invariably does with uncomplicated adolescent torticollis. Third, it has recurred frequently. Fourth, she had constant pain between episodes. Fifth, there was no cause.

Objective Examination

On observation there was a torticollis rotating her neck to the right. Any attempt at correcting this torticollis caused severe pain and spasm. Left rotation was impossible, being restricted by severe spasm and reproducing pain in the left upper neck. Right rotation was painless and full range. Flexion was full range and painfree. Extension was very painful and limited to about 30° by spasm. Right-side flexion was full range and painless. Left-side flexion was severely limited by spasm and produced severe pain.

There were no neurological deficits. Light compression was painful. Posteroanterior pressures were negative. She was extremely tender to palpation over the right neural arch of the third cervical vertebra.

How would you diagnose and treat this patient?

Please turn to page 409 for solutions.

A High-Speed Rear-End Collision

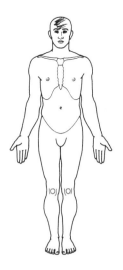

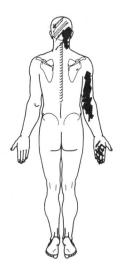

Subjective Examination

A 60-year-old man is referred a week after being involved in a motor vehicle accident. He complained of right upper neck pain and right occipital headaches and another more diffuse headache that is felt deeper and more centrally. He is experiencing pain in the posterior aspects of the upper and lower right arm and paresthesia in the right three middle digits. He also complains of dizziness.

He was rear-ended at high speed (80 kph or 50 mph) while unprepared. He was looking to the left, attempting to make a left turn. He did not strike his head nor suffer any other direct trauma.

He experienced onset of neck pain and occipital headache within 15 minutes of the accident. The occipital headache was continuous but varied in intensity, being worse when he was overactive and when his neck was particularly painful. The cervical pain was intermittent. He woke each morning with neck pain and increased headache. The cervical pain also worsened with rapid and unguarded movements.

The more diffuse onset of headache started 3 days after the accident and had been worsening. It was present at all times and was not made better or worse with movements or position of the neck. The headache was a little worse now than it had been after the accident.

The paresthesia began the day after the accident and had remained stable. It was worsened whenever the patient bent his head backward and sometimes on waking in the morning.

On direct questioning, the patient experienced two different types of dizziness, the type 2 dizziness with lightheadedness, nausea, and unsteadiness in quality, and the type 1 dizziness, feeling that he was spinning to the right. The type 2 dizziness became noticeable when his head was rotated and extended to the right. The vertigo was present when turning his head suddenly to the right and often occurred with the type 2 dizziness but also occurred alone. The vertigo lasted for about a minute after its onset and was accompanied by severe nausea, which lasted for about an hour after the vertigo terminated.

He had no history of neck pain but did have periodic headaches for no apparent cause about once a month.

What are you thinking at this point? How will you proceed with the examination? ☞

Cervical Case 21 Continuation

This man's most important symptom is the diffuse headache. The concern here is with intracranial bleeding. The headache is worsening and is atypical of cervicogenic headaches. In addition, the impact velocity had been sufficient to cause intracranial bleeding. If the patient relates any problems with mental acuity such as drowsiness, concentration difficulties, or anything similar, he must be referred back to the physician immediately.

The second most potentially serious symptoms are the two types of dizziness. The worry here is that the dizziness is due to vertebrobasilar insufficiency. The patient must be questioned about cranial nerve symptoms (such as blurred vision or other visual deficits, hypoacusis, tinnitus, facial and perioral numbness, dysphagia, dysarthria, or dysphonia) and long tract symptoms (such as hemilateral, bilateral, or quadrilateral paresthesia, and ataxia). However, the absence of these symptoms cannot exclude vertebral artery pathology.

The near immediate onset of cervical pain raises concerns about profound tissue damage such as fractures and ligamentous damage. Careful testing is required to exclude this possibility.

His prognosis is not good. The following aspects of his presentations indicate a poor prognosis: his age (the older patient does less well all things being equal), an immediate onset of pain, the presence of neurological symptoms (upper limb paresthesia), and the existence of preaccident headaches.

Objective Examination

The fracture tests were negative, except that he had very severe limited movements and multi-directional spasm end feels. The cranial nerve tests were negative. Craniovertebral stability tests were negative.

On dizziness testing, body-head tilting backward and to the right with the head and neck stabilized reproduced the patient's vertigo. Body rotation to the left under the stabilized head did not reproduce vertigo but did cause mild type 2 dizziness, which was also reproduced with head right rotation and extension. Hautard's test was negative.

All ranges were very restricted. Flexion was about 50% and reproduced upper cervical pain. Extension was only about 10% of the expected range and reproduced the headache, the upper cervical pain, and the paresthesia. Right-side flexion was only a few degrees and produced upper arm paresthesia. Left-side flexion was about 50% of the expected range and produced upper cervical pain. Right rotation was about 30° and caused arm paresthesia and upper cervical pain. Left rotation was about 45° and produced mild upper cervical pain.

There was decreased pinprick sensation over the dorsal aspect of the forearm and the middle three fingers. Elbow extension and wrist flexion was slightly weak and abnormally fatigable. The reflexes were normal. The extensor-plantar response was normal as were the ankle and knee jerks.

He stated that he had no cognitive problems.

Do you have a diagnosis and treatment plan or do you want to refer this patient back to his physician? If so, why? Also, do the objective findings support or weaken the poor prognosis?

Please turn to page 409 for solutions.

Vertebral Artery Injury: Was it Preventable?

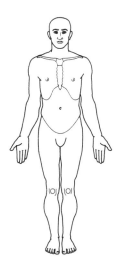

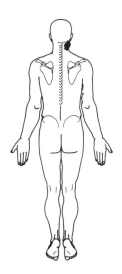

Subjective Examination

A 22-year-old woman complaining of moderate cervical pain attended a chiropractic clinic complaining of neck pain. The pain had been present for about 2 weeks and had no obvious cause. The patient did not relate any neurological symptoms, and did not suffer from dizziness or any other symptoms that might be ascribable to vertebrobasilar ischemia. This episode was her only experience with neck pain, although she suffered occasionally from low-back pain.

Aggravating and relieving factors were not documented, except to say that the pain was worse with activity. No current or past medical conditions were noted except two episodes of mononucleosis. Otherwise she was healthy. She had not received any past chiropractic care.

Objective Examination

Due to the lack of neurological or quasi-neurological symptoms, the practitioner did not carry out either a neurological or neurovascular examination.

He noted that there were restrictions at C6/7, T1–3, T5/6, and both sacroiliac joints.

Treatment

This particular chiropractor handed over her treatment to a colleague, who relied on the first assessment and a verbal summary of the examination findings from the initial practitioner. Manipulative treatments of multiple segments now also including the craniovertebral joints and the lumber joints were continued for 6 months.

On the next to last treatment (her nineteenth treatment), the cervical pain had increased substantially. The atlantooccipital and atlantoaxial joints were manipulated in addition to all of the other joints usually treated. On the next treatment 2 days later, she was still complaining of acute pain. Her mother said that the evening after the manipulation she was also complaining of clumsiness, dizziness, and nausea as well as an acute increase in her pain. The chiropractor subsequently and under oath denied what the patient's mother had said.

According to the chiropractor, the final treatment was a gentle side flexion manipulation of the C5/6 segment. Immediately after this, the patient began crying and saying that she under a lot of stress. The chiropractor noted that there was upwards and lateral deviation of the left eye. An ambulance was called and while waiting for the ambulance, the patient became unconscious and began decerebrate and decorticate posturing.

She died 3 days later of medullary compression caused by cerebellar tonsillar herniation, resulting from nonhemorrhagic infarction. The right vertebral artery was hypoplastic being only about one-fourth the average size (1 mm). The left vertebral artery, which was a little larger than usual (5 mm) and suffered intramural tearing. This tearing is believed to have occurred on the next to last manipulation and a number of emboli were thrown off. Thromboembolysis cleared emoboli in the vertebral and basilar artery but did not affect the one in the left posterior inferior cerebellar artery.

What if anything could have been done to prevent this tragedy from occurring?

Please turn to page 420 for solutions.

70-Year-Old Patient with Chest Pain

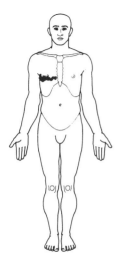

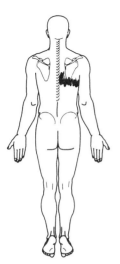

Subjective Examination

A 70-year-old woman attends complaining of severe burning pain and paresthesia running around the right side of her chest from the middle of the thoracic spine to the xiphoid process. The pain had started 2 days earlier, without apparent cause, as a sharp pain that turned into the current pain within a few hours. No movements or positions aggravated or relieved the constant pain. Any pressure on the painful area caused severe shooting pains around the trunk.

She had no history of similar pain, although she did have a history of occasional mild low-back pain if she spent too much time in the garden. She was also diabetic.

Her physician ordered X-rays, which were negative. Her diabetes was under control.

What are you thinking at this point? How will you proceed with the examination? 🖝

Thoracic Case 1 Continuation

The pain the patient describes is neurological in nature. It is also segmental running around the seventh or eighth thoracic dermatome. However, no cause is given for the pain and the pain does not appear to be mechanical in origin because it is constant and does not change with position or movement. The patient's age is cause for concern when there is no obvious underlying cause for her pain, and neoplastic disease is possible. At this point in the examination it seems to be neurological pain from a nonmusculoskeletal cause.

Objective Examination

The patient had full range thoracic movements, none of which altered her underlying pain. She was extremely sensitive to light or deep palpation anywhere along the painful region, and posteroanterior pressure over the eighth thoracic spinous process caused lancinating pain around the chest.

Sensation could not be tested because either light touch or pinprick caused too much pain for her to be aware of any sensation changes.

Neck flexion, straight leg raising, and slump testing were all negative as were deep inspiration and coughing.

How would you diagnose and treat this patient?

Please turn to page 412 for solutions.

Anterior Chest Pain

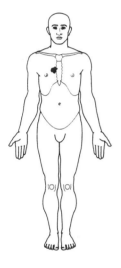

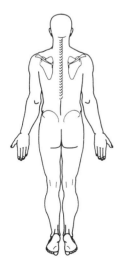

Subjective Examination

A 29-year-old female competitive white-water kayaker attended complaining of pain in her right anterior chest. The onset was 6 weeks earlier when she was using the paddle to backwater against a very strong eddy. She felt a sudden sharp pain in her right posterior chest at the mid-scapular level. This pain disappeared quickly and did not bother her again during the event. However, the next morning she woke with pain near the costochondral junction at about the fourth rib level. This anterior pain eased off over the next few days with rest but as soon as she started working out with weights it recurred.

The patient's physician referred her to a physical therapist with a diagnosis of costochondritis. The therapist treated the patient for 4 weeks with ultrasound to the costochondral junction, stretching exercises for the pectoralis major, and progressive strengthening exercises for the back extensors. The therapist's reasoning was that muscle imbalances had allowed the tight pectoralis major to disturb the costochondral joint. In this case, treatment did not help because as soon as the patient started to lift heavier weights, the anterior pain recurred.

The patient has now been referred to you for treatment of her anterior chest pain. What are you going to do?

What are you thinking at this point? How will you proceed with the examination? ☞

Thoracic Case 2 Continuation

First, you should examine the patient.

Objective Examination

On observation the patient was a healthy looking woman with no obvious postural deficit.

The patient had full range of thoracic movement with slight anterior pain on right rotation overpressure. The end feels were normal. Her cervical spine was also full range and painfree.

The slump tests, neck flexion, and scapular retraction were negative. There were no neurological deficits.

Compression, traction, and posteroanterior pressures were all painfree.

Anteriorly, there was no swelling or thickening over any of the costochondral or chondrosternal junctions. However, anteroposterior pressure over the right fourth costochondral joint reproduced the patient's pain.

Where do you go from here? Can you make a diagnosis or eliminate any? Do you have a treatment plan in mind?

Please turn to page 412 for solutions.

60-Year-Old Patient with Low Thoracic Pain

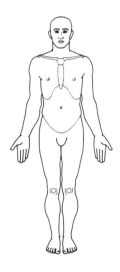

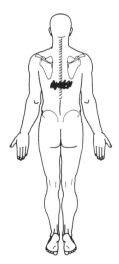

Subjective Examination

A 60-year-old woman complains of central lower thoracic pain of unknown etiology. The onset was 3 weeks earlier and sudden. Upon waking one morning she felt an ache across her lower thoracic area, which worsened a little that day, but then improved. She has had no history of similar pain. The pain is worse when sitting and easier when lying. The pain was neither constant nor consistent from day to day. Her X-rays were negative, and she was taking Tylenol 3 with some effect for the pain.

The patient is a retired nurse and has no medical history of significance. She used to have mild low-back pain, which had not troubled her since retiring.

Objective Examination

There was nothing remarkable on observation. She was a robust woman who looked slightly younger than her years.

Thoracic flexion was full range but painful. Both rotations and side flexions were negative. Extension was full range but slightly painful.

Slump testing was negative. There were no neurological signs. Posteroanterior pressures over T8 and T9 were moderately painful. Compression reproduced her pain, whereas traction had no effect.

Because there was nothing to hang a diagnosis from, a type of biomechanical examination was undertaken. This was position testing of the thoracic spine. The position tests revealed an ERSL at T8; that is, positionally, T8 was relatively flexed rotated and side flexed. Pressure was applied the left transverse process of T8 to try to glide the superior facet of the left zygopophyseal joints superiorly and anteriorly as it would move during flexion. A hard end feel was encountered that was interpreted as being the result of a subluxation (pathomechanical hypomobility).

What are you thinking at this point? How will you proceed with the examination? ☞

305

Thoracic Case 3 Continuation

Diagnosis My diagnosis of this patient was an extension subluxation of the left zygopophyseal joint. This was based on the position and the positive glide.

Treatment There did not seem to be any real indication of osteoporosis. Her ribs were nice and resilient. She had no history of pathological fractures or anything that might suggest them.

The patient was manipulated three times. Each time she reported improvement immediately after in that she was almost painfree when her movements were tested. However, each time she came back, she reported that the pain had recurred within an hour or two and was bad as ever.

How should her treatment proceed?

Please turn to page 413 for solutions.

Pain After Playing Squash

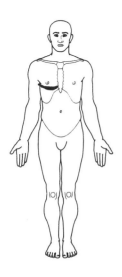

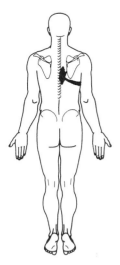

Subjective Examination

A 32-year-old woman is referred complaining of pain in the right paravertebral midthoracic area with lancinating pain running around to the right anterior chest just lateral to the sternum. The onset occurred while playing squash a week earlier when she twisted violently to hit a ball going to her right. She felt a sudden onset of pain in the posterior midthoracic area that was worse a few hours later. The next morning she had severe posterior pain with lancinating pain around the right chest. The pain was present to some degree at all times but was severe with unguarded movements of the trunk, arm overhead movements, and coughing. Deep inspiration was painful, and she tended to breathe shallowly to prevent any pain from breathing.

Sharp posterior somatic pain woke her in the night when she turned onto her right side. She was unable to stay in any one position for very long, although she was more comfortable lying on her left side and least comfortable while standing and sitting.

She had no history of any similar pains nor did she have any medical history of note. She was currently off work as a police officer.

Her physician diagnosed her as suffering from thoracic facet syndrome and prescribed Naprosyn and physical therapy in the form of ice, ultrasound, and exercises.

Objective Examination

The patient was in obvious distress and guarding her movements very carefully. There were no deformities, although she did tend to stand a little flexed and left rotated in her thorax.

She had almost no movement in the thoracic spine. Flexion was limited to a few degrees and she deviated to the left. Extension was zero in that she was unable to move out of her slightly flexed position. Right-side flexion was 0° and left-side flexion about 15°. Right rotation was 0° and left about 30°. Her lancinating pain was reproduced on extension and right rotation. Sharp somatic posterior right midthoracic pain was experienced with the other movements. Neck flexion and the slump test provoked sharp posterior pain.

There were no neurological signs.

Posteroanterior pressures over T5/6 caused sharp posterior pain as did traction and compression of the thoracic spine.

Do you have a diagnosis and treatment plan?

What are you thinking at this point? How will you proceed with the examination? ☞

Thoracic Case 4 Continuation

Diagnosis It is unlikely that this is a "facet syndrome." The pain that the patient is experiencing is neurological. It is possible that the zygopophyseal joint did become inflamed or even fractured by the injury. The nerve has been inflamed by contact with an inflamed tissue, but the pattern of restriction of motion is not typical of even very acute zygopophyseal arthritis. The delay in the onset of immediate severe somatic pain until the next morning would tend to argue against a fracture.

The lancinating pain indicates neurological inflammation and/or adhesions. The delay in the onset of the lancinating pain suggests that inflammation is the more likely cause. The site of the lancinating pain indicates that a spinal nerve or nerve root is compromised. The degree of articular restriction plus the mode of onset would suggest mechanical compression of the nerve by disk prolapse. The level of the compression is probably the thoracic fifth or sixth segments given the location of the radicular pain and the pain reproduction with posteroanterior pressures at these levels.

The lack of neurological signs is not uncommon in this part of the spine. Weakness and sensory loss are difficult if not impossible to detect at this level of the spine. However, there is an outside chance that Beevor's test (abdominal contraction causing umbilical deviation) might be positive if the sixth thoracic myotome is playing a part in the innervation of the abdominals. However, this is unlikely.

The diagnosis is midthoracic (T5/6 or T6/7) disk prolapse with nerve root compression.

Treatment In this case there are no red flags to suggest a serious disease but the presence of a disk prolapse in itself requires careful treatment. Perhaps initially, the best course of action would be to try to decrease the degree of inflammation present. To this end, the physician's request for ice and ultrasound can be complied with. Additional treatment could involve interferrential current therapy, acupuncture, TENS, and other such pain-reducing modalities. Taping the area often helps to cue the patient to avoid exacerbating movements and was used in this patient. The patient must be advised on resting positions and the need to minimize the frequency of the episodes of lancinating pain.

In this case, a week of such treatment had no effect. What course of action would you take now?

Please turn to page 414 for solutions.

Pain After the Flu

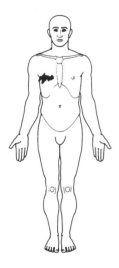

Subjective Examination

A 58-year-old woman complains of right lateral and anterior mid-chest pain of 8 day's duration. She had a sudden onset of pain while coughing during a bout of flu. The pain, which was severe, was felt mainly when she turned in either direction, on coughing, and on deep inspiration. It woke her suddenly during the night, but she had no difficulty in getting to sleep.

She had no history of thoracic pain, and she denied any medical history of note.

From this lady's history, do you have any provisional diagnosis?

What are you thinking at this point? How will you proceed with the examination? ☞

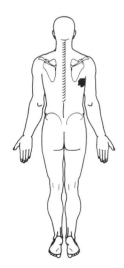

311

Thoracic Case 5 Continuation

Prolonged fits of coughing can cause mechanical disturbances of the spinal and/or costal joints and may also cause rib fractures. Given this patient's age and the sudden onset of the pain, this must be the primary consideration.

Objective Examination

Because of the possibility of a rib fracture being present, no overpressures were applied after the active movement tests. Both active rotations were severely limited (about 25% of the expected range). Active flexion and extension were full range and painfree. Right-side flexion was very painful and left-side flexion was moderately painful.

Careful isometric tests in the neutral position elicited painful weakness in both rotations and right-side flexion.

No neurological deficits were found. Among the neuromeningeal tests, neck flexion and the slump test were negative, whereas deep inspiration reproduced her pain.

Are you still leaning toward a diagnosis of rib fracture? If so, are there any other tests that might support your diagnosis? Or, do you have some other diagnosis in mind or other tests that you would like to do?

Please turn to page 414 for solutions.

"Tietze's Syndrome?"

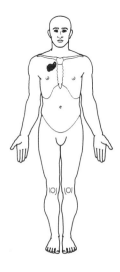

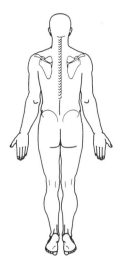

Subjective Examination

A 23-year-old man complaining of very localized anterior chest pain about 2 inches right of lateral to the sternum is diagnosed with "Tietze's syndrome" (costochondritis). The pain had been present for 3 weeks and came on gradually with no specific incident precipitating it, although the day before he was competing in a white-water kayaking competition. The pain was present when he thought about it, but was worse on heavy exertion, he was unable to kayak strenuously or work out with weights if it involved his shoulders.

He had no history of similar pain and had been kayaking competitively for about 5 years, the last 2 at national and international level. He denied any medical history of significance.

Objective Examination

There was very local and acute tenderness over the costal cartilage of the third right rib. There was very slight palpation over the chondrium, and posterior pressure on the sternum reproduced the pain as did isometric bilateral horizontal adduction of the arms.

Do you agree with the physician's diagnosis? If so, what will your treatment plan consist of? If you do not agree, do you have a diagnosis? If not, what other tests would you like to do?

What are you thinking at this point? How will you proceed with the examination? ☞

Thoracic Case 6 Continuation

Given the site of the pain, the very local and acute tenderness, the swelling and the positive isometric test for the pectoralis major (this causes compression), the diagnosis does seem to be correct. However, we are not ready to treat the problem, because a cause has not been established, even though it seems obvious. Local treatment is likely to fail or at best be temporary if we do not do something about the presumed ongoing stress to this area. If we are going to argue that it was the kayaking, then the question must be why now after all these years? Why this particular costochondrium? And why the chondrium in any case? This is not a common source of pain, and it seems likely that the posterior joints would have suffered before the anterior joints as they usually do.

Where do we look?

Please turn to page 415 for solutions.

Visceral Pain?

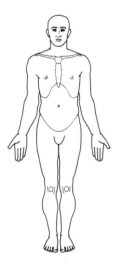

Subjective Examination

A 57-year-old woman presents with right posterior and lateral chest pain and left posterior chest pain at the midthoracic levels. The pain is felt as a continuous ache but is worse with movements of the trunk, especially if unguarded. The onset of her condition followed helping her sister move a large trunk. The pain started a few hours later and reached its present level by the next day.

The patient's medical history included congestive cardiac disease and a bout of right lobar pneumonia 15 years earlier. She had shortness of breath on exertion but otherwise was functioning well.

Objective Examination

Right and left trunk rotations reproduced her pain and were limited by spasm. Right-side flexion was full range and painfree, whereas left-side flexion was full range but provoked her pain. Flexion and extension were full range and negative. But flexion combined with left-side flexion was painful.

There were no neurological deficits.

Do you have a diagnosis and treatment plan or do you need further information?

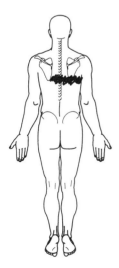

What are you thinking at this point? How will you proceed with the examination? ☞

315

Thoracic Case 7 Continuation

Some elements about this case should make you uncomfortable. These include the patient's age and history of cardiac and pulmonary problems. On the other hand, there was a definite incident related to the onset of the pain.

The scan examination did not provide enough information to determine a treatment plan and so a biomechanical examination was necessary.

Position testing showed an ERSR (the right transverse process was posterior in flexion suggesting a flexion hypomobility of the right zygopophyseal joint). This patient was seen in the days when I was playing with position testing and a true biomechanical examination, which includes passive physiological movements and joint glides was not carried out.

Diagnosis was segmental hypomobility of T6/7. Treatment should have been mobilization of the affected segment and conditioning exercises. Do you agree with the diagnosis and treatment?

Please turn to page 415 for solutions.

Post-MVA Neck and Back Pain

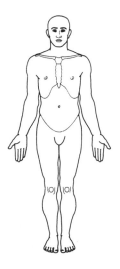

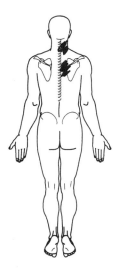

Subjective Examination

A 23-year-old woman is referred complaining of right lower cervical and right interscapular pain following a motor vehicle accident 3 weeks ago. The car that she was driving was hit from the rear at high speed (estimated to be 45 mph or 70 kph). She did not strike her head nor was she knocked unconscious. She could remember everything about the accident. She stated that she was unprepared for the impact and was looking forward when her car was hit.

The scapular pain was immediate and severe, even though the worst cervical pain was delayed until the next morning upon waking. Since the accident, she had been taking anti-inflammatories and until last week was off work. The pain had improved generally over this period until she returned to work as a waitress. Then the thoracic pain increased to its immediate postaccident level. The neck pain, although a little more sore at the end of the work day, had actually improved somewhat since returning to work.

She denied any history of neck or upper back pain. She also denied any paresthesia. She had no medical history of relevance.

From the history do you think that the interscapular pain is from a local source or referred from the cervical spine? (This case could have easily gone into the cervical section as the thoracic section.)

Does she have a good or bad prognosis?

What are you thinking at this point? How will you proceed with the examination? 🖅

Thoracic Case 8 Continuation

The source of the interscapular pain is most likely local. The onset was not only separate from the cervical pain's onset but was immediate even though the cervical pain's onset was delayed. Although somatic referred pain can, unusually, be more severe than the pain at its source, it is usually spontaneous with or secondary to the source pain, not leading it. Additionally, the cervical pain made better gains than the interscapular pain during her rest period. Generally as things improve, the referred pain either starts to centralize or diminishes. Also the exacerbation caused by the return to work increased the interscapular pain but not the cervical pain. It seems fairly clear that the association between them is tenuous at best.

The prognosis is mixed in this case. The immediate onset of severe interscapular pain may suggest structural damage. As a consequence, a delayed recovery should not surprise anybody. Added to this is the relapse when she returned to work, suggesting that the condition causing the interscapular pain is going to take considerably longer before it will allow the region to tolerate her normal stresses. The cervical spine on the other hand had a delayed onset and recovered and did tolerate her working stresses. Although she was unprepared for the impact, which may afford a poor prognosis, she did not have her head rotated or extended, which bodes well.

Objective Examination

On cranial nerve testing and segmental testing, she demonstrated no neurological signs.

In the cervical spine, right rotation and extension reproduced her low cervical pain and extension additionally provoked her interscapular pain. Right rotation was limited to about 70° and extension to about 50% of the expected range. Flexion pulled in the interscapular region but was full range. All other cervical movements were painfree and full range.

Compression and traction tests were negative. Posteroanterior pressure over C5 and C6 produced local pain. Her thoracic movements were all full range and painfree. Right shoulder elevation was about 160° and produced pain on top of the shoulder. Left shoulder elevation was negative. Compression and traction were negative and posteroanterior pressure over T3 was tender.

Do the results of the objective examination support or refute your ideas on the association between the cervical and interscapular pains? Are you ready to make a diagnosis and treatment plan, or do you require further information? If so, what clinical tests are required?

Please turn to page 416 for solutions.

A Rugby Injury

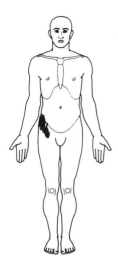

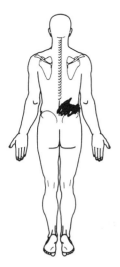

Subjective Examination

A 28-year-old man complains of right upper to lower lumbar pain with radiation around the right iliac crest to reach the outer groin and upper thigh. The onset of the pain was sudden but moderate 2 weeks earlier. He stated that he had been hit in the lower back while playing rugby. The initial pain was felt in the lower back and was worse the next morning. While working that day as an electrician, the pain had increased and spread to the area as described. Recently the pain in the back had localized to the right side but apart from that, there had been no change except when provoked.

The patient stated that prolonged standing, working overhead, and rapid walking all worsened the symptoms especially in the lumbar region. Sitting and side lying eased the pain, whereas supine or prone lying increased the symptoms.

He had no history of lumbar pain or of any significant health problems. There was no bladder or bowel dysfunction. The patient is a graduate student who admits to smoking and drinking to excess at times.

Objective Examination

The patient is healthy looking, of average weight for his build, and stands in a "normal" posture with no atrophy or unusual creases in the lumbar region.

Extension and right-side flexion were both limited to about 25% of their expected ranges. Both reproduced mid to low lumbar pain with a spasm end feel. Flexion, both rotations, and left-side flexion were mildly painful at the ends of their ranges with normal end feels. Compression was negative, but the general torsion test reproduced lumbar pain and spasm when tested into right rotation. Posteroanterior pressures over L3 and L4 were locally painful and produced some spasm. Isometric testing of the trunk muscles was negative.

The sacroiliac primary stress tests were negative but on testing the sacroiliac kinetic tests, the right ipsilateral step (Gillette's test or Stork test) and the right standing flexion tests were postive. Neurological tests

were all negative.
Diagnose, prognose, and treat.

What are you thinking at this point? How will you proceed with the examination?   ☞

Case 1 Continuation

Diagnosis As with all cases of traumatic onset, fracture must be suspected. In this case, transverse process fracture is the most likely fracture, if it is a fracture. However, from the history, the peak onset of pain was delayed. This delay suggests that a fracture, which generally will cause immediate severe pain, is not present. In addition to this, isometric hip flexion carried out during the neurological tests was negative. If a transverse process had been fractured, painful weakness would probably have resulted.

Another consideration is soft tissue bruising due to contusion of the erector spinae and/or quadratus lumborum muscles. However, no bruising was observed and isometric testing of the trunk was negative. Additionally, if these muscles were injured, you could expect to find contralateral side flexion being painful when it stretches the damaged tissues; in fact, ipsilateral side flexion was painful and reduced.

The negative primary sacroiliac stress tests and the location of the pain tend to rule out sacroiliitis. Positive sacroiliac kinetic tests suggest sacroiliac dysfunction; however, these tests are often falsely positive in the presence of lumbar spine problems. As a consequence, their only value at the moment is to indicate that the sacroiliac joint should be assessed once the lumbar spine has been cleared.

The levels affected are probably L3/4 and L4/5 given the presence of positive anteroposterior pressures over L3 and L4. The spasm end feel on these pressures suggests an acute lesion, probably arthritis. The loss of extension and right-side flexion with a spasm end feel could also suggest traumatic arthritis of the zygopophyseal joint(s). The general torsion test may be positive due to compression of the inflamed zygopophyseal joints rather than due to instability.

Because no definitive diagnosis can be made from the results of the examination, it is very unlikely that there is severe damage. The most likely diagnosis is posttraumatic arthritis of the L3/4 and/or L4/5 levels.

The patient requires a biomechanical examination to obtain further information about the lumbar and sacroiliac joints. The biomechanical assessment demonstrated that combined segmental extension and right-side flexion of the L3/4 segment was severely limited with a spasm end feel, whereas the L4/5 segment moved through its full range. Passive testing of the sacroiliac joints was negative. The biomechanical assessment supports the hypothesis of posttraumatic arthritis and localizes it to the L3/4 segment and to the right zygopophyseal joint specifically.

How would you treat this patient and what is his prognosis?

Please turn to page 417 for solutions.

Too Long Driving!

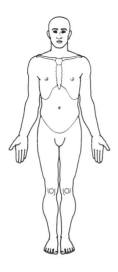

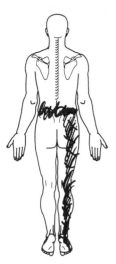

Subjective Examination

A 39-year-old man complained of a severe aching pain across his lower back, with radiation into the right buttock, posterior thigh, calf, and lateral foot and two toes. He also complained of severe lancinating pain into the posterior right leg on trunk flexion, which disappears on standing upright but increases in the lower back, buttock, and leg for a few minutes afterwards. Paresthesia in the posterolateral calf and lateral plantar aspect of the foot and two toes was also experienced when sitting.

The onset of the symptoms was 2 weeks earlier with right low-back pain after driving for 6 hours without a break. Over the next few days the pain increased due, the patient believed, to further sitting at work as a computer program designer. The back pain increased and spread to both sides of the back. The ache began first in the buttock and gradually over a day or two spread down the leg. The lancinating pain and paresthesia had been a recent development starting 2 days earlier. The paresthesia was associated mainly with prolonged sitting and for an hour or two after experiencing the lancinating pain. The pain was worse with prolonged sitting especially in a soft chair and was painful for the first few minutes on standing from sitting. Walking was difficult, especially the first few steps, and had to be done slowly. He was most comfortable in right-side lying with the hip and knees flexed.

This man has a history of minor back pain after comparatively heavy exertion such as prolonged yard work but nothing that had caused more than a few hours discomfort or that required treatment.

The patient denied any medical history of significance and appeared in good health. He reported no recent change in health status. He does not smoke or drink alcohol. He has no problem with bladder, bowel, or genital function.

Objective Examination

The patient is healthy looking but slightly obese and looks young for his age. He stands with a moderate kyphosis and a rotoscoliosis convex to the right with the right knee slightly flexed.

The patient had severe restriction of lumbar movement. Flexion was limited to about 30° from his kyphotic start position if the right knee was kept flexed. If he attempted to straighten the knee, trunk flexion was zero. In both cases, attempted flexion produced lancinating pain in the posterior aspect of the right leg. Extension and right-side flexion was unobtainable and caused a sharp pain in the back, radiating into the right buttock and posterior thigh. Left-side flexion was about 25% limited and produced a moderate ache into the right lower back. Compression testing reproduced back, right buttock, and posterior thigh pain. Posteroanterior pressure over L4 and L5 were painful and provoked a spasm end feel.

The right SLR was unobtainable because the patient was unable to extend the knee without lancinating pain in the posterior right leg and hamstring spasm. Flexing the hip to 90° and extending the knee (Lasegue's test) allowed only 100° of knee flexion before the onset of radicular pain and spasm. Right ankle dorsiflexion in this position reproduced the lancinating pain. The left straight leg raise was limited by spasm to 55° and produced right low-back, right buttock, and posterior thigh pain. Neither neck flexion or left ankle dorsiflexion in conjunction with the SLR affected the patient. The slump/sitting SLR test reproduced the effects of the other SLR tests without change. Prone knee flexion was negative on both sides. Although the sacroiliac stress tests were negative, all of the sacroiliac joint kinetic tests on both sides were positive.

Dermatomal testing revealed some pinprick loss over the lateral border of the right foot and toe and over the skin of the posterolateral right calf. Myotomal tests demonstrated pronounced weakness of the right ankle plantar flexors and evertors. There was no change in the deep tendon reflexes of either leg. Spinal cord tests were negative.

List your concerns, if any. Then diagnose and treat.

What are you thinking at this point? How will you proceed with the examination? ☞

Lumbopelvic Case 2 Continuation

Diagnosis The onset, severe articular limitations, and neurological findings make this a fairly clear-cut case of uncontained (large prolapse or extrusion) herniation of the fifth lumbar disk with isolated compression of the first sacral spinal nerve and dural sheath causing sensory and motor paresis. Various studies have suggested that the most indicative test results for an uncontained disk herniation are severe articular signs, severe loss of straight-leg raise, a crossover straight-leg raise, and the presence of lancinating pain. Other studies have found that the spinal nerve only produces lancinating pain or causalgia and to do this, there must be either inflammation or preexisting neural adhesions.

From the crossover SLR and the unaffected adjunct neck flexion test, an axillary prolapse may be possible, although this is far from proven. The kinetic tests are irrelevant and should not have been carried out. With this degree of lumbar dysfunction, these tests almost have to be positive.

There are no red flags for this case as such, but there are plenty of yellow ones. A disk herniation can easily get worse. With the lancinating pain and neurological signs, the need for caution is being screamed by this patient's presentation. Progression to a cauda equina syndrome is possible.

Treatment Although manipulation has been advocated for disk herniation, mainly by chiropractors, the success rate is not very high, whereas the risk of exacerbation and worsening is. Even if this progression is a natural one, independent of your intervention, you are in close proximity and likely to be blamed.

Correcting the shift a la McKenzie is not likely to be very successful with a herniation as obvious as this one. More likely the attempt will cause spasm and possibly reproduce the patient's symptoms. However, a trial attempt is unlikely to be dangerous and, if it fails, do not waste time by repeating this. Similarly, exercises alone are not likely to be curative. However, if you are going to try exercises, make sure that they do not reproduce the patient's symptoms.

Rest is always an option in acute cases. There is evidence that the lancinating pain and even the neurological symptoms may be caused by chemical irritation and/or simple contact with the escaped nucleus pulposis material rather than simple compression. Simple spinal nerve or root compression has been demonstrated to produce motor and sensory paresis and paresthesia but not pain, unless the compression is against the dorsal root ganglion, which of course is a possibility in this case. However, rest is still a good and safe bet. Let the patient select his own position, providing that it does not produce pain either at the time or afterward. Changing positions is almost invariably required, and selected careful painless activities and exercises are useful. Being guided by the

pain, especially the lancinating pain, will reduce the contact with the irritated nervous tissue and should help to lessen the inflammation. In
general, the patient should avoid sitting, bending, and lifting and should
be shown how to use pillows to support the legs while lying.

Mechanical traction may be used with caution in the position of deviation. Usually if the traction tends to correct the deviation, the patient
has serious trouble when the traction lets off. These notorious cases can
take hours getting a patient off of traction. If this is an axillary prolapse,
traction may be more effective, if it is reversed; that is, the pull is from
the thorax rather than from the pelvis.

Prognosis Unless rest produces remarkable results (which it does sometimes), this patient is in trouble. The degree of neurological involvement,
especially when combined with movements other than flexion causing
lancinating pain, does not suggest a good prognosis with physical therapy. This patient may require surgery.

Having selected your treatment and administered it on four treatment
sessions, the patient returns on the third visit to tell you that although
the lancinating pain and aching are unchanged, the paresthesia has disappeared. What is your reaction?

Please turn to page 418 for solutions.

A Nurse with Back and Leg Pain—How Unusual

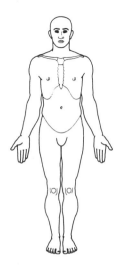

Subjective Examination

A 36-year-old female charge nurse with left low-back pain and left-sided nonlancinating sciatica of 3 months' duration. Onset was apparently without cause and was initially felt in the lower back a month before it radiated down the posterior left thigh, leg, and lateral heel and foot, with the leg pain becoming worse than the back pain. She had been treated by her physician with rest, analgesics, and a back support. She had recently received five sessions of chiropractic treatment with no improvement in her condition. She was able to continue work but was unable to do heavy lifting.

She complained of increased low-back pain when sitting for more than a few minutes, especially in a soft chair. If she sat for longer than half an hour, she experienced pain in the leg and foot. Walking did not increase the pain. In fact, it gradually eased the leg pain after sitting. She had no pain or problems with sleeping. She has no history of low-back pain or sciatica, and no relevant medical history. She does not smoke, but does drink alcohol socially.

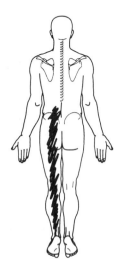

Objective Examination

Lumbar flexion was about 50% of her claimed normal range and reproduced low-back pain and posterior thigh and calf pain. Extension was 75% of the expected range and reproduced mild to moderate low-back pain. Right-side flexion was full range and painfree. Left-side flexion was about 75% of right-side flexion and reproduced low-back pain. Right straight leg raise was 80° and painless. Left straight leg raise was 60° and produced radiating left posterior thigh and calf pain. The neurological tests were negative. General torsion, compression, and traction tests were negative. Posteroanterior pressure was moderately painful over L5 and less so over L4.

Diagnose, prognose, and treat.

What are you thinking at this point? How will you proceed with the examination? ☞

Lumbopelvic Case 3 Continuation

Diagnosis The only yellow flags here are the lack of previous history or any obvious cause. The lack of radicular pain and neurological deficit would suggest the moderate nature of the condition. The straight leg raise limitation and the radiation of pain into the foot would tend to argue against an isolated zygopophyseal joint problem as would the extent of the pain referral. The possibility of a disk protrusion or small prolapse would tend to be supported by the relief of pain with extension activities (walking) and its worsening by flexion postures (sitting). The level could be the lumbosacral junction given the increased pain on posteroanterior pressure over L5. The most likely diagnosis is disk protrusion or herniation impinging on one of the dural sleeves of a lower lumbar spinal nerve or root. MRI demonstrated a posterolateral disk bulge to the left at L5/S1.

Treatment Given the relief of pain she experiences with walking, an extension program is indicated. Extension exercises of careful abdominal muscle reeducation and traction is recommended together with advice on sitting only in straight back chairs (and then only to a minimum), avoiding bending for prolonged periods, and reducing lifting to a minimum (and when lifting is required to do so without flexing the spine). Muscle stimulation to try to encourage extension of the segment may help. As the patient improves (if she improves), more strenuous exercises using the principles of stabilization therapy and also moving into flexion can be carefully initiated to reeducate movements in all directions. However, the move toward a flexion exercise program must be made cautiously. The pain should be confined to the back and buttock. She should be able to sit without any problems and the straight leg raise should be normal or near normal.

Manual therapy may be a possibility but it must be done carefully, avoiding rotation. The fact that the chiropractor had not done any harm suggests that it will not help even though it is unlikely to worsen her condition. It might be best to try some of the alternatives listed above before manipulating this lady. In this case, treatment over a 6-week period helped. The leg pain disappeared and the back pain was reduced to a mild ache after prolonged sitting. However, 2 months after discharge from physical therapy, the lumber pain suddenly worsened for no apparent reason and became almost continuous, with relief only to be had when she laid in the fetal position. Radiating pain was felt in the right posterior thigh. Radicular pain was experienced 4 days later while attempting to bend and was felt in the posterior thigh, leg, and lateral foot. She complained of paresthesia in the heel, lateral border of the foot, and lateral two toes. She had not worked since the onset of the radicular pain.

Objective Examination

She was mildly kyphotic and deviated to the left. Lumbar extension was impossible and reproduced radicular pain. She was able to flex about 20° from her kyphotic position so that her hands could reach to about mid thigh when there was severe radicular pain in the right leg. Both side flexions were limited to about 50% of their range and produced leg pain. The left straight leg reached about 60° and reproduced back pain. The right straight leg raise was 30° and reproduced the radicular pain. There was moderate fatigable weakness of the right hamstrings and gastrocnemius and reduction of the ankle jerk on the right. The patient reported decreased sensation to pinprick over the lateral border of the heel, foot, and the lateral two toes. Compression increased her back pain but did not affect her leg. Traction had no effect, whereas both torsions reproduced back pain. Posteroanterior pressures over L4/5 were both extremely painful locally and evoked spasm.

Diagnose, treat, and discuss any concerns.

Please turn to page 418 for solutions.

Too Long Standing!

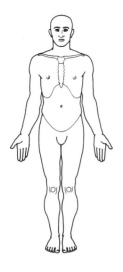

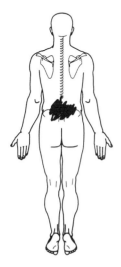

Subjective Examination

A 48-year-old man complained of central low-back pain of 3 weeks' duration. Onset followed prolonged standing while watching his son's baseball game. The initial onset occurred during the game and worsened over the next day to reach its current level of intensity that he described as moderate with exacerbations with rapid walking. The pain improved to a mild ache while sitting. He was unable to lay supine unless his hips and knees were flexed. He was often sore upon waking in the morning. He had no neurological symptoms or referred pain.

This was the fourth episode of this type of problem in the last year; the onset of the first two was associated with prolonged standing and the third onset occurred upon waking. Each episode had lasted about 4 weeks, gradually improving to become painfree when he avoided the postures and activities provoking the pain. He had not sought medical attention before this episode.

The pain had been improving for the last week but he saw the physician at his wife's urging to find out what the problem was and to try to prevent this from happening again.

The patient works as an insurance actuary with most of his duties involving sitting. His leisure activities include cross-country skiing and hiking although he had discontinued hiking since the onset of his back problems.

The physician had ordered x-rays, which showed mild to moderate disk narrowing and degenerative changes at L4/5 and L5/S1.

He has no medical history of relevance. He smokes heavily and drinks alcohol moderately.

What are you thinking at this point? How will you proceed with the examination? ☞

Lumbopelvic Case 4 Continuation

The behavior of the symptoms just about eliminates a diagnosis of disk herniation. Extension is the causative and aggravating factor of the symptoms, whereas flexion reduces them. Central stenosis behaves in this manner but there are no leg symptoms in this case and the patient is a little too young for this condition. A possible diagnosis is spondylolisthesis, which produces stenosis both lateral and central.

Objective Examination

On observation, the patient is overweight, but not seriously obese, carrying most of his excessive weight in his abdomen. He is more lordotic in the lumbar spine than average but otherwise appears healthy.

He had full range movement in all directions with mild pain on extension. Recovery from the fully flexed position was accomplished by deviating to the right and extending his hips before extending his lumbar spine so that he came up with a rounded back, which he straightened near the vertical position. At full flexion, the lumbosacral segment was rounded instead of straight or concave. Posteroanterior pressures over L5 were painful centrally but had normal end feels.

There were no neurological deficits. Both straight leg raises and prone knee flexion tests were negative.

Diagnose, prognose, and treat.

Please turn to page 419 for solutions.

Buttock Pain After Gardening

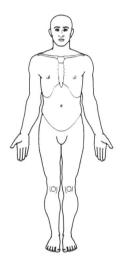

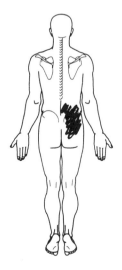

Subjective Examination

A 50-year-old man complaining of right low-back and right buttock pain of 2 weeks' duration attends for treatment. The onset of pain occurred a couple of hours after gardening. The pain was initially felt in the right low back and spread to the buttock by mid-morning of the next day after sitting in his office for 2 hours. The patient had tolerated the pain for the first 3 days but sitting, and therefore work, increased his pain. He was finding it increasingly difficult to do his job, which was almost entirely sedentary. He saw his family doctor who prescribed analgesics and muscle relaxants, but these barely took the edge off the pain. Sitting increased his pain in both areas, whereas standing and walking improved it. He was sleeping well and had no increased pain in the morning. There was no radicular pain or paresthesia and no referral below the buttock, as well as no bladder problems.

He has a history of occasional low-back pain (never into the buttock before) over the previous 2 years, usually associated with prolonged driving or remaining in a bent position for some time. The pain had been until now self-limiting within a week or so, and he had never received any treatment prior to this. He has no medical history relevant to this pain. The patient does not smoke but does drink an occasional beer.

Objective Examination

The patient did not show any postural abnormalities or deformities. Flexion was limited to his fingertips reaching just below the knees when normally he could touch his toes. Flexion also caused strong right low-back pain. Extension was mildly limited and reproduced mild right low-back pain. Right-side flexion was a little less than left, producing a discomfort in the right low back. The other movements were full range and painfree. There were no neurological deficits in the form of weakness, and sensory or reflex changes. The right straight leg raise produced pain in the right low back and was limited to 60° by spasm. Neck flexion and dorsiflexion of the ankle were negative because they did not alter the patient's straight leg raise pain. The left straight leg raise and both prone knee flexion tests were negative. The slump with right straight leg raise test provided the same result as the right straight leg raise.

Posteroanterior pressures over L4 and L5 were locally painful. Compression, traction, and torsion tests were negative.

What are you thinking at this point? How will you proceed with the examination? ☞

Lumbopelvic Case 5 Continuation

This case is typically difficult to diagnose. Everything about it looks like a disk lesion but in miniature. The articular and dural signs are marginal and there are no neurological signs or symptoms. Diagnosis could be a contained herniation (internal disruption) or a small protrusion. It could also be a zygopophyseal joint problem or a sacroiliac joint dysfunction.

A biomechanical examination of the spine and sacroiliac joint should provide further information even if that information is negative.

In this case, passive physiological intervertebral movement (PPIVM) extension and right-side flexion were limited at L4/5 with a springy end feel, but the passive accessory intervertebral movement (PAIVM) had a normal end feel. Flexion and left-side flexion were normal.

The right sacroiliac joint kinetic tests were positive because anterior rotation (extension) of the right ilium was limited as was extension of the left side of the sacrum. The passive movements of the sacroiliac joints were negative.

For those of you not versed in segmental examination, where would you go from here?

Please turn to page 419 for solutions.

Lancinating Thigh Pain

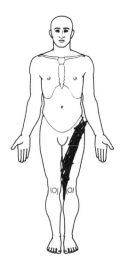

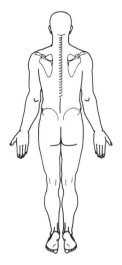

Subjective Examination

A 40-year-old man complaining of severe radicular (lancinating) pain and paresthesia in the anterolateral aspect of his left thigh is referred by his physician. The pain and paresthesia extend from an area just lateral to the anterior superior iliac spine in a band about 5 inches wide to the anteromedial aspect of the thigh just above the knee. The pain had been present for 2 weeks and had followed unaccustomed physical activity (he cleared his basement out). He felt the pain the same evening when he stood up from watching TV for an hour or so. He had no pain in the back at any point. An x-ray and CT scan were taken of his lumbar spine; both were negative.

Any unguarded movement caused severe leg pain. He was only comfortable in lying but he was able to move about slowly and carefully.

The physician's diagnosis, in the light of the negative CT scan, was atypical meralgia paresthetica and the treatment requested was ultrasound and pain-reducing modalities. The patient was taking analgesics that were not helping very much.

The patient's medical history is unremarkable. He does not smoke and drinks alcohol on social occasions.

What are your thoughts at this point? How will you proceed with the examination? ☞

Lumbopelvic Case 6 Continuation

The patient is suffering neurological pain along the second lumbar dermatome not the area of the lateral cutaneous nerve of the thigh, which is an oval area on the anterolateral aspect of the thigh. Disk herniations in the upper two lumbar levels are believed to be rare and we are taught to always suspect neoplastic disease when encountered. However, the mechanism of injury is very typical for a disk herniation but the lack of lumbar pain at any point in the history of the condition is atypical.

Objective Examination

The patient walked in with a severe antalgic gait favoring the right leg by keeping the hip and knee flexed. He stood in a slightly flexed posture and slightly deviated to the right, again with the hip and knee of the right leg flexed.

Range of movement testing disclosed that the patient was unable to move very far in any direction without severe thigh pain. Right-side flexion and flexion were his best movements but these were only about 10° out of his posture before they produced leg pain. All other attempts at movement were impossible and caused thigh pain.

Strength testing in side lying produced severe thigh pain when the hip flexors were tested and no conclusion was reached about their strength. The other muscles were normally strong. Sensation was tested and disclosed hyperesthesia and dysesthesia (tingling) on pinprick testing over the painful region. There were no changes in tendon reflexes.

A modified straight leg raise was tested in side lying and reproduced the thigh pain at 70° on the left and was negative on the right. The prone knee flexion was tested in the same position and with the hip flexed to about 60°. Left knee flexion reproduced his pain at 90°. The right prone knee flexion test was positive at 120°.

Posteroanterior pressures in the side lying position were negative.
What is your diagnosis, prognosis, and treatment?

Please turn to page 421 for solutions.

Leg Aching

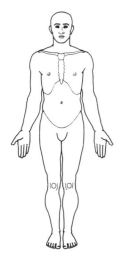

Subjective Examination

A 68-year-old man complaining of low-back and bilateral leg pain is referred to you with a diagnosis of low-back pain and a prescription for abdominal exercises. The back pain was felt centrally and was intermittent, coming on with fast walking for more than a few minutes, prolonged standing, and occasionally in the morning upon waking. The leg pain was posterior and equally bilateral and is an ache rather than a sharp pain provoked by the same activities and postures as the leg pain. The leg pain generally starts just after the onset of the back pain. After walking, sitting or flexing the trunk eased the pain, usually in about 15 minutes.

The pains had been present for about 10 years. The patient could not remember a specific onset or cause, but felt that the pains had gradually progressed. He had tried various medications and chiropractic treatments, all without relief. He had self-limited to those activities that did not provoke the pain. He was trying physical therapy as a last resort.

Where are your thoughts about a diagnosis, prognosis, and treatment? What do you expect the results of the objective examination to be?

What are you thinking at this point? How will you proceed with the examination? ☞

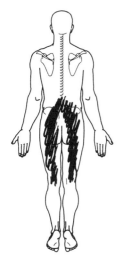

Lumbopelvic Case 7 Continuation

The pattern of provoking factors (extension postures and activities) suggest a stenotic problem of some kind. The bilateral sciatica would indicate a central stenosis of the lower lumbar spinal canal. The patient's symptoms and the relief gained by flexing the spine tends to support a diagnosis of central stenosis.

Developmental central stenosis, as opposed to that caused by spondylolisthesis, tends to have very little to see in the way of articular dural or neural signs. Most of the symptoms are produced by compression of the dural sleeves of the spinal nerves and roots or by ischemia of these structures and/or of the neural tissues themselves. If this were developmental central stenosis, I would not expect to see substantial articular, dural, or neurological signs.

Objective Examination

The patient is a thin man with no obvious deformity. The lumbar spine was hypolordotic compared with the average.

All lumbar movements were generally stiff with little extension occurring in the spine. Most of trunk extension was the result of hip flexion. Flexion was better but he was only able to reach to his knees. Both side flexions were equally limited to about 50% of their expected range. Both rotations were mildly limited. None of the movements were painful, although extension did produce some discomfort.

Both straight leg raises and prone knee flexion tests were negative. There were no neurological deficits.

Posteroanterior pressures over all of the lumbar vertebrae were painless but had a very stiff end feel. Torsion, traction, and compression tests were all negative.

What will be your diagnosis, prognosis, and treatment?

Please turn to page 421 for solutions.

Too Long Sitting, Two!

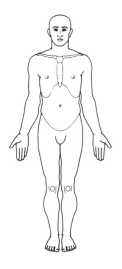

Subjective Examination

A 42-year-old man attends complaining of severe low-back pain, greater on the right than on the left, of a week's duration. The onset followed driving for 6 hours, an unusual activity for this patient. He was unable to get out of the car without extreme difficulty due to the pain. On sitting or bending, he had some radiation of pain into the right buttock and upper thigh. He was not experiencing any radicular pain or paresthesia and had no problems with his bladder. The pain had leveled off but was still intense if he bent forward or sat. He saw a chiropractor the day after the onset of pain, but two sessions of manipulation made the pain worse. He has a history of 10 years of episodic low-back pain that was unpredictable in its onsets. He had received treatment in the past from chiropractors with good results. The patient is a controlled diabetic, who otherwise has no medical history of note. He neither drinks nor smokes.

Objective Examination

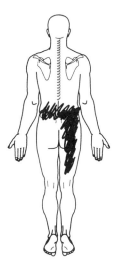

The patient was deviated so that his shoulder was shifted to the left with little curvature to the deviation. He was slightly flexed at the hips. Flexion was extremely limited to about 10°, and he flexed in line with the deformity, that is, to the left. He was able to extend his hips to bring the trunk vertical but little more than this. Left-side flexion was about 50% of the expected range and produced central low-back pain, whereas right-side flexion was limited to neutral and produced right low-back and buttock pain. Both rotations were almost full range with left rotation being painfree and right rotation causing minor central low-back discomfort. The right straight leg raise was limited by spasm to 40° and reproduced the back and buttock pain. Neck flexion did not affect the pain. Left straight leg raising was negative. Right straight leg raising in sitting was more painful and more restricted than when tested in lying.

There were no neurological deficits.

Compression reproduced the central low-back pain, but traction and torsion had no effect. Posteroanterior pressures over L4 were very painful and moderately painful over L5. The pressure over the L4 vertebra produced spasm.

What are you thinking at this point? How will you proceed with the examination?   ☞

Lumbopelvic Case 8 Continuation

Diagnosis This patient may be suffering a contained disk herniation (protrusion) that is not compromising the neural tissues but is irritating the dural sleeve of a lower lumbar spinal nerve or root. The severe articular signs and restriction of the right straight leg raise support this diagnosis, as does the exacerbation caused by flexion postures. However, this is far from proved because there are no neurological signs or symptoms. It is safer though to assume disk herniation than assume an acute zygopophyseal joint dysfunction or some other minor lesion. From the pain and spasm caused by posteroanterior pressures, it seems likely that the affected level is L4/5.

Treatment On the face of it, this patient may benefit with the McKenzie deviation correction maneuver. The deviation should be tested for its ability to correct. If it is correctable manually, it should be done as quickly as possible. The usual formula is then to follow the shift correction with extension exercises and the maintenance of an extension posture and avoidance of flexion and sitting.

However, in this case, attempting to correct the shift resulted in severe low-back and buttock pain and spasm. This was not unexpected in this case given the severity of the signs and symptoms.

How are you going to treat this patient?

Please turn to page 422 for solutions.

A Running Injury?

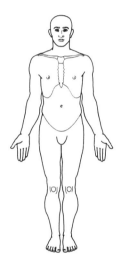

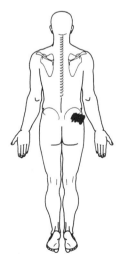

Subjective Examination

A 23-year-old woman stumbled while running and felt an immediate stab of pain in the right buttock. The stab of pain was short lasting and she continued her run without further incident. Upon waking the next morning she had an ache in the right buttock that became sharper when she put weight on her right leg. When she continued to move around, it improved, and by the time she had her shower, there was no pain. She went to work as a medical technologist without any further symptoms. She decided to take a couple of days off from running and had no further symptoms. Three days later she ran again and within a mile, the buttock was aching and a mile after that, it forced her to stop running. The pain eased after taking a hot bath, but the next morning her buttock was very sore. There was improvement that day but it did not completely clear as it did before. Two days later the buttock was still painful. She saw her physician who referred her to physical therapy. When asked to locate the pain, the patient pointed to a small area medial to the right trochanter over the piriformis muscle.

Her main exercise activity was running 5 miles four times each week.

She has no history of low-back pain and no medical history relevant to this condition. The patient is very concerned with her health and does not drink alcohol or smoke.

What are you thinking at this point? How will you proceed with the examination? ☞

Lumbopelvic Case 9 Continuation

Currently piriformis syndrome is a popular diagnosis for this type of pain. Its most common meaning is entrapment of the sciatic nerve in the piriformis muscle. The diagnosis for this case cannot be piriformis syndrome, because there are no neurological symptoms that you would expect if neural tissues were compromised.

Could the piriformis muscle itself be damaged? Because it is a muscle, it has the ability to tear. However it does not seem too likely that the tear would clear so completely after the first injury only to recur without a specific injury the second time. This is one of the only sites in the body where we say here is a pain and it is over such and such a muscle, therefore it must be such and such syndrome. We would not dream of diagnosing a patient with pain over the deltoid as a deltoid injury, and we should not do so here. We can certainly test it and we should test it.

Other possible causes are zygopophyseal or sacroiliac joint dysfunction. The examination should proceed as normal.

Objective Examination

There was nothing remarkable on observation. The patient is a fit young person.

Right-side flexion was the most restricted movement being limited to about 75% of left-side flexion and reproducing the patient's pain. Flexion and left-side flexion were painfree; full range rotation was slightly painful and minimally limited. Extension appeared to be full range but had an abnormal end feel (possibly jammed). Combined extension and right-side flexion was restricted to about 50% of the left and produced her buttock pain. The other combined movements were negative. Straight leg raising and prone knee flexion tests were negative, as was the slump test. There were no neurological deficits. Compression and traction were negative. General torsion testing was positive into right rotation in that it reproduced her pain. Posteroanterior pressure over L5 was slightly painful locally. The sacroiliac primary stress tests (gapping and compression) did not reproduce pain. Isometric testing of the piriformis was negative, as was stretching the muscle.

Have you a diagnosis and treatment plan in mind?

Please turn to page 422 for solutions.   ☞

Acute Sciatica

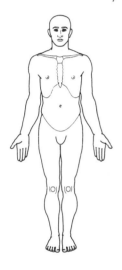

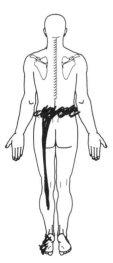

Subjective Examination

A 25-year-old man complaining of acute low-back pain and acute radicular sciatica with causalgia is referred for treatment. The pain was felt centrally and to the left in his low back. Lancinating pain went down the back of his left leg when he flexed. He is also complaining of paresthesia in the lateral border of the left foot and two toes. He has a history of 6 months of episodic back pain that was unpredictable in its onset but often related to heavy physical exertion. This is his first episode of sciatica and has been present for a week since the onset of this current bout of low-back pain. This time the onset of pain had followed a workout in the gym, but he could recall no specific incident that might have injured his back.

The back and leg pain was aggravated by sitting and by fast walking for more than a few minutes. It was eased by lying down on his side and by standing from a seated position.

Previously the pain had cleared up with a day or two with rest, but this episode was not improving and might even have been worsening. The patient has no bladder, bowel, or genital problems.

He has no medical history of note. He is a student physical therapist and does not drink excessively or smoke.

From this information, can you provisionally diagnose, prognose, and treat?

What are you thinking at this point? How will you proceed with the examination? 🖝

347

Lumbopelvic Case 10 Continuation

From this information, this looks like a fairly typical disk herniation compressing the first sacral nerve. Most aspects of the objective examination would support this diagnosis including the weakness of the plantar flexors and knee flexors, and the positive left straight leg raise. However, other features argue against a disk herniation. The patient's age is a little young for the typical onset, although it is not unknown by any means. The lack of causal factors, especially in such a young patient, is also unusual.

Objective Examination

Observation of the patient's posture revealed nothing remarkable. He is a fit looking young man, who is, if anything, a little underweight.

Trunk flexion allowed him to reach just below his knees; normally he could easily touch his toes. This movement caused low-back and leg pain. A few seconds after standing straight increased his foot paresthesia for a few more seconds. Extension was full range but painful in the low back. Both side flexions and both rotations were full range and painfree.

Left straight leg raising caused low-back and left leg pain and was limited to 40°. The right straight leg raise was negative. When neck flexion was added to the straight leg raise, the patient experienced paresthesia through the trunk and into both legs. Prone knee flexion was negative. Neck flexion alone caused trunk and bilateral lower extremity tingling. There was moderate weakness in the plantar flexors of the left ankle and the flexors of the left knee. Mild weakness was detected of the right knee extensors and dorsiflexors of the right ankle. The deep tendon reflexes and sensation were normal.

Compression, traction, and torsion were negative. Posteroanterior pressure over the L5 spinous process reproduced mild central low-back pain.

What is your most likely diagnosis?

Please turn to page 424 for solutions.

A Disk Prolapse on MRI

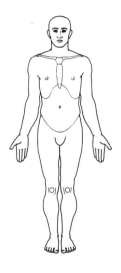

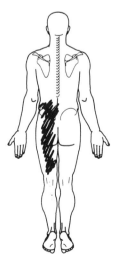

Subjective Examination

A 34-year-old man complains of acute left low-back pain with nonlancinating pain into the left buttock and posterior left thigh. The onset was 2 weeks earlier when he lifted a heavy, awkward box from the trunk of his car. The initial pain was mild low-back pain that became considerably more painful that evening when he sat watching TV. He described the pain as moderate but not disabling. Over the next 2 days, the pain became sharper and more intense. The buttock and leg pain was first felt 2 days later. The patient described it as a "natural progression of the back pain." The pain was more intense when sitting for more than 15 minutes and on standing from sitting. It eased with walking, provided he did not walk too far or too fast. Sleep was not disturbed and he awoke feeling refreshed with only a mild backache.

The x-ray was negative but an MRI demonstrated a disk prolapse to the right at L5/S1.

The patient has neither history of low-back pain nor any medical history of note. The patient is a family physician. He does not smoke and drinks wine socially.

Objective Examination

There was no deviation or deformity observed.

Flexion was limited to the point where the patient was able to reach just below his knees with his fingertips. Before the onset of pain, he could reach his toes. Flexion produced pain in the low back and buttock but not the posterior thigh. Extension was full range and painfree. Left-side flexion was full range and painfree, whereas right-side flexion was about 25% of left-side flexion and produced right low back pain. Both rotations were full range—left rotation was painfree, and right rotation produced mild right low-back pain.

There were no signs of neurological deficit.

The right straight leg raise was limited to 50° and reproduced the patient's back and buttock pain. Neither neck flexion nor ankle dorsiflexion affected the straight leg raise limitation or the pain produced. Straight

349

leg raising in sitting was equivalent to that in lying and produced the same pain. The left straight leg raise was full at 90° and painless. Torsion, compression, or traction did not affect the pain. Posteroanterior pressure over L5 reproduced the patient's right low-back pain.

Do you have a diagnosis?

What are you thinking at this point? How will you proceed with the examination? ☞

Lumbopelvic Case 11 Continuation

For the moment, ignore the MRI result. A number of studies on asymptomatic subjects demonstrate that prolapses are a relatively common finding on MRI. It will be better if you carry out your examination in ignorance of any objective test results and integrate the results of both after you have a clinical impression. Any discrepancy between the two must be rationalized before undertaking treatment. Because we are not in the habit of treating patients from radiographs, CT scans, or MRIs, the clinical impression must take precedence unless the objective test is unequivocal.

In this case, the absence of radicular pain or neurological signs tends to exclude compromise of the neural tissues. However, the positive straight leg raise and its reproduction of the patient's low-back and buttock pain indicate compromise of the dura, whereas the adjunct test of neck flexion and ankle dorsiflexion do not support this (nor do they refute it).

The limitation of trunk flexion was approximately to the same degree as the straight leg raise restriction and produced similar pain. The pattern of restriction of movement did not preclude a disk prolapse, but on the other hand it could easily be due to a zygopophyseal joint hypomobility or even muscular inextensibility.

The reproduction of pain with compression would strongly suggest a disk source but its absence does not exclude the disk as the villain. The provocation of the patient's pain with anteroposterior pressure over L5 would suggest the lumbosacral segment as the site of the lesion.

Another possibility that cannot be dismissed out of hand is sacroiliac joint dysfunction or arthritis. However, the sacroiliac joint primary stress tests (anterior and posterior gapping) did not reproduce pain. For a sacroiliac joint to be able to limit the straight leg raise to such a degree, there usually has to be a degree of inflammation present that can be detected by primary stress tests. However, a minor biomechanical dysfunction of this joint cannot be ruled out completely until it is examined biomechanically.

All things considered, this patient's condition could be disk related. It might, at least initially, be wise to proceed on that assumption. It does not seem likely that, even if a disk lesion is the cause of the patient's symptoms, it is a prolapse and even less likely an extrusion.

Diagnosis In order of probability and in order of significance the diagnosis could be: L5/S1 contained disk herniation or protrusion with compression of the right dural sleeve of the fifth lumbar or first sacral spinal nerve or root, right L5/S1 zygopophyseal joint flexion hypomobility, or minor right sacroiliac joint dysfunction.

What is your first treatment plan and what is your prognosis?

Please turn to page 424 for solutions. ☞

Episodic Pain over 5 Years

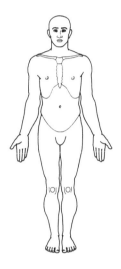

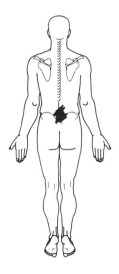

Subjective Examination

A 40-year-old man complaining of episodic central low-back pain attends at the request of his physician. He has a history of central low-back pain for the last 5 years. The original onset followed a rugby injury when the scrum he was in collapsed and a player fell across his back and hyperextended his lumbar spine. He had immediate severe pain and had to stop playing. This initial pain was felt only in the central low back and lasted 2 months, the first 3 weeks of which were so acute that he had to take this time off work and spend most of it in bed. Since then, he has had ongoing pain in the same area of the spine in an episodic fashion. The provoking factor was sometimes obvious and included running and sudden unexpected twisting movements. But more often, there was no apparent cause; the pain came on slowly and built up to a peak that prevented him from running, his favorite activity. Between episodes he was painfree and could do any activity he wanted. During an episode, walking, running, and prolonged standing were painful and could cause ongoing pain for hours after the provocation. Initially the episodes occurred every 4 months or so, but over the last 2 years he was experiencing them once every 6 weeks on average with each episode lasting about 3 weeks. As a result he was in pain for the same amount of time as he was painfree.

Over the years, he had received chiropractic treatment and physical therapy. Chiropractic treatment had initially helped in the first few episodes but then failed to be of much use. Physical therapy in the form of manual therapy (mobilization), mobility exercises, and stretching provoked his pain as frequently as it helped him. The most beneficial thing that the patient could do for his problem was to stay active. Whenever he took time off from running, the pain would recur. The patient had a history of various sports injuries including a torn and repaired right anterior cruciate ligament 10 years earlier and recurrent left shoulder problems for a period until he stopped playing racquetball 6 years earlier. On attendance, he had been having pain for a week and decided to give physical therapy one last shot.

353

He has no relevant medical history. He is a university professor and has been able to do his job during the episodes. He smokes the occasional cigar and drinks on social occasions.

What are you thinking at this point? How will you proceed with the examination?   ☞

Lumbopelvic Case 12 Continuation

Almost every element of this patient's history is typical of instability.

A traumatic onset causing immediate severe pain that lasted a considerable time to be followed by gradual recovery is strongly indicative of significant tissue damage.

Unpredictable episodic pain with minor or no apparent cause is commonly due to instability as is a sensitivity to a reduction in exercise levels.

The previous physical therapy may have failed due to a poor selection of treatment. The use of stretching and mobilizing exercises in a case of instability should be questioned.

Objective Examination

The patient is a healthy looking man with no obvious deformities or postural defects.

He had full range trunk movements but extension and both side flexions reproduced his back pain, whereas the other movements were painfree.

He had no neurological deficits. Both straight leg raises and prone knee flexion tests were negative.

Compression, traction, and the sacroiliac stress tests were negative. Both general torsion tests were painful like posteroanterior pressures over L4/5.

Essentially, the differential diagnostic examination was negative, although full range motion in the presence of ongoing pain and disability is often indicative of instability. A biomechanical examination should be carried out. Mobility testing of the intervertebral segments demonstrated a painful extension hypermobility of L4/5. Intersegmental stability testing was negative.

Do you have a diagnosis and treatment?

Please turn to page 425 for solutions.

Ankle Pain

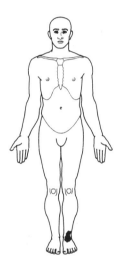

Subjective Examination

A 30-year-old man complaining of anterior left ankle pain attends. The pain had been present for 2 weeks. There was no apparent cause and the onset was gradual, becoming worse over a period of 3 days. He has no history of pain or injury to his ankle and no history of any lower limb or lumbar pain. The pain came on during walking just before heel lift and when he stretched his calf muscles prior to running.

He has no medical history of note. He is a graduate student and likes to run about 4 miles a day during the week. Other activities include softball and kayaking. He neither smokes nor drinks.

Objective Examination of the Ankle

Dorsiflexion range was greater in the left ankle than the right and had a soft capsular end feel but was painfree in non-weight bearing but painful in weight bearing. Other movements were full range and painfree.

The isometric tests were negative except for moderate weakness of the left plantar flexors.

Collateral ligament stress tests were negative, but stressing the inferior tibiofibular joint reproduced the patient's pain and some movement was felt during the test.

Given that this is a lumbopelvic case study, can you offer a provisional local diagnosis and a remote cause?

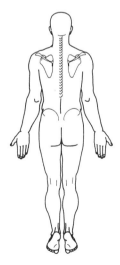

What are you thinking at this point? How will you proceed with the examination? ☞

Lumbopelvic Case 13 Continuation

The anterior ankle pain tends to exclude a ligament sprain as does the lack of trauma in the history. Anterior ankle pain may be due to an anterior subluxation of the talus or inferior tibiofibular joint/ligament pain. Both will be more painful during weight-bearing dorsiflexion, but generally both are traumatically induced. But the ankle had full range movement (and more) so a subluxation can be eliminated, leaving an unstable inferior tibiofibular joint, a diagnosis supported by the stress test.

The question now is how did this instability come about? There had to be failure of one or more restraining structures. This was confirmed by the inferior tibiofibular stress tests. However, there was no trauma, so direct ligament damage was not a factor. Cumulative stress is an option, but the patient really was not doing anything that would come into that category, his running being within reasonable bounds. This leaves the calf muscles; if these are insufficient, the ligament takes more stress than it may be able to tolerate. The patient would have remembered tearing his calf muscle and there is nothing in the history to suggest this. This leaves hypotonicity and/or weakness, which was discovered in the objective examination of the ankle.

Therefore, the next question is where did the weakness originate? It cannot be weakness due to a partial or complete tear; again, there is no history. Disuse weakness is not reasonable, considering the amount of exercise the patient gets. Central neurological or peripheral nerve disease is also a possibility, but there is no reason to select the least likely cause until the most likely appears impossible. The most likely cause and the most easily tested is a first sacral nerve or nerve root palsy.

Objective Examination of the Lumbar Spine

The patient had full range motion with no pain on cardinal movement testing but combined extension/left rotation/left-side flexion was limited. The straight leg raise and prone knee flexion tests were negative. The left plantar flexors were weak and the Achilles deep tendon reflex was slightly reduced compared to the right. There was no sensory loss. Compression, traction, torsion, and posteroanterior pressures were negative.

Diagnose and treat.

Please turn to page 426 for solutions.

Bilateral Sciatica in a Police Officer

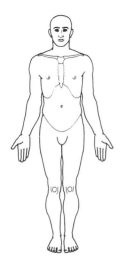

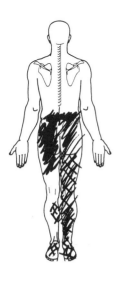

Subjective Examination

A 36-year-old man complaining of acute low-back pain and bilateral sciatica of 2 weeks' duration attended at the request of his physician with a diagnosis of "lumbar disk herniation" and a request for traction and extension exercises. The pain was felt across the low back with pain into both buttocks and down the posterior thighs. In the right leg the pain went into the calf and the plantar and dorsal aspects of the foot. In the left leg it only reached the knee. There was paresthesia in both legs. In the right leg it was felt in the posterior thigh, calf, and foot (plantar and dorsal aspects). In the left leg the paresthesia was sketchy, being felt on the medial aspect of the calf and the dorsum of the foot and the heel. There was no lancinating pain.

The onset of pain started in the back, buttock, and left posterior thigh after he had been involved in a work accident. He is a policeman, who had been involved in trying to suppress a drunk who wanted to fight. He had been bent over trying to grab the drunk's legs when another policeman had dived in and forced him into flexion. The pain had been immediate and had worsened and spread over the next 4 hours when he continued his shift. By the next day the pain was in both legs, and he took the day to see his doctor. He was taken off work and was told to rest in bed with prescribed muscle relaxants and analgesics. Ten days later, the pain had improved to the point, when he returned to work after driving his car for an hour, the pain had recurred in the back and both legs. He came off work and saw his physician who concurred with his coming off work again and continued with the same medication. By the next morning, he was feeling worse and the paresthesia had made its presence felt. He returned to his doctor, who arranged for an orthopedic surgical consultation 2 weeks later, and suggested that he start physical therapy. He was comfortable in supine lying with the knees flexed over two or three pillows or by sitting forward on a chair and supporting his weight on his arms.

359

He has had no problem with his bladder or bowels. When asked about genital function, he said that he had been so uncomfortable that he had not given sex any thought.

He has a history of knee injuries at work including a torn left anterior cruciate but nothing otherwise. He smokes and drinks moderately.

What are you thinking at this point? How will you proceed with the examination? ☞

Lumbopelvic Case 14 Continuation

The forced flexion injury and the immediate pain would suggest the possibility of profound tissue damage. The extension of the pain from the left to the right leg is expanding pain rather than shifting pain. This type of pain is frequently due to enlarging lesions, neoplasms, infections, and externalizing disk lesions. The first two conditions are unlikely given the mechanism of onset. The bilateral location of the pain suggests a posterior herniation. The presence of the paresthesia indicates that neural tissue is involved. The ease with which the condition recurred suggests that the condition is unhealed and unstable. From his preferred positions (lumbar flexion) it seems likely that there is sufficient posterior herniation of the disk that any positioning or movement toward extension pinches and forces it further backward.

Because of the bilateral paresthesia and pain, the main concern is cauda equina compression. The lack of bladder, bowel, and genital symptoms tends to argue against this, but the absence of these symptoms may simply mean that the S4 spinal nerve roots are not yet being compressed.

Objective Examination

The patient was slightly flexed and deviated to the right. Flexion was about 30° allowing him to reach his upper thighs, and followed the line of deviation to the left. Extension was less than 0°, and he could not move out of the slightly flexed position. Both side flexions were restricted to about one-fourth of what was expected. Both rotations were about 60% of the expected range. All movements were painful. Extension reproduced the paresthesia in both legs and low-back and buttock pain. Flexion caused back, buttock, and posterior thigh pain in both legs and posterior calf pain in the right. Both side flexions caused central low-back pain, with additional left leg pain on left-side flexion. Both rotations reproduced low-back pain. The right straight leg raise was limited to 25° by spasm and produced low-back, right buttock, and right leg pain and foot paresthesia. Neck flexion increased the patient's pain in the same areas. The left straight leg raise was limited to 40° and produced left back, buttock, and posterior thigh pain, with neck flexion increasing these symptoms. Right prone knee flexion was limited to 100° and caused pain in the dorsum of the right foot. Left prone knee flexion was limited to 120° and caused pain in the left back. Neurological testing revealed profound weakness in the right great toes and ankle dorsiflexors, evertors, plantar flexors, hamstrings, and gluteus maximi. Reflex testing demonstrated areflexia in the Achilles tendon and tibialis posterior and hyporeflexia in the tibialis anterior, extensor hallucis brevis, and peroneus longus. In the left leg, there was weakness of the hamstrings, plantar flexors and evertors and the great toe extensors. The left Achilles reflex was reduced and the extensor hallucis brevis reflex was absent. There was reduced sensation to pinprick over the anterior medial aspect of the left lower leg and dorsum of the foot. Sensation was also reduced over the skin of the posterior right calf, heel, lateral foot and toes, and the dorsum of the foot. Compression increased the back and buttock pain and was limited to getting the hips flexed to 90° by spasm. Traction had no effect. Posteroanterior pressures caused spasm and reproduced back and right leg pain at L4/5. Both torsion tests reproduced back pain. Because of possible cauda equina syndrome, pinprick was tested in the perineal region and found to be normal on both sides.

What are your thoughts on diagnosis, treatment, and prognosis?

Please turn to page 427 for solutions.

A Fall onto the Buttocks

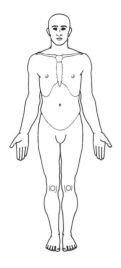

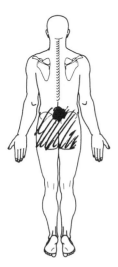

Subjective Examination

A 35-year-old man skating with his child fell directly onto his buttocks with his legs straight out in front of him a week ago. He had immediate severe mid to low lumbar pain and was unable to move in any direction. He was taken to the emergency room, x-rayed, and released, the radiograph being negative. He was told to take a week off work and take analgesics. At the end of the week the pain was still severe, so his physician referred him to physical therapy.

The pain was there almost all of the time but was worse with sitting and standing and better with lying. There was no referred pain to the legs, even though he had developed bilateral buttock pain the day after the injury.

He has no history of back pain or any medical problems of note. He does not smoke and drinks only on social occasions.

Objective Examination

On observation the lumbar spine did not have a lordosis, and the patient stood with slightly flexed hips and knees.

The patient had severe limitation of movement in all directions, being able to move only a few degrees in any direction. All movements reproduced the back pain and spasm on gentle overpressure.

There was no neurological deficit. Both straight leg raises and prone knee flexion tests were negative.

Compression was extremely painful and spasm prevented the hips being flexed to 90°. Torsion in both directions was very painful. Posteroanterior pressures over L3,4, and 5 were extremely painful, especially over L4, and all produced strong spasm.

Are there any other tests you would like to do or can you make a diagnosis and treatment plan?

Please turn to page 428, Part III, Diagnosis and Resolution to Cases.

Severe Calf Pain

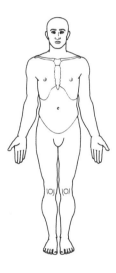

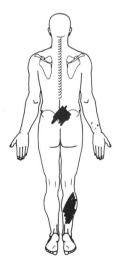

Subjective Examination

A 48-year-old man complaining of central low-back pain and right calf pain of 3 days' duration attends. The pains started when standing up from his seat in an airplane after an 8-hour flight. He found that he had to limp on the toes of his right foot with his knee flexed because of the calf pain. The back pain had improved since the onset, but the calf pain was about the same (an estimated 7 on a scale of 1 to 10). The back pain was not severe (about a 3), but was worse (4) on sitting. The leg pain was absent if he rested it by lying down but increased to its usual intensity if he tried to walk normally or if he tried to straighten his knee when sitting, standing, or lying.

The patient has a history of the same type of low-back pain that goes back 10 years. The pain usually began with prolonged sitting, remained confined to the low back, and cleared spontaneously within a week or so of the onset. It was never severe enough to disable him or to have him seek treatment. He had never experienced the leg pain before this episode. He had not had his back pain treated before this attendance.

His medical history includes gout and diabetes, both of which were well controlled with medication. He smokes and drinks moderately. He is an automobile engineer and spends most of his time in a supervisory capacity where his time is equally divided between sitting and walking. He had not returned to work since the onset of the pains.

What are you thinking at this point? How will you proceed with the examination? ☞

Lumbopelvic Case 16 Continuation

The temptation in this case is to think that the calf pain is part of the patient's lumbar problem (which of course it could be) and that the behavior of the leg pain can be explained in terms of neuromeningeal tension. However, a number of things should make you pause.

First, this is the first episode of calf pain and even though it has to start at some point, the lack of a history of any pain might mean the first onset of a new condition. Second, the onset and offset of the calf pain is not associated with the increase and decrease in back pain. The calf pain is worse when walking (at least on trying to walk normally), whereas the back pain is worse on sitting. Third, there has been no change in the intensity of the leg pain over the 3 days even though the back has improved.

There is a good chance that these two pains are unconnected, and a separate examination of the ankle and knee may be required. From the lumbar examination, the tests that will probably give us the greatest insight into what is going on with this patient are the neuromeningeal tests.

Objective Examination

The patient stood with the lumbar spine flexed and side flexed to the right. The right hip and knee were bent and the patient stood on his toes. Any attempt to straighten the knee and the hip caused severe calf pain.

Allowing the patient to stand in this posture, his range of lumbar motion was assessed. Flexion was full range with low-back pain reproduced. Extension, both side flexions, and both rotations were full range and painfree.

The right straight leg raise was not testable because of reproduction of calf pain on straightening the knee, which was flexed to about 160° (about 20° short of full extension). Lesague's test permitted 160° of knee extension with the hip at 90° of flexion. Dorsiflexion of the ankle in this position caused severe calf pain, while neck flexion did not affect the pain. The left straight leg raise was negative and reached 90°. The slump test replicated the results of the right leg tests. Prone knee flexion on both sides was negative. The patient did not exhibit any neurological signs although the strength of the right plantar flexors and dorsiflexors was not tested due to the amount of pain that the attempt caused.

Lumbar compression, traction, torsion, and posteroanterior pressures were all negative.

Do you have a diagnosis and treatment, or are there any other tests that you would like to do?

Please turn to page 428 for solutions.

Lumbar Sprain?

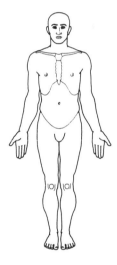

Subjective Examination

A 34-year-old man complaining of right low-back pain is referred with a diagnosis of lumbar sprain. The pain had been present for 2 months, initially as a low-grade ache after running more than 2 or 3 miles and more recently as a more intense pain in the same area. The pain was intermittent and more easily provoked than it had earlier been, being felt after running very short distances and prolonged walking. Occasionally he would experience a twinge in the right low back, of short duration but usually followed by an ache in the same area that would last for some minutes. The pain did not interfere with his work as a telephone services salesman but did interfere with his leisure activities—cross-country skiing and running, both of which he had been doing without change for 6 or 7 years.

There is no obvious cause for the problem, and he denies any history of back pain.

Objective Examination

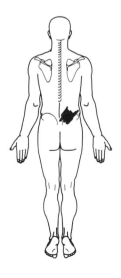

On observation he is a healthy looking man with no obvious deformities. Trunk flexion was limited allowing him to reach his ankles with his fingertips, whereas normally he was able to touch his toes. Overpressure increased the pain but otherwise gave a normal end feel. He felt mild pain in the right low back. Recovery from flexion included a "glitch" in the movement, which consisted of slight deviation to the right. Trunk extension was full range but painful in the right low-back area with some spasm on overpressure. Right-side flexion was full range and painful, and left-side flexion was restricted slightly compared to the right side but painless. Both rotations were full range and painfree.

There were no neurological deficits. The straight leg raise (90°) and prone knee flexion tests were negative. Lumbar compression and traction tests were negative. Right torsion testing produced pain in the relevant area especially when localized to L5/S1. Posteroanterior pressures over L5 were painful and provoked slight spasm. The primary stress tests for the sacroiliac joints were negative.

The findings do not generate a strong diagnosis, so a biomechanical assessment was carried out. This determined that a right anterior torsional instability was present at L5/S1.

Are you ready to make a diagnosis and generate a treatment plan?

What are you thinking at this point? How will you proceed with the examination? ☞

Lumbopelvic Case 17 Continuation

There are no red or yellow flags here apart from the causeless onset. But this is of course a common presentation and should not be regarded as a flag unless there are other features in the examination that make you worry.

Diagnosis This patient has a functional instability at the lumbosacral level. The twinges followed by aching would suggest pathomechanical movements resulting in low-grade inflammation. The abnormal recovery from flexion would support the idea of instability as would the two most painful movements being full range. The torsion test tends to confirm the diagnosis and the biomechanical tests specify the direction of the instability and its level.

Treatment We are not ready to treat this patient because the cause of the problem has not been determined. If we treat him with stability therapy at this point, any improvement we might make will almost certainly be temporary because the underlying cause has not been dealt with.

Where do we go from here?

Please turn to page 429 for solutions.

Another Fall onto the Buttocks

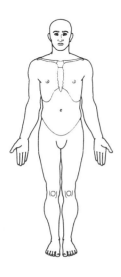

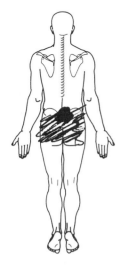

Subjective Examination

A 28-year-old man fell onto his buttocks while playing ice hockey. He experienced immediate strong (7–8 on a scale of 1 to 10) pain across the sacroiliac region and into both buttocks forcing him to stop playing. He saw his doctor the following afternoon when he found he was unable to work as a computer software designer. He said that he had a continuous dull throbbing pain unless he sat, in which case it was severe, or if he walked more than a hundred yards, then it was extremely strong. His best position was lying on either side with his hips and knees semi-flexed. When his x-rays were negative, his physician prescribed Tylenol 3 and told him to stay off work until he was able to sit. He stayed off work over the next 10 days, at which time the pain had subsided to a level where he could sit using a cushion.

Even though he was able to work with some discomfort, he was unable to skate or even walk quickly due to increased pain in the left buttock. This pain was now central and situated left of center. When it flared up, the pain was quite intense (7) and remained a problem until he lay down, when it would settle in an hour or so.

He attended physical therapy 15 days after the injury and stated that the joint flared up after walking to the clinic from his home, a mile away.

Objective Examination

There were no obvious deformities on observation.

Trunk flexion was limited to the point where the patient could reach his knees with his fingertips; normally he was able to touch his toes. Using a modified Schober's test, it was apparent that the spine was moving during trunk flexion. Trunk flexion reproduced moderate sacral and left buttock pain, which was increased with overpressure. There was no spasm on overpressure but the test was stopped by the increase in pain level.

The other cardinal lumbar movements were full range and painfree.

There were no neurological deficits in the patient's sensation or reflexes. However, many of the proximal muscle tests reproduced strong

371

pain. Hip extension was painful with consequence weakness, and apart from the ankle tests and quadriceps, which were normal, no decision could be made concerning strength.

The left straight leg raise was limited to 50° and reproduced left buttock pain, which prevented further elevation of the leg.

Lumbar compression and traction tests were negative. The prone lumbar torsion tests were painful, especially when localized to L5/S1. Posteroanterior pressures over L5 and the sacrum were painful.

The primary stress tests for the sacroiliac joints (anterior and posterior gapping) were positive over the left sacroiliac region and in the center of the back. He was very tender in the left sacral sulcus and sacum.

Do you have any concerns? Are you happy with the tests you have done or do you feel you need more? If you feel there has been enough testing, do you have a diagnosis, a treatment plan, and a prognosis?

What are you thinking at this point? How will you proceed with the examination?   ☞

Lumbopelvic Case 18 Continuation

A fall onto the buttocks is the classic cause of a sacral cranial subluxation (the upslip). However, other more serious things might have occurred. So let's look at the results of the examination so far.

The trunk flexion seems likely to be limited by something other than vertebral column given the reasonably normal Schober's test and the negative (except for L5 and the sacrum) posteroanterior pressures. In addition, the other cardinal lumbar movements were negative, which is unusual with this degree of pain and disability, if it were coming from the lumbar spine.

The straight leg raise was limited by pain, an empty end feel, and painful weakness of the hip extensors and knee flexors. The patient has what appears to be the sign of the buttock. Further testing of the hip revealed that hip flexion was limited to about 70° by pain, whereas medial and lateral rotation with the hip in neutral were full range and painfree.

Although the positive sacroiliac tests might suggest sacroiliitis, they of course also increase pressure on the sacrum itself and the central pain they produced also suggest sacroiliitis.

The possibility of the sign of the buttock being present indicates that an examination of the hip is more essential than a biomechanical examination of the sacroiliac joint.

Have you a provisional diagnosis and treatment plan now?

Please turn to page 431 for solutions.

A 20-Year-Old with Buttock Pain

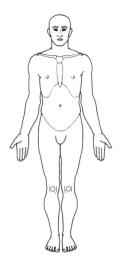

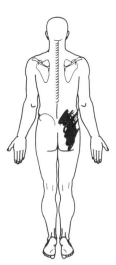

Subjective Examination

A 20-year-old man attends complaining of right low-back pain with radiation into the right buttock. The pain had been present for 4 weeks and had no apparent cause, although it did start the day after he had played touch football with some friends. The pain was always there to a minor extent, but on exertion it would become worse going from a 2 (on a 1 to 10 pain scale) to an 8. The exacerbation would last for between 2 hours and 8 hours, depending on how much provocation it had. Provoking activities included running, prolonged fast walking of more than a mile, wrestling with his younger brother, and once after working overhead putting up a lamp over a pool table.

If it had been exacerbated, it disturbed his sleep, waking him with a sharp stab of pain he associated with rolling over in bed. While it was flared, he was unable to walk or stand without pain.

He has no history of back pain and he denies any medical history of significance. X-rays were negative.

Objective Examination

There were no obvious deformities with this man.

Trunk flexion was full range and painfree. Trunk extension was full range but reproduced his pain. Right-side flexion was full range and painful. All other movements were painfree and full range.

There were no neurological deficits. The right straight leg raise was full range but mildly painful to the right low back at full range (70°). Prone knee flexion testing was negative. Lumbar compression, traction, torsion, and posteroanterior pressures were negative. Flat-footed hopping on the right foot produced his pain when unsupported, but if a sacroiliac belt was applied, it was almost negative. The right anterior gapping primary sacroiliac stress test reproduced pain over the right sacroiliac joint region. He was tender over the dorsal sacroiliac ligament.

Have you a diagnosis? If so, what treatment do you initiate? If you do not have a diagnosis, what tests would you like to follow up with?

What are you thinking at this point? How will you proceed with the examination? 👉

Lumbopelvic Case 19 Continuation

The pattern of restriction and pain-producing movements suggest sacroiliac joint pain. The positive primary sacroiliac stress test tends to support this and makes a more specific diagnosis of sacroiliitis. The tenderness in the sacral sulcus (Fortin's finger test) would also suggest sacroiliitis. The gender, age, and insidious onset should have you concerned that this man is suffering from ankylosing spondylitis. However, he is not immune to the nonsystemic causes of sacroiliitis.

The "positive" straight leg raise was not positive in the range usually attributed to dural compromise but near the end of the range where it would have maximally rotated the innominate bone, potentially causing sacroiliac pain.

What other tests could you utilize to provisionally confirm or refute a provisional diagnosis of ankylosing spondylitis?

Please turn to page 432 for solutions.

Neural Adhesions?

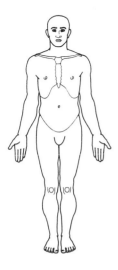

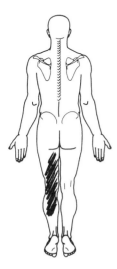

Subjective Examination

A 44-year-old woman complaining of left posterior thigh and calf somatic pain attended with a diagnosis of neural adhesions. The pain has been present for 6 weeks, coming on one month after she had undergone surgery for a prolapsed L5/S1 disk causing an S1 radiculopathy.

Prior to the surgery she had suffered low-back pain radiating to the posterior thigh and calf on sitting. She also suffered severe lancinating pain in the left posterior upper and lower leg with paresthesia and objective numbness in the lateral border of the foot and lateral two toes when bending forward or backward. Leading to the surgery, she had a history of episodes of acute low-back pain and left somatic sciatica for 2 years for a total of six episodes, each lasting approximately 4 weeks. The last episode occurred 3 months before the surgery after she helped a friend move house. She experienced a sudden severe onset of low-back pain and left radicular pain while lifting a heavy box. In the interval between this onset and her surgery, she had undergone numerous imaging and electrical investigations and had taken physical therapy without any apparent relief.

Initially after the surgery, she had only mild pain in the low back and left buttock and some numbness and paresthesia in the lateral two toes. She felt that the surgery had been successful until the left leg pain resumed after she went on a bicycle ride lasting 3 hours. She felt that she was still much better than she had been prior to her surgery.

For the last 6 weeks since the resumption of the pain, she had been experiencing left posterior thigh and calf pain whenever she bent over. The toe paresthesia remained unchanged.

Objective Examination

Trunk flexion was limited, allowing her to reach her knees, whereas before this resumption of leg pain she had been able to reach her mid shins, which was still less than her normal reach. She experienced severe lancinating pain at the end of her range.

Extension, both side flexions, and both rotations were negative with all producing normal end feels.

There were no neurological deficits.

The left straight leg raise was about 40° and produced the somatic sciatica pain. Neck flexion while the straight leg raise was held in the painful range reduced her pain. The right straight leg raise was about 90° and painless. Sitting straight leg raise was positive on the right at 40°. Slumping the spine made no difference but adding neck flexion decreased the sciatica. Both prone knee flexion tests were negative.

Compression, torsion, traction, and posteroanterior pressures were all negative. The primary sacroiliac stress tests were negative.

Do you agree with the physician's diagnosis? If so, why and what will be your treatment? If you do not agree with the diagnosis, what do you think is causing the pain? Do you need any further tests?

Please turn to page 433, Part III, Diagnosis and Resolution to Cases.

Multiple Back Surgeries

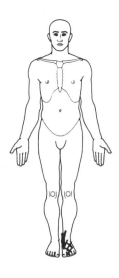

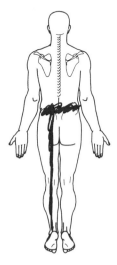

Subjective Examination

A 42-year-old woman attends complaining of bilateral low-back pain and lancinating radicular pain in the left posterior thigh, calf, and the medial aspect of the dorsum of the foot. She also complained of paresthesia in the dorsum of the foot when the lumbar pain was particularly bad. The pain was always present to some degree in the low back, but was intermittent in the leg. Prolonged standing exacerbated the lumbar pain and walking, although walking shorter distances could help the back pain. Bending over provoked the lower limb radicular pain and sometimes standing from sitting when she was not careful about this movement.

Her medical history includes four lumbar surgeries, three laminectomies, a fusion, and a revision. All surgeries were carried out on the L4/5 segment between 1988 and 1992. The original onset followed a fall at work. She had a sudden onset of lumbar pain, which was accompanied by a "pop." Posterior leg pain followed within a few days and her first surgery within 2 months. She only did well after the fusion, and has been functional with minimal to moderate discomfort since that time, until now.

This episode of pain followed falling flat on her back at home 3 weeks ago. The back and leg pain started immediately and has become severe. She is only able to relieve her pain by lying down and taking medication.

Objective Examination

Apart from the surgical scars, there are no unusual presentations on observation.

Trunk flexion was full range but reproduced lancinating posterior left thigh and calf pain. Extension was extremely limited to a few degrees and caused strong low-back pain. Left-side flexion was full range and painless. Right-side flexion was limited to about 75% of left-side flexion. Both rotations were full range and painfree.

On neurological testing, the entire left leg was weak. She had pinprick and light touch reduction over the medial aspect of the dorsum of the foot and absence of both sensory modalities. Her deep tendon reflexes were absent in both Achilles tendons and normal in all others.

Straight leg raise in sitting was limited to 60° of knee flexion and in supine to 40° of hip flexion. Both produced lancinating posterior left thigh pain.

The slump test was positive in the same way that the seated straight leg raise was positive. Slumping the spine made no difference to the leg pain, but neck flexion relieved the leg pain. Both prone knee flexions were negative.

Anterior and posterior primary sacroiliac stress tests were negative. Both general torsions were painful. Compression and traction did not exacerbate or provoke any of her pains. Posteroanterior pressure over the fourth and fifth lumbar vertebrae produced local pain and spasm.

What are you thinking at this point? How will you proceed with the examination?   ☞

Lumbopelvic Case 21 Continuation

The weakness in the leg is difficult to assess for relevance because it involves all muscle groups. The likelihood is that at least some of the weakness is due to deconditioning and anxiety. It is also possible that some neurological weakness is hiding in there.

There were neurological signs and symptoms, decreased sensation, and radicular pain. And neuromeningeal signs were also very positive. So, is this a disk herniation? Probably not! Flexion was full range and extension, while being severely limited, cannot produce radicular pain.

Her provoking factors would also tend to argue against a disk herniation being the cause of her pain. Prolonged flexion, prolonged standing, and walking were painful in the lumbar spine.

An alternative diagnosis could be neural adhesions. The lancinating pain would support this diagnosis, as would the full range of trunk flexion and the results of the neuromeningeal tests, particularly the relief of her leg pain with neck flexion, which has been observed clinically. The multiple surgeries would explain where the adhesions came from.

However, this diagnosis should not be made until a biomechanical examination is carried out. Segmental testing demonstrated that there was no motion at L4/5, and testing did not produce spasm. There was presumed extension hypermobility at L5/S1 due to the presence of spasm at the end of range. Testing also reproduced her back pain but not the leg pain.

Develop a diagnosis and treatment.

Please turn to page 434 for solutions.

Degenerative Disk Disease?

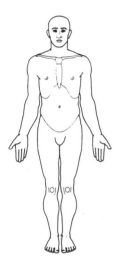

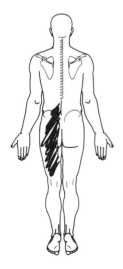

Subjective Examination

A 38-year-old man complaining of left low-back, buttock, and posterior thigh somatic pain attends with a referral of degenerative disk disease and a treatment prescription of mechanical traction and extension exercises. The onset of pain was 8 days earlier and occurred while playing rugby when the scrum collapsed on the patient who was flexed at the time. He felt immediate central back pain and continued playing. At the end of the game, the pain was a little better and by the next morning almost gone.

Two days later, he was working on his car, bent over the hood for about 20 minutes. When he tried to straighten up, he had severe low-back pain. He went in the house, took aspirin, and lay down for the rest of the day. By the next morning, the pain was much improved, so he went to work in his office. The pain gradually increased as he sat at work and he returned home at lunch-time and lay down again. The next morning, the pain was still present in the left low back and was also felt in the posterior aspect of the left leg. He noticed at this time that he was bent forward and to the right. Then he went to his physician, who prescribed rest, analgesics, and physical therapy.

He had no paresthesia in the legs or bladder or bowel dysfunction.

He denies any history of similar back pains or any medical history of relevance. X-rays showed degeneration of the two lower lumbar levels.

Objective Examination

On observation the patient is kyphotic and deviated to the right and stands with his left knee flexed.

Trunk flexion was limited to about 20° and produced back and left leg pain. No extension was available in the lumbar spine and the attempt produced low-back pain. Right-side flexion was full range and painfree. No left-side flexion was present and again the attempt reproduced the back and left leg pain. Compression and traction were negative, whereas posteroanterior pressures caused pain and spasm when applied over the fourth and fifth lumbar vertebrae.

385

The right straight leg raise was negative. Left straight leg raising was limited to 30° and produced low-back and left thigh pain. Neck flexion increased the leg pain. The slump test results were no different from the straight leg raise results.

There were no neurological deficits.

From the subjective and objective examinations does it seem likely that the physician's diagnosis was correct? If so, is the treatment prescribed appropriate?

What are you thinking at this point? How will you proceed with the examination? ☞

Lumbopelvic Case 22 Continuation

Technically, degenerative disk disease is not a painful condition and is a universal process linked with aging. Degradative disk disease would be a more precise and quite possibly an accurate diagnosis. The kyphosis combined with lateral shifting is sometimes the result of disk herniation or a transverse instability through the segment allowing fixing of the superior vertebra in a shifted position.

The very positive straight leg raise would suggest the former, that is, disk herniation with compression of the dural sleeve. The absence of neural signs or symptoms would argue against compression of the nerve root. From this examination, it is difficult to state which level is affected especially in view of at least one study refuting the idea that shifting can only occur at the L4/5 segment. A biomechanical examination might help to pin down the level but because our treatment is likely to be initially regional, there is no need to examine each segment.

Any attempt at shift correction by stabilizing the pelvis and pushing the trunk across to the left provoked very strong pain and spasm. When the pressure was maintained, it produced paresthesia into the anterior and medial aspect of the lower leg and into the medial aspect of the dorsal foot and into the great toe.

What now?

Please turn to page 434 for solutions.

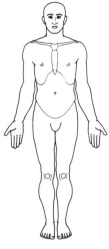

LUMBOPELVIC CASE 23

Very Local Back Pain

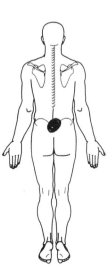

Subjective Examination

A 60-year-old man was referred for low-back pain. He complained of pain in a small area the size of a golf ball in the dead center of his back at about the lumbosacral level. There was no referral or spread of the pain from this area although the intensity was now worse than earlier in its course.

The pain had been present for many years, starting very gradually and with no obvious cause. He works as a lathe operator and first felt the pain after being bent over doing intricate work. The pain would go away on straightening. Over the last few years the pain came on immediately when straightening from flexion and not while flexed. The pain was additionally felt while turning in bed and would usually awaken him once or twice a night.

He had no pain when sitting or walking and was able to stand for indefinite periods without symptoms.

From the history do you have any thoughts on a diagnosis and treatment plan?

What are you thinking at this point? How will you proceed with the examination? ☞

Lumbopelvic Case 23 Continuation
Objective Examination

Flexion was full range and painfree. The return from flexion was painful, especially on initiation. There was no abnormal quality to either flexion or its return. All other movements were full range and painfree.

Compression, traction, and posteroanterior pressures were painfree. The sacroiliac pain provocation tests were negative.

There were no neurological deficits. The straight leg raises and prone knee flexion were negative as was the slump test.

Does this help with your diagnosis? If you need further tests, which do you think are most likely to clarify the situation?

Please turn to page 435 for solutions.

Sacroiliac Pain?

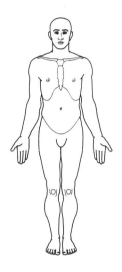

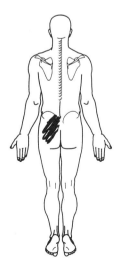

Subjective Examination

A 36-year-old woman is referred with low-back pain of 2 days' duration. The pain is felt over the left sacroiliac area and buttock. The onset followed a long run in training for a triathlon and was felt initially while running but was a good deal worse a hour or two later. The pain was felt mainly in the area directly inferior to the left posterior inferior iliac spine and it spread from here to the buttock. The pain had not really changed in intensity or location since the onset and was intermittent, being present whenever she tried to run or walk fast.

She had no pain sitting or standing for prolonged periods. Her sleep was not disturbed and she woke without pain. She denied any paresthesia.

She has no history of back pain and no medical history relevant to her pain. Her history included a sprained left ankle about 6 months earlier that also occurred while running. She had been running for 10 years with few problems except for an inversion injury that had sprained her left ankle.

Objective Examination

Flexion, right-side flexion, and right rotation were painfree and full range. Extension was slightly limited and reproduced sacroiliac area pain. Left-side flexion and left rotation were full range but also reproduced left sacroiliac area pain.

There were no neurological deficits. The straight leg raise and prone knee flexion tests were negative as was the slump test.

Compression and traction were negative. Posteroanterior pressures over L5 were locally mildly painful.

The primary sacroiliac stress tests (pain provocation tests) were negative. Fortin's finger test was positive; the patient pointed to an area inferior and medial to the posterior inferior iliac spine as the main pain area.

What are you thinking at this point? How will you proceed with the examination? ☞

391

Lumbopelvic Case 24 Continuation

This patient's problem could either be due to a lumbar or a sacroiliac joint dysfunction. Fortin's finger test has a high degree of sensitivity but a relatively low degree of specificity, so it will pick up most cases of sacroiliac pain but it will also be quick to pick up other conditions. In addition, the more minor lesions of the sacroiliac joint such as biomechanical dysfunction are not always painful, but over stress other structures, which then become painful.

Probably this condition is a sacroiliac joint dysfunction. The pain area and pain provocation factors, such as walking and running, are commonly found with sacroiliac joint problems. This is supported by the pain produced when testing extension and ipsilateral side flexion. From this, the patient either has a sacroiliac joint dysfunction or a low lumbar zygopophyseal joint extension hypomobility or hypermobility.

The scan was negative for either, so a biomechanical examination must be done. Examine the lumbar spine biomechanically first, otherwise many of the sacroiliac tests will be positive through altered muscle tone caused by any lumbar dysfunction that might be present. Once the spine has been cleared, the sacroiliac joint can be examined with more confidence in its outcome.

The lumbar examination demonstrated a painless extension hypermobility at L5/S1. The examination of the sacroiliac joint showed that ilium was hypomobile into flexion or posterior rotation, that is, jammed into anterior rotation or extension.

What are your plans for treatment? Do you need to test anything else?

Please turn to page 435 for solutions.

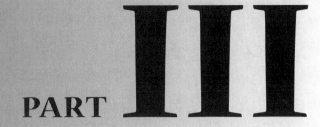

PART **III**

Diagnosis and Resolution to Cases

Cervical Case 1 Discussion

Diagnosis

The results of the objective examination strengthen the hypothesis that the most likely cause of the dizziness is cervical joint dysfunction. The most likely source is the C2-3 cervical joint extension hypomobility (subluxed or jammed in flexion). The upper cervical levels are intimately associated with balance and experimentally have been shown to cause dizziness when dysfunctional.

Treatment

The best treatment is manipulation; second best is nonrhythmic mobilization followed by either segmental stability testing and stability therapy, if appropriate. Whether stable or unstable, the neck must be treated with functional reeducation movement exercises.

The patient should be assessed for balance because this seems to be affected in many long-term cervical injury cases. If disequilibrium is found, exercises to optimize balance should be given.

Cervical Case 2 Discussion

There are a number of reasons why treatment, particularly manual treatment, helps initially but not over the long term. These include the following:

1. Insufficient, inadequate, or inappropriate exercises being given
2. The therapist treating the obvious joint dysfunction but failing to find the root cause of the problem
3. The therapist failing to change adverse environmental factors
4. The patient failing to comply with the exercise program or suggested changes in the environment

In this case, the foam pillow should be changed to feather or artificial feather and the patient should be warned about spending too much time reading or watching TV while sitting. The exercises were reviewed and corrected, and the patient was painfree after three treatment sessions.

Cervical Case 3 Discussion

Diagnosis

This case is almost certainly cervical disk compression with a C6 motor and sensory radiculopathy. Normal reflexes in the presence of motor and sensory deficits are a little uncommon but do occur and probably indicate a better prognosis than if the reflexes were reduced or absent.

Treatment

Reducing the presumed inflammation is of paramount importance. This can be accomplished best by making sure that the patient is not continuously reinjuring it with unguarded movements. A hard collar will prevent this; as a general rule, if any cervical movement produces lancinating pain or paresthesia, a collar is indicated. In addition, the patient needs to be instructed in rest and nonpainful exercises and anti-inflammatory modalities can be applied.

Because traction did not increase the pain on testing, it can be cautiously applied, but I would suggest that the effect of the above treatments be evaluated first. If there is significant inflammation present, traction may exacerbate it. If the patient's condition resolves rapidly with the initial measures, then traction is unnecessary. If there is partial or minimal improvement, traction may be required to try to relieve any pressure on the neural tissues.

In this case, the use of the collar, rest, and anti-inflammatory modalities eliminated the lancinating pain in 10 days but failed to affect the neck pain, arm ache, paresthesia, or neurological deficits. Mechanical traction was applied over 10 treatment sessions. This appeared to substantially reduce, but not eradicate, the neck and arm symptoms and left the neurological deficits unchanged. At this time the patient was discontinued from treatment by the physician and returned to work.

It seems likely that the collar, rest, and modalities were effective at reducing the inflammation as demonstrated by the elimination of the lancinating pain. The traction possibly reduced some of the compression from the spinal nerve but was not able to completely clear it. Alternatively, there may have been some spontaneous reduction in compression force and the traction did nothing. When neurological deficits are established, gaining full recovery with physical therapy is difficult.

Ideally, once the more acute pain had subsided and there was no further improvement with traction, a biomechanical examination would have been carried out and biomechanical treatment initiated, if appropriate. However, in this case, the physician unexpectedly discharged the patient.

Cervical Case 4 Discussion

Diagnosis

This lady appears to be suffering from a mild posttraumatic arthritis of the lower cervical region, probably C5-6. There may be some underlying biomechanical dysfunction, but it may not be possible to assess this until the inflammation has resolved. From the isometric tests, there also seems to be a minor injury to the left sternomastoid; palpation along its length will confirm and localize the lesion.

Treatment

The patient should be instructed to do nothing that reproduces the pain, because this will retard the resolution of the inflammatory processes. Because she seems to be functioning well, the need for a collar is debatable, and I would try to avoid this if possible. However, there is a little worsening at the end of the work day. If this continued or if there was failure to improve with treatment, a hard collar for work for a few days or alternately a week off work might be indicated. Otherwise treatment can be reasonably aggressive, providing the patient's symptoms are not brought on by the treatment.

Anti-inflammatory modalities such as ultrasound and interferrential currents aimed at the C5-6 segment region can be applied but it is not likely to have a dramatic effect given the low level of inflammation present. Exercises both for the neck and for the segment (segmental PNF) should help maintain muscle coordination while the inflammation resolves.

In this case, it was necessary to manipulate or mobilize the right zygapophyseal joint into flexion once the inflammation had resolved.

The sternomastoid injury would almost certainly have resolved itself, but ultrasound applied over the injured area probably speeded healing.

The minor range of motion loss in the neck and the absence of neurological signs strengthen the good prognosis. This patient became painfree in 2 weeks with six treatments.

Cervical Case 5 Discussion

It is unlikely that this patient is suffering from vertebrobasilar insufficiency, because there has been a distinct absence of neurological signs on cranial nerve testing while he was dizzy. More likely the vertigo felt on lying down and on extending and turning the head to the right is benign paroxysmal positional vertigo possibly due to displacement of otoconia (cupulolithiasis or canalolithiasis). In any event, it should be diagnosed and treated as ongoing vertigo. This condition makes it difficult, if not impossible, to recover cervical movement, especially those movements that cause the vertigo. The reason for this is that, even though the therapist is encouraging painfree movement, the patient is trying to avoid moving the head in order to prevent the onset of vertigo.

The type 2 dizziness is likely due to cervical mechanoreceptor problems resulting from the movement dysfunctions in the upper neck. Again, the lack of cranial nerve signs or other neurological symptoms tend to preclude the vertebrobasilar system as a cause of this dizziness. It would have been nice, from a diagnostic perspective, if the posteroanterior pressures or any of the segmental tests had reproduced this dizziness, but typically they did not.

The fracture tests (compression and isometrics) were negative, but they should be by this point in time. There is no concern with craniovertebral stability, the tests were negative, and a dense fracture will cause much more distress than this patient has suffered and would have been picked up by this point. Tearing of the transverse ligament is rare, except as part of fracturing, and again, there is no evidence of this.

That the range of motion losses at the atlantooccipital and atlantoaxial segments were eliminated with hold-relax techniques demonstrates that the restrictions were caused by excess muscle tone or guarding, not articular restriction or spasm. Movement loss of this type in the presence of vestibular dysfunction causing vertigo is often due to reflex guarding to prevent the head moving and causing dizziness. This phenomenon is well known to vestibular rehabilitation therapists, who commonly find range of motion increases when the vestibular problem begins to resolve with treatment.

The biomechanical tests demonstrated an articular pathomechanical restriction (the so-called subluxation) of extension at the right C2-3 joint (demonstrated by loss of right-side flexion in extension and of inferior gliding of the right zygapophyseal joint). The lack of findings in the lower neck strongly indicates that the disk bulging seen on the MRI is asymptomatic and irrelevant, because many of these are.

Diagnosis

1. Paroxysmal vertigo (needs to fully diagnosed) from labyrinthine concussion

2. Extension pathomechanical hypomobility (subluxation) at the right C2-3 zygopophyseal joint

3. Cervical spine induced nonvertiginous dizziness from the C2-3 subluxation

Treatment

1. Referral back to the physician for further referral for vestibular examination and rehabilitation therapy if indicated

2. Spinal manipulation or mobilization

3. Neck exercises to re-educate movement

This patient was referred back to his family practitioner for further investigation of the vertigo. The patient's physician then referred him to an otolaryngologist, who diagnosed him as suffering from benign positional paroxysmal vertigo due to cupulolithiasis. He was then referred to a vestibular rehabilitation therapist for treatment.

The vestibular rehabilitation therapist performed Epply's maneuver successfully, and the patient was vertigo free within a week. When seen again by the orthopedic therapist, extension, right-side flexion, and right rotation had increased to almost full range; flexion, left-side flexion, and left rotation were full range and painfree. Extension, right-side flexion, and right rotation were still painful in the right suboccipital area. The patient continued to complain of type 2 dizziness on left rotation, although this was less than previously experienced.

The C2-3 right zygapophyseal joint, which remained restricted, was manipulated into extension, after which the patient had full range of motion in the neck in all directions. He still had some pain on extension and right rotation, but this was considerably less than before the manipulation. He was given general exercises for neck movement and treated with segmental (as specific as possibly) PNF techniques over the next 2 weeks. He remained off work during this period. At the end of this period, he was almost painfree except for a mild headache upon waking some mornings. There had been no recurrence of his vertigo or dizziness.

When he returned to work, the neck pain and occipital headache recurred in 2 days. He was remanipulated and became painfree immediately. However, work the next day caused the condition to relapse once more. A functional capacity examination was arranged for him, which he underwent after again having the C2-3 segment manipulated. The functional assessment demonstrated that without the helmet on, the patient was capable of doing his job, but with it on, the symptoms recurred quickly and he was unable to perform.

The patient was offered and accepted vocational retraining in sales by his company. He has minor relapses once or twice a year, usually caused by unguarded movements, and responds well to remanipulation.

Cervical Case 6 Discussion

Diagnosis

The patient was referred to a neurosurgeon, who ordered a magnetic resonance angiogram (MRA). The MRA demonstrated indentation and reduced filling of the right vertebral artery. The diagnosis was now disk prolapse with radiculopathy and compression of the vertebral artery.

Both the therapist and the physician had ignored the vertigo, because it was short lived and the patient did not make a fuss about it. This case demonstrates a need for a routine examination of the balance system in any patient who manifests any symptoms of a disturbance in the system. This is especially important in those patients who may have damaged the system of its arteries through trauma or when treatment is a potential threat to the vertebral artery. The patient should have undergone a cranial nerve examination and general dizziness reproduction testing before range of motion testing.

A symptomatic vertebrobasilar accident is a rare occurrence and even rarer when it results from this type of indirect trauma. However, it is a possibility, and at the very least, the patient should have been asked about central neurological symptoms. Has there been any diplopia, visual field defects, other forms of dizziness/nausea, taste disturbances, hearing difficulties, dysphagia, and other such conditions? A cranial nerve examination could have been carried out, which might or might not have reproduced signs, although it is probable that occlusion would have to have been present for this. Vertebrobasilar patency testing in the clinic is certainly required in some form, even if this was only having the patient go through the range of cervical motion while observing for central neurological signs and symptoms and retesting some of the cranial nerves.

Cervical Case 7 Discussion

I have never encountered this situation, but a few possibilities arise.

1. There could be a frank partial rotatory dislocation at the atlantoaxial segment.
2. Infection-causing inflammation of the cervical glands can irritate the sternomastoid, but this usually occurs in younger children.
3. Primary bone cancer may cause acute torticollis.
4. The traction technique is poor and is tending to correct the deformity. This makes matters worse.
5. Traction is insufficient as a technique, and manipulation needs to carried out. However, the failure to recover quickly is unusual in this age group and further investigations need to be carried out prior to undertaking manipulative therapy. These investigations should include x-rays, at a minimum, and MRI, CT scans if readily available.

Cervical Case 8 Discussion

The symptoms appear to be linked with his posture, not because he has a head forward posture but because the symptoms are worse when he is in a head forward posture such as during standing and driving. In this theory, the angulation that occurs at the hypermobile C5/6 segment with the increased lordosis closes down the intervertebral foramen and produces symptoms on the side that is predisposed to stenosis by increased degenerative changes.

The link can be demonstrated by having the patient sit in an exaggerated head forward position until the pain and perhaps the pins and needles begin, which should be sooner than in normal sitting. "Correcting" the posture should relieve the symptoms faster than would normally occur. In this case, the link was established, and treatment was aimed at improving the patient's posture and so relieving the stress on the C5/6 segment.

The upper thoracic spine was examined for hypomobilities that may have been contributing to the problem. These were manipulated. The craniovertebral joints, particularly the atlantooccipital, were mobilized to increase flexion. The patient was then instructed in total body correction to bring the head more vertical in both static and dynamic working postures.

With practice, the patient was able to reduce the pain and paresthesia, provided that he remembered to avoid the head forward posture. When he did go into this position, the pain recurred.

Prognosis

If the patient can remember to maintain an optimal posture, then there should be no major recurrences. What does recur should be quickly remedied by the appropriate postural correction.

Cervical Case 9 Discussion

This case is loaded with red flags:

1. There is no apparent cause. This is especially significant in children because cumulative stress (repetitive strain) has not had a chance to make its presence felt.

2. Childhood pain in nonathletes is always something to be careful with, especially in the absence of trauma.

3. The pain is continuous, which is a pain state that could indicate inflammation or something more serious.

4. There has been no improvement in her condition. Children generally shake off minor musculoskeletal problems quickly. This persistence is not a good sign.

Diagnosis

Palpation of the right cervical glands demonstrated swelling and extreme tenderness. This young girl had an upper respiratory tract infection that involved her cervical glands. She was referred back to her physician, who put her on antibiotics that cleared the torticollis in 2 days.

Cervical Case 10 Discussion

The absence of cranial nerve signs and the negative "vertebral artery tests" exclude, as far as possible, vertebrobasilar compromise as a source of her symptoms. However, it does seem clear that she should be assessed for traumatic brain injury due to the presence of her ongoing diffuse headache, lack of concentration, lack of motivation, and general fatigue. She should also be assessed for vestibular function. Although she does not complain of vertigo, the ongoing dizziness could be due to a central vestibular dysfunction as evidenced by the Hallpike-Dix test. However, this test involves considerable stress through the neck. The dizziness might be cervicogenic, even though positioning the neck in extension and rotation failed to produce dizziness unless the body was laid horizontally. This can easily be checked during treatment. If the neck is causing the dizziness and its pain improves, then the dizziness should likewise improve. If it does not, it is unlikely that it originates from the neck.

The musculoskeletal dysfunction that is the cause of the neck pain and headache seems to be a flexion "subluxation" causing extension hypomobility of the left atlantooccipital joint. The source of most of the pain cannot be this joint because it is on the wrong side of the body although the minor left upper neck pain may be from this joint. A reasonable hypothesis is that the left hypomobility has caused undue strain on the right joint, and this has become symptomatic. The lower cervical biomechanical dysfunction is probably unrelated to the patient's symptoms. Asymptomatic articular hypomobilities are often seen on manual therapy courses and the same can be expected of the general public.

Diagnosis

1. Left atlantooccipital pathomechanical extension hypomobility
2. Probable posttraumatic head injury syndrome
3. Possible vestibular hypofunction

Treatment

The atlantooccipital dysfunction must be treated with either manipulation or mobilization. General stretching did not help in the past and there is no reason to expect it to help here. Once the joint is moving again, exercises should be given to reeducate movement. However, it must be remembered that a similar treatment had been tried previously by the chiropractor with limited success. The failure to gain long-term recovery may have been due to poor localization of the manipulative technique so that the dysfunctional joint was not affected. It may be that no exercises were given or that the exercises were inappropriate. It may also be that the possible vestibular dysfunction prevented long-term recovery due to its restricting effect on the cervical movements. This is a case of try it and see.

In this case, manipulative treatment and exercises failed to produce any long-lasting improvement after four treatments. The patient was referred back to her physician with a request for vestibular evaluation and a neuropsyche evaluation.

The neuropsychological evaluation stated that she was at the lower end of normal but because no baseline was available, it was difficult to know if there had been a reduction in her intellectual abilities.

The result of the vestibular evaluation was that she did have a central vestibular lesion, so she was referred to a vestibular rehabilitation therapist, who got in touch with the orthopedic therapist when vestibular rehabilitation was not having much of an effect. Combined manual therapy and vestibular rehabilitation therapy gradually improved her condition. She was almost painfree in the neck and occipital region within 6 weeks of beginning combined treatment and had no problems with her dizziness except on Hallpike-Dix testing. The diffuse headache was unaffected by any of the treatments but disappeared gradually over a 12-month period.

Cervical Case 11 Discussion

The cause of the vertigo still has not been found. In fact we have not been able to reproduce it, which is not a good sign because it suggests that its onset is dependent on the thrust rather than on the position.

The most stressful clinical vestibular test is the Hallpike-Dix. However, this should not be carried out in the standard manner until the vertebral artery has been eliminated as a diagnosis, which so far it has not. Another modification that is more stressful than the body tilt test but less stressful on the neck can be carried out. In this modification the patient's head is not dropped over the end of the bed but laid upon it so no extension occurs. The bed end can be tipped in order to extend the thorax rather than the neck, which simulates the test even more closely. In this case, the patient's head was dropped on the bed so that the neck remained in neutral but the head did fall below the body's level, the requirement for the full test. No vertigo occurred and no nystagmus was seen (Frenzel glasses were not used so there may have been nystagmus), strongly suggesting that the vertigo that followed cervical manipulation did not originate from the vestibular structures but may have been caused by ischemia of the neural projections in the vestibular system.

Diagnosis

Diagnosis is cervicogenic headaches from a left atlantooccipital flexion hypomobility and postmanipulative vertigo of unknown source.

Treatment

The biomechanical dysfunction requires manipulation or mobilization but the source of the vertigo is unknown. I worry when I am unable to reproduce the patient's symptoms. In this case, the problem was discussed with the physician, and he was offered two choices:

1. Treat the patient with careful mobilization, avoiding thrust techniques.
2. Refer the patient for vertebral artery studies (MRAs were unobtainable so Doppler or angiographic studies should be performed).

The physician thought both approaches were reasonable—to carefully treat the patient with nonthrust manual therapy and to see a specialist.

Mobilization brought about a rapid resolution of her headaches. She became painfree in three treatments. There was no recurrence of her vertigo during or after the treatment. So, when she saw the specialist, he decided to leave well enough alone and did not order any tests.

It was more than possible that this patient had an anomaly of one of her vertebral arteries that made her susceptible to the thrust of manipulation. She was advised by the specialist to never have her neck manipulated again.

Cervical Case 12 Discussion

Isolated orbital pain is not typical of cervical headaches regardless of her past history of neck-head pain. If she had been experiencing neck pain, then the eye pain would have been acceptable. In addition, there was no correlation between head and neck postures and/or movements and her eye pain, which was always present regardless of the posture of the head.

The important tests for this lady will be the cranial nerve tests. If the cranial nerve tests turn out to be negative, then the patient should have an ophthalmic examination if positive, a neurological one. During this examination, the therapist immediately noticed that the right pupil was dilated and when tested, failed to respond to light. The patient was advised to go to the emergency room. This she did and was immediately prescribed another migraine medication and given an eye patch. Within days, the aneurysm ruptured and the patient suffered a third nerve palsy.

This is a case in which there was a very unusual symptom—not the orbital pain, which is relatively common, but isolated orbital pain whose usual causes are ophthalmic or neurological. Uncommon pains generally have uncommon causes.

Cervical Case 13 Discussion

There should be some concerns with this case, but to be honest, this one escaped me.

The lower cervical dysfunction is simple enough—a symmetrical flexion subluxation (jamming) causing a pathomechanical extension hypomobility. The treatment consisted of traction manipulation that afforded immediate and complete relief from his lower cervical pain and gave him full range of motion. The prognosis should be good. The pain onset was delayed. It was a flexion rather than an extension injury. There were no referred pains (except possibly the headache). There was no pre-existing headache before the accident. He is young and there was nothing seen on the x-ray.

He was treated three times because there was slight and diminishing recurrence of the lower neck pain between treatments, and he maintained a painfree state in the cervicothoracic region for a week after the third treatment.

The headache is another matter. There were no clinical findings that would explain the headaches. They did not improve with treatment so the idea that they were being referred from the lower cervical dysfunction, a real possibility, was unlikely to be true.

The patient was referred back to his physician. I had no idea what was causing the headaches but I was reasonably sure that they were not emanating from his neck.

I did not see the patient again. About a month later, the emergency room physician phoned me asking what I had done with this patient. The patient had suffered a hind brain stroke as a result of a vertebral artery injury. Instead of seeing his physician when I sent him out, he had seen a chiropractor, who had started a course of manipulation for craniovertebral subluxations, which I had not found. He had four sessions of manipulation, and about 10 days after the final treatment, he had stoked from a ruptured vertebrobasilar pseudoaneurysm.

This case occurred many years ago before I tested routinely for vertebral artery compromise. At this time, only those patients relating symptoms of brainstem functional compromise were tested by me. I learned much from this case. First, you do not need dizziness or any other nonmusculoskeletal symptoms to have a damaged vertebral artery. Second, all patients need to be tested for vertebral artery sufficiency before manipulative treatment or any other therapy that may threaten the hind brain vascular system. Third, be careful of pains that do not have an obvious association with other symptomatic areas and where local joints do not have movement dysfunction. Fourth, if the possible source of the referred symptoms is improving and the referred symptoms are not, the chances are that the symptoms are not referred from here.

Would testing the vertebrobasilar system have demonstrated the insufficiency and thereby prevented the stroke? There is no way of knowing. However, the best way in preventing the stroke for this patient would have been to treat only those clinical signs that are obvious. My feeling is that the chiropractor, who probably was not using a biomechanical assessment, depended on the headache to determine what spinal levels required treatment. In my opinion, in the absence of pain provocation when these levels were tested and the absence of biomechanical findings, the craniovertebral joints were not a viable target for treatment.

On the other hand, either the chiropractor did some damage to a previously undamaged vertebral artery or the artery was damaged at the time of the injury and my assessment was inadequate. With hindsight and the current thoughts on testing for neurovascular sufficiency, my examination was certainly less than it could have been. Whether it would have demonstrated arterial damage is another matter. However, two principles come through in this case. Do not treat an area unless you can find objective evidence of an underlying dysfunction (that is, do not treat symptoms biomechanically). In fact, be downright suspicious of it. Second, if treatment is failing to improve the condition quickly, reconsider your premise.

Cervical Case 14 Discussion

I would not (nor did I) return her to work at this point. She had already had one poor experience with too early a return to work, especially considering what work she would be doing and the position (neck flexion) that she would be doing it in. Additionally, the presence of the nerve root signs and symptoms especially of the ongoing paresthesia would suggest that her condition is precarious and could easily slide back into its former acute state.

There does not seem to be much point in continuing with the traction. The range of motion is almost normal. The neurological signs have for the most part disappeared, and she has not noted recent improvement with this treatment.

So what treatment do we initiate? There is not enough information to make this decision, so further information must be generated from the biomechanical examination. We also have to wonder about the ongoing paresthesia after the articular signs have optimized. This may be the time to carry out the upper limb neuromeningeal mobility tests.

The biomechanical examination demonstrated a left C2-3 zygopophyseal joint extension hypomobility with a pathomechanical end feel. This suggests a flexion subluxation of the left C2-3 zygopophyseal joint. The other cervical joints were biomechanically normal.

The lack of biomechanical findings at the lower cervical levels removes a mechanical dysfunction as the cause of the paresthesia. This led to upper limb tension testing. The results of this were that paresthesia was produced with right neck flexion, abduction and extension of the shoulder, and extension elbow. The paresthesia was significantly worse when the wrist was flexed in this position.

Diagnosis

C2-3 flexion subluxation is suggested by the movement restriction and the pathomechanical end feel. The absence of arm pain and biomechanical signs in the lower cervical levels together with the paresthesia and the radial nerve upper limb tension test would suggest adhesions or edema of the sixth spinal nerve (presumptive based on the initial compression).

Treatment

The biomechanical dysfunction at the left C2-3 zygopophyseal joint was treated with manipulation (nonrhythmical end range mobilizations could have been used). Movement was regained immediately with an immediate subsidence in the neck pain and its complete disappearance over the next couple of days.

The paresthesia was treated with careful and graded stretches for sixth cervical spinal nerve and roots and its continuation into the arm. The paresthesia disappeared within 10 days of starting the stretches on an alternate day basis. In addition to the neural stretches, she was also treated with progressive resisted exercises and work conditioning.

The patient returned to work 6 weeks after accident and had a relapse within a week. A phone call from her told me that all of the original pain recurred. However, this time she also experienced severe radicular pain in the left arm to the thumb. An MRI at this time confirmed the presence of a left posterior to posterolateral herniation of the C5/6 disk with compression of the C6 root. Eventually, she had surgery.

Cervical Case 15 Discussion

The patient's history is one of unfamiliar overuse. The biomechanical signs in the neck are not at segments that are likely to be involved in tennis elbow. Diagnosis is epicondylar tennis elbow of local origin. Not everything is spinal in origin. Treatment was tennis elbow support, avoidance of pain-provoking activities, modalities, frictions, stretches, and strengthening.

Cervical Case 16 Discussion

The onset of the headache after the examination supports the contention that it is referred from the cervical spine.

The restriction of general range of motion was in a pattern that could be due either to inflammation of one or more joints on the right side of the neck or to a biomechanical dysfunction into extension of one or more joints on the right. The absence of spasm would argue against inflammation as a cause of the restriction, whereas the pathomechanical end feel suggests that a more mechanical explanation is probable. The rapid reduction of inflammation suggests a good prognosis. The mechanical basis for the neck pain tends to argue against the need for a collar.

Treatment

Treatment could initially consist of mobilizing or manipulating the dysfunctional C2-3 articulation. However, because she is improving rapidly on her own, it would be advisable to leave well enough alone. In this case, she was initially treated with advice on rest and activity and painfree exercises. She improved over the following days, but she did not get rid of the headache until the C2-3 joint was manipulated.

Cervical Case 17 Discussion

If this was a Pancoast syndrome, elements of Horner's syndrome can be expected to be found. Among these elements are ptosis, anhydrosis (absent or reduced sweating on one side of the face), facial flushing, enophthalamus (eyeball retraction), and miosis (pupil constriction).

Potential causes are apical lung cancer (Pancoast's tumor) or breast cancer infiltrating the lower brachial plexus and inferior cervical ganglion.

Diagnosis

In this case, the patient did have a minor ptosis and miosis. When he was sent back to his physician, he was x-rayed, and an apical lung tumor was found.

Cervical Case 18 Discussion

It seemed probable that the neck was playing a role in this man's symptoms. The level of involvement as determined from the biomechanical examination was appropriate. The reproduction of the symptoms during the upper limb tension tests when the neck was side flexed contralaterally seemed to confirm this.

The patient was successfully treated with local treatment to the wrist (interferential currents and ultrasound) and manual traction to the cervical spine.

Cervical Case 19 Discussion

Diagnosis

1. Infraspinatus tendonitis
2. Extension hypomobility T1/2

3. Extension hypermobility C6/7 and C7/T1 with segmental facilitation leading to restricted shoulder movement

Treatment

The infraspinatus can be treated with a variety of modalities including deep transverse frictions, ultrasound, interferential currents, muscle stimulation, and strengthening and stretching exercises.

The neck should be treated with mobilization or manipulation for the hypomobile segment in order to relieve the stress on the hypermobile joint.

In this case, the shoulder movements, with the exception of medial rotation/extension, became full range and painfree after manipulating the neck. The medial rotation/range improved gradually when frictions were applied to the tender area of the infraspinatus tendon. At the end of six treatments, she had full range, painfree shoulder and neck movements.

Cervical Case 20 Discussion

No diagnosis was made except to send the patient back to the physician querying inappropriate pathology and to ask for further objective investigations.

Another x-ray revealed an osteoblastoma of the left lamina of the third cervical vertebra. When the earlier x-rays were reviewed, it was visible.

This patient was referred back almost solely on the basis of her history. The torticollis itself behaved like a normal torticollis and afforded little information.

Cervical Case 21 Discussion

The prognosis remains poor due to the presence of neurological signs.

Diagnosis

The diagnosis is C7 cervical radiculopathy. From the provocative factor of extension, the paresthesia is due either to an inflamed C7 nerve root or a root that has been damaged by the hyperextension. If it is simple inflammation, the paresthesia should resolve fairly quickly. If the accident actually damaged the nerve root, then recovery will take much longer.

In addition, there may be undetermined structural damage to the craniovertebral joints. This will require a biomechanical examination.

The type 2 dizziness is related to the neck, due to either the joint dysfunction or an injured vertebral artery. It seems probable that the dizziness is due to cervical joint dysfunction, but there is always the possibility of it being neurovascular.

The vertigo is probably due to inner ear disturbances, most likely otoconia displacement.

The diffuse headache appears not to be related to the cervical condition nor does it seem to be part of intracranial bleeding, given the absence of intellectual impairment. However, during its early days, the patient must be watched carefully. Another possibility that would explain this headache is postconcussion syndrome. Although he does not remember being knocked unconscious, it is possible that he was. He requires more careful questioning regarding amnesia.

Treatment

The patient needs to be referred back to the physician because of the vertigo alone. This needs to be assessed and if necessary treated by a vestibular rehabilitation therapist before much can be expected in terms of recovery.

Meanwhile treatment can be initiated. Manual therapy at this time is probably to risky for the likely gains. The patient should be watched for progression of symptoms.

This particular patient was treated with Epley's maneuver for his vertigo, which was diagnosed as BPPV due to otoconic displacement. Essentially this maneuver shakes the displaced bodies in the vestibular labyrinth and moves them to a position of unimportance. The patient did well with this treatment, and the vertigo disappeared with one treatment.

The paresthesia and hypoesthesia did not improve and was present on discharge 6 weeks later. The type 2 dizziness improved when the cervical pain improved with modalities and painfree exercises.

The patient was discharged with some remaining upper cervical pain, which was easily exacerbated with overactivity and paresthesia in the forearm and hand.

Cervical Case 22 Discussion

This accident may have been unavoidable, but we will never know. A number of things done and not done may have alerted the practitioner to the possibility that all was not well with this patient.

1. Never rely on the examination by another therapist when treating a patient, especially if that treatment involves significant risk.

2. Do not rely on the history to definitively exclude neurological or neurovascular complications. Every patient should be routinely assessed for neurological deficits, both segmental and central nervous systems prior to treatment being undertaken.

3. Every patient having manual therapy, whether manipulation or mobilization, should be examined using Hautant's, minimized Wallenberg's (de Klyne), or some other positioning test at a minimum. These should be done at the beginning of every treatment session.

4. If there is any hint from the history or another part of the examination that there is a central nervous system disorder, a full neurological examination, including cranial nerve and long tract tests, should be undertaken.

5. If dizziness is related, a progressive dizziness-testing protocol should be initiated.

6. Any patient with definite central nervous system signs or symptoms must be referred to the physician or emergency room.

7. Any patient who develops dizziness or other nondefinite signs or symptoms that are potentially central must be kept in the clinic until the symptoms are gone. Or if they remain for more than 15 minutes with no improvement or they worsen, the patient should be sent to the emergency room by ambulance.

In this case there was conflicting evidence about the presence of neurological symptoms. However, the fact that the symptoms were worse during the course of her treatment program should have caused the chiropractor to undertake a complete re-examination of the patient.

There is conflicting evidence about the efficacy of the positioning tests. Thiel[1] and Cote[2] both cast doubts on the validity of the rotation-extension position as a screen for vertebrobasilar pathology. However, in neither study was there a single patient with this pathology as an established diagnosis. Rather it was presumed because their vertigo was otherwise unexplained. On the other hand, a case cited by Combs and Triano[3] demonstrated that the test was positive in a case of vertebrobasilar pathology. Until the invalidity of these positioning tests has been definitively demonstrated, this test should not be eliminated from our examination techniques. It is quick, relatively safe, if done progressively in suspect patients, and known to be appropriately positive in some patients. In this particular case, the test may have been useful because the patient on whom Combs and Triano found the test to be positive had a hypoplastic artery, the same circumstances as with the patient in this case.

1. Thiel H, et al.: Effect of various head and neck positions on vertebral artery blood flow. *Clin Biomech* 1994; 9:105–110.
2. Cote P, et al.: The validity of the extension-rotation test as a clinical screening procedure before neck manipulation: A secondary analysis. *J Manip Physiol Ther* 1996; 19(3):159–164.
3. Combs SB, Triano JJ: Symptoms of neck artery compromise: Case presentations of risk estimate for treatment. *J Manip Physiol Ther* 1997; 20(4):274–278.

Thoracic Case 1 Discussion

Diagnosis

Diagnosis is neurological pain of nonmusculoskeletal origin.

Treatment

The absence of movement restriction or reproduction of pain with trunk movements removes this patient from the scope of the physical therapist until the physician has made a more definitive diagnosis. The patient should be referred back to the physician for further testing. This patient was referred back to the physician. By the time he saw her, a rash of vesicles had appeared and the diagnosis of Shingles (herpes zoster) was made.

Thoracic Case 2 Discussion

Certainly, given the reproduction of the patient's symptoms with palpation, the costochondral junction seems to be the source of the pain. But is it the cause of the pain? There is no swelling, which is a usual accompaniment of costochondritis. The thickening that is usually seen after the resolution of this type of inflammation is absent. However, perhaps the resolution was rapid and complete and no thickening resulted. But in this case, why the recurrences? In any case, if 4 weeks of treatment to this area failed to resolve the problem, 4 more weeks of the same are unlikely to do any better.

I was unable to make a diagnosis, apart from costochondralgia (which is simply a regurgitation of the patient's symptoms), and require further information. Consequently, a biomechanical examination was carried out.

Results of passive intervertebral movement testing of the thoracic spinal segments were negative. The posterior rib joints were examined, and the right fourth articular complex was found to have lost all of its glides.

Diagnosis

Right fourth costotransverse and/or costovertebral joint subluxation (jammed) causes abnormal stresses to be imparted on the costochondral junction and results in costochondralgia. It is a relative common observation that the hypomobile joint is asymptomatic (why is not well understood), but may cause symptoms in another joint that its hypomobility is stressing. There is some support for this hypothesis from the history when the patient related that the original pain had been posterior. The theory can be tested easily by manipulating or mobilizing the posterior rib joint and by assessing the degree of change in the anterior pain and the patient's level of function.

Treatment

The right fourth posterior rib articular complex was manipulated. The pain that was felt on right trunk rotation disappeared, but the costochondral junction was still tender. The patient was asked to resume normal weight lifting in a week (to allow any costochondral inflammation time to subside) and then see what happens.

The patient was able to lift without pain, although on examination, the posterior joint did seem to have subluxed once more and was re-manipulated. The patient began kayaking again a month later without problems and was at her full functional level within another 2 weeks.

Prognosis

Given the unpredictability of the sport of white-water kayaking, it would be foolhardy to say that this problem will not recur. If it happened once, it can happen again. But a reasonable statement would be that for normal function the prognosis is good, but that sudden and severe forces applied to the joint may cause a recurrence.

Thoracic Case 3 Discussion

The patient's physician phoned me 2 days after I had last seen her and asked if there had been anything unusual about her. I said no and asked why. He said that he had seen her the day before, which is the day after I had last treated her. She was fine, still painful, but otherwise fine, but today she was admitted as a spastic quadriplegia and was waiting to have exploratory surgery. The surgeons removed a large neurofibroma from her spine. She recovered fully, which is more than I can say for me.

A number of points should have made me suspect that all was not as it should be. These include:

1. The patient's age
2. The lack of causative factors
3. The lack of response to treatment

This case illustrates that not all cancers fall into the pattern of signs and symptoms often taught, that is, severe, constant, intractable pain worsens at night. This pattern is more characteristic of advanced bone cancer than anything else.

I learned from this patient the need to carry out a proper biomechanical examination, not just position testing with a half-baked arthrokinematic tests. And I learned that the combination of an older patient and pain with no obvious etiology or history is something of which to be wary.

Congratulations to those of you who were brighter than me.

Thoracic Case 4 Discussion

We disagree with the physician's diagnosis. The treatment requested by the physician has made no difference to the patient so we should be planning to change treatments. At this point, the physician must be informed of our opinion and the need to change treatments and the proposed change. It is also probable that given the degree of pain that the patient is in and our difference of opinion with the diagnosis afforded by the physician, the physician might want to order other tests, particularly an MRI. In this case, no MRI was taken but the physician agreed to a change in treatment.

Treatment

The original treatment should be maintained. The inflammation is still present and its resolution is a priority. However, it is possible that it cannot be resolved because of ongoing compression. The most obvious method of trying to reduce this is with manual traction but traction in the examination increased the patient's pain. When traction was reapplied more carefully, making sure that the traction was not correcting the patient's deviation, she was able to tolerate it without any increase in symptoms. A more aggressive treatment would be traction manipulation but, given the intensity of the patient's symptoms and the degree of restriction of motion, this can wait until later and be used if necessary.

The patient was treated with manual traction on a daily basis. Gradually the pain subsided and her range of motion increased. The lancinating pain was suddenly absent one morning 3 weeks after starting traction and did not reappear. At this point she returned to work. Six weeks into treatment when she was being seen three times a week, she stopped progressing. She had no deviation and moderate restriction of right rotation and extension; a traction manipulation was applied that gave her full range of motion and almost no pain. Two days later she was painfree.

Thoracic Case 5 Discussion

Nothing from the objective examination has changed my mind that a rib fracture is a real possibility. The active movements would argue against a disk herniation or a zygopophyseal joint dysfunction because both of these would have more involvement of flexion and extension. There is the possibility of a rib subluxation or a transverse subluxation of the vertebral segment, both of which might present with similar patterns of restriction. However, they are found through the biomechanical tests and we have yet to clear the medical conditions.

Although deep inspiration did reproduce her pain and is considered by many to be a neuromeningeal test (the lateral rib movement pulling the intercostal nerve and its roots and their dural sleeves laterally along the foramen), it also stresses the rib.

Of course, the positive isometric tests stress the rib, but there is also the real possibility that if a fracture did occur, one or more intercostal muscles were lacerated. This is only likely to occur with a displaced fracture.

We need to test the rib carefully. This can be done by palpating for tenderness, gently applying compression along the long axis of the rib, and by using a low-frequency tuning fork along the length of the rib. I would suggest the tuning fork and palpation and compression only when these two turn out to be negative.

In this case, the fracture tests were positive, so the patient was referred back to the physician, who had x-rays taken that demonstrated the fracture.

Thoracic Case 6 Discussion

The first place to look is always the closest, both geographically and functionally. In this case, it is to the posterior joints. From personal experience and from the literature,[1] one possible etiology of Tietze's syndrome is mechanical dysfunction of one or more of the posterior joints, either the spinal or the costal. The mistake in this patient's case was to diverge from the normal examination protocol, short-cuts are often much longer and, worse yet, can lead to inappropriate treatment.

Objective Examination

All trunk movements were full range and painfree except left rotation, which reproduced the anterior pain in mild form. None of the movements produced posterior pain.

Isometric trunk resisted tests were negative.

A biomechanical examination was clearly indicated, which demonstrated an anteriorly subluxed third rib on the right side. This was assumed to be the immediate cause of the patient's symptoms and was manipulated. It was assumed that the right rotation was stressing the rib enough to produce symptoms, whereas the other movements were not.

On reexamination, the biomechanical tests were negative but he could still feel the low-level anterior pain. However, left rotation was painfree. It was believed that the remaining pain was due to low-level inflammation

---

1. Grieve GP. Thoracic musculoskeletal problems. In: *Grieve's Modern Manual Therapy*, 2nd edition. Edinburgh: Churchill Livingston; 1994:428.

and the patient was asked to avoid all pain-provoking activities for a week, then reattend. Anti-inflammatory modalities could have been utilized, but it was believed that the inflammation was such a low grade that they would not be very effective and, in any case, that they were unnecessary.

The patient reattended the following week and had been painfree from the day following the manipulation. However, it was recognized that the root cause had still not been discovered.

Stability tests on the third costotransverse joint (for a detailed and pictorial description of some of these mobility and stability tests, see Lee[2]) demonstrated anterior instability, but again did not elucidate a cause.

The patient was treated eight times with stability exercises. However, it was recognized that this treatment still did not address the underlying problem and that it might not be possible to determine the real cause. The patient's coach was asked to assess his technique and correct it if necessary.

The patient resumed weight training 2 weeks into treatment and kayak training 2 weeks later. He competed without problems 4 weeks later and has not had a relapse.

Thoracic Case 7 Discussion

In retrospect, no! Mobilization and muscle energy treatments produced pain relief for about 2 hours for each of the three treatments I gave this lady, but each time her pain returned to its previous level spontaneously. Naturally I initially blamed her for the relapses, telling her that she had not been doing the exercises or had been overactive against my advice. But she consistently denied these accusations and by the fourth visit, I was forced to accept that it was the treatment that was at fault. I asked her to return to her physician, who auscultated her chest. He found pleural sounds and deduced that she had pleural adhesions from the prior attack of pneumonia.

From this case, I learned that position testing alone is not a sufficiently specific examination process and that a complete biomechanical examination is required. It is likely that if this had been done properly, the joint glides would have been found to be normal, which might have cued me to distrust a musculoskeletal diagnosis.

Thoracic Case 8 Discussion

The objective examination results strengthen the contention that the thoracic pain is from a thoracic rather than a cervical source. Even though cervical extension did reproduce her interscapular pain and the thoracic

2. Lee DH. *Manual therapy for the thorax: A biomechanical approach.* Delta, BC: DOPC Publishing; 1994.

movements did not, this is not uncommon. The upper thoracic spine may be stressed more with cervical motion than with thoracic. Elevation causing shoulder pain that had not been previously experienced by the patient is another indication that there is a dysfunction in the upper thoracic spine. This limits shoulder elevation and puts increased stress on the tissues of the shoulder, which is not painful until the shoulder is taken to extreme.

This lady requires a biomechanical examination. This examination demonstrated hypomobility into extension of the right zygopophyseal joint at C5/6 and an extension hypomobility of both zygopophyseal joints of T3/4.

She was treated with cervical and thoracic manipulation (mobilization can be used if the therapist is not manipulating) and immediately recovered full and painfree ranges in the spine although the shoulder that now was full range was still painful at the extreme of elevation. She was taught upper body and upper limb exercises to maintain range and reeducate movement. On reattendance a week later, the cervical spine remained painfree, but the interscapular pain recurred with working. She was remanipulated and taped for proprio-ceptive cueing and did well at work until the tape was removed whereupon the pain returned.

When stability was tested, she was found to be painfully unstable anteriorly at T3/4. Stabilization therapy was initiated and she was told not to work without the tape on. In addition, she was advised to be careful about her posture and to not spend more time than necessary in neck flexion. After 6 weeks, she was allowed to remove the tape. She managed to work a week without pain at which point she was discharged.

Lumbopelvic Case 1 Discussion

Treatment

The biomechanical examination was not strictly necessary to arrive at the diagnosis of posttraumatic arthritis and because no manual therapy is indicated (except for possibly general pain modulation techniques) it does not help to determine treatment. However, it is nice to have the diagnosis confirmed by other tests.

Treatment should consist of facilitating the resolution of the inflammation, avoidance of activities or postures that cause pain, anti-inflammatory modalities, and gentle, nonpainful exercises. The patient is more likely to be comfortable in flexion postures, which should not be discouraged even though frequent posture changes should prevent painful stiffness. The exercises will stimulate mechanoreceptors thereby providing pain modulation and also helping to reduce venous congestion.

Prognosis

Given the patient's age and condition and the traumatic nature of the onset, prognosis is very good. If full resolution does not occur within a week or two, patient compliance must be questioned. If this appears to be acceptable, the diagnosis might be incorrect. Then a fracture or other severe traumatic pathology must be reconsidered.

Lumbopelvic Case 2 Discussion

There are two probabilities here. The patient is recovering, which is demonstrated by the absence of the parasthesia. Or the patient is worsening and the parasthesia has been replaced by increased sensory paresis, indicating increasing pressure on the spinal nerve or posterior root. The patient may not be aware of decreasing sensation or may not be volunteering information.

In either case, the neurological signs must be reassessed in detail. If they have worsened, treatment should be discontinued and either another tried or the patient referred back to the physician. If there is no change in the neurological signs or if improved, continuation of the same treatment is indicated.

With very difficult problems, there is a tendency to take the most optimistic view of generated information especially subjective information. Be critical. Subject the patient to clinical testing and fairly pointed questioning. In this case, such questions as "Has the feeling in your leg changed?" or "Do you feel stronger or weaker than when I last saw you?" may give a hint about progress.

Lumbopelvic Case 3 Discussion

Things have obviously gotten much worse with this lady. The presenting signs and symptoms strongly suggest a much larger disk lesion with compression of the S1 and perhaps the S2 spinal nerve/root. The patient now has neurological signs that include deficits of all three of the measurement criteria—strength, sensation, and reflexes. The presence of radicular pain indicates either inflammation or adhesions of the spinal nerve or root or its contact with nuclear material. In any event, the nerve is affected. The right straight leg raise is very limited and produces radicular pain; neither aspect is encouraging. The loss of both flexion and extension and the fact that both reproduce the radicular pain also strongly suggest a large herniation of the disk substance. The switch from the left to the right leg would suggest an unstable disk, possibly with sequestrated material.

Diagnosis is L4/5 or L5/S1 disk prolapse or extrusion with possible sequestration causing a right S1 radiculopathy.

Prognosis is not good. It is unlikely that physical therapy will substantially help this patient in anything but the extreme short term. She must be advised about the best resting position. A lumbar support might help her to remember not to straighten up or bend down. If any treatment is going to be attempted, it should be in neutral, neither trying to flex nor extend her. She should be referred as soon as possible to a surgeon.

A second MRI at this time revealed a lumbosacral disk herniation with sequestration and compression of the right dural sleeve of S1.

Lumbopelvic Case 4 Discussion

Diagnosis

Diagnosis is developmental lumbosacral spondylolisthesis. The patient's weight problem and the hyperlordosis support this diagnosis. Also the lumbosacral junction should not flex during trunk flexion to the point where it is rounded; this can indicate an anterior instability. In addition, the paradoxical recovery from flexion when the spine extends after the hips also suggests that instability is present.

Treatment

Because the condition has a history of spontaneous improvement and seems to be doing just that right on schedule, this would be a good time to do nothing. Allow the patient to fully recover from the condition, giving advice on what to avoid as he does so. Once recovery has occurred, then stability therapy is the appropriate treatment. Flexion exercises producing a kyphosis can be given as a means of reversing any tendency toward spondylolisthesis. Trunk stability exercises should be taught and practiced to ensure that the extensor and abdominal muscles are firing appropriately to prevent a hyperlordotic position occurring during activities and static positions. Quasisegmental PNF exercises calling for concentric and eccentric contractions of the muscles at and near the dysfunctional segment should be administered.

Prognosis

With attention to detail and persistence with his exercises, this patient should have a good prognosis. He may have to limit or change his leisure activities but his job should not present any problems in either the long or the short term.

Lumbopelvic Case 5 Discussion

The passive biomechanical tests eliminate the sacroiliac joint as a player in this patient's conditions. The pelvic position tests are completely unreliable because the starting positions of the pelvic bones are unknown and are almost never symmetrical. The positive kinetic tests are probably a function of the lumbar dysfunction because they were not supported by the passive movement tests.

The spinal biomechanical tests show a right extension hypomobility caused by a segmental structure. The normal end feel on the zygopophyseal joint glides excludes an articular restriction and the springy end feel would suggest a small disk bulge. The absence of any mechanical findings in flexion would suggest that the flexion restriction has an extra-segmental origin, probably dural irritation when flexion pulls the dura onto the disk bulge.

A nonbiomechanical approach to the ongoing examination of this patient could be the McKenzie approach. In this case, I would ask the patient to repeat extension initially in standing. If reduction or centralization of the pain occurs, then this would be the patient's treatment. If there was no change, I would have the patient repeat extension in standing. If this failed to improve the condition or if prone extension increased the pain, I would ask the patient to repeat flexion. In this case, repeated prone extension, which I used after the biomechanical examination, improved both the intensity and location of the pain.

Diagnosis

Diagnosis is small L4/5 disk protrusion or contained herniation with right posterolateral L4/5 or L5/S1 dural sleeve compression.

Prognosis

This patient should do well because this is his first major episode and the signs are minimal.

Treatment

The patient is advised to avoid sitting for a week (which means taking time off work). If this is not possible, make sure that his lumbar spine is well supported into extension. He should not be lifting or bending for about a month if possible.

Passive prone extension exercises (half push-ups) were advised and the patient was instructed to do 10 of them every hour. He was seen daily for a biomechanical exam to ensure that the exercises were not hyperextending the normal segments. He continued to improve over the week until he was painfree and had full range movement in the cardinal planes of flexion, extension, side flexion, and rotation. However, combined extension and right-side flexion was limited and slightly painful.

The prone extension exercises were discontinued and asymmetrical extension exercises substituted. This had the patient bending backward and to the right. After 3 days of this exercise, he had full and painfree asymmetrical extension. The patient was instructed in sitting, lifting, and bending. He was put on a fast walking program to replace the exercises and asked to come back in 6 to 8 weeks for a progression of his treatment.

Once things had stabilized and the patient had been painfree for 7 weeks, he returned and was instructed in abdominal and extensor exercises for muscle conditioning and reeducation and flexion and torsional exercises to begin strengthening the segmental tissues. Once these exercises had been learned, the patient was discharged after being told to discontinue these exercises in about 2 months.

Lumbopelvic Case 6 Discussion

Diagnosis

This patient has all the hallmarks of a lumbar disk herniation with compression of the second spinal nerve or nerve root except for low-back pain. However, far lateral (foraminal or extra-foraminal) disk herniations (Cyriax termed these primary posterolateral protrusions) present in this manner and at these levels produce similar symptoms to those complained of by the patient when it compresses the dorsal root ganglion or the nerve root. High-resolution CT scanning or MRI examination will normally disclose the herniation so it is possible that the resolution was not sufficient.

Treatment

There is disagreement in the diagnosis. The physician should be informed of your opinion before anything else is undertaken with this patient if you are considering changing the treatment from that on the prescription. In any event, it will be almost impossible to do anything with this patient except make him comfortable. With that in mind, travelling to and from the clinic seems somewhat counterproductive.

The physician was contacted and agreed to order an MRI, which disclosed foraminal compression of the second lumbar nerve root by the L1/2 disk.

Lumbopelvic Case 7 Discussion

Diagnosis

Diagnosis is low lumbar central developmental spinal stenosis. This is frequently caused by hypertrophy of the zygopophyseal joint capsules or osteophytosis. Usually there is a predisposing factor in the form of a trefoil spinal canal or otherwise congenitally narrow spinal canal. It could be multisegmental bilateral lateral stenosis but the chances of it affecting two levels bilaterally and equally are fairly remote. In any event, it makes no real difference, the treatment will be the same.

Treatment

Because this condition is due to structural changes, treatment is really management. The patient is instructed in things that he almost certainly already knows about daily activities—avoid extension postures that occur during prolonged standing or overhead work, and extension activities such as fast walking. Flexion exercises can be helpful in reversing the symptoms and mobilizing the spine over a very protracted period. Occasionally, lumbar traction increases the patient's tolerance to extension and the patient can be shown how to do this at home by lying supine, putting his calves on a chair, and contracting the hamstrings. This produces some minor lumbar traction, which can sometimes have a therapeutic effect out of all proportions to the mechanical effect. In addition, some patients receive long-lasting relief (a few weeks or months) with mechanical lumbar traction applied in flexion or neutral.

Prognosis

Any therapeutic effect will be temporary. The patient must persist with the exercises and/or have treatment on an intermittent basis permanently, or at least until the treatment stops having an effect. In this case, the patient, who was avoiding extension activities as much as possible, did well on a flexion exercise program and self-traction being able to relieve any symptoms that arose faster than before.

Lumbopelvic Case 8 Discussion

Shift correction can still be attempted but much more slowly. The patient was laid on his left side so that the pelvis tended to fall toward the bed. The patient was supported so that he could not roll forward or backward. A muscle stimulator was used to stimulate the left erector spinae muscles and a hot pack was strapped to the patient's back to relax him. He was left for 15 minutes and told to take up the same position at home for 15 minutes every hour. In addition, he was warned about flexing and sitting. To reinforce this, his back was taped lightly in a diagonal cross.

When he was seen 3 days later, the deviation was a little less and his movements a little better. But the pain was still acute. However, on retesting the mobility of the deviation, it was found that it could be partly corrected without provoking severe pain or spasm. Treatment consisted of shift correction in the clinic and self-correction plus prone extension exercises at home.

The patient continued to improve over the next week and by the end of the week was standing straight. He was painfree in 2 weeks. The usual instruction on prophylaxis and activity was given.

Lumbopelvic Case 9 Discussion

The piriformis muscle as a source of the pain was eliminated with the contractile tests and by stretching the muscles. Neither test reproduced the patient's pain.

I think we can eliminate any serious disease processes or disk herniations from the differential diagnosis. The pain is definitely linked to mechanical stress, which lessens the possibility of it being caused by visceral disease or primary bone cancer. There are no dural or neurological signs and the articular signs, while very definite, are minor. It also seems likely that this is not due to a sacroiliitis because the primary stress tests for the sacroiliac joint were negative.

This appears to be a biomechanical dysfunction of either the lumbar zygopophyseal joint or the sacroiliac joint.

On intervertebral mobility testing, L5/S1 was found to have reduced physiological and arthrokinematic extension and right-side flexion movements with a jammed end feel. All other movements and segments had normal ranges. Passive mobility testing of the sacroiliac joints was negative.

Diagnosis

This case demonstrates the typical easy manual therapy patient. She has a flexion subluxation of the right lumbosacral zygapophyseal joint, which limits extension. This dysfunction is a very real problem for her because she needs this motion to be able to run efficiently and painlessly.

A larger question, which is beyond the scope of this book, is why this happened. The investigation of cause will take in the entire lower quadrant.

Treatment

Manipulation is the most efficient and effective method of dealing with this problem. One treatment proved to be sufficient to regain full range painfree motion in the spine.

If you are not manipulating, then erratic mobilizations to try to shake loose the jammed joint are next best. Poorest will be exercise into extension and side flexion hoping to be able to move the joint.

Prognosis

This is difficult to assess at this time. It might be that this was a simple aberration and the stumble was in precisely the right (or wrong!) direction to cause the subluxation to occur. If so, then her prognosis is good and she need not worry unless she stumbles in the same direction again. However, if this was the last straw on the camel's back, the future does not look so rosy.

It will be necessary to see how she reacts to running over the next few weeks. If the problem recurs, then a thorough clinical examination of the whole lower quadrant will have to carried out.

In this case, the pain did not recur during a 2-month period and she was running without problems.

Lumbopelvic Case 10 Discussion

The objective examination gives us more to worry about. Neck flexion, with and without the straight leg raise neck flexion, produced tingling in the trunk and legs. Although this may be acceptable during the straight leg raise, it must be viewed with suspicion when it occurs in isolation. The production of trunk paresthesia with neck flexion is definitely not associated with a lumbar disk herniation. We must also be concerned with the presence of weakness in the nonpainful leg.

This patient is definitely out of the scope of the orthopedic therapist. He has L'Hermitte's sign (tingling in the trunk and limbs on neck flexion), which is a manifestation of nerve damage and is found on peripheral nerve and spinal cord injury and disease. The presence of neurological signs in the absence of pain or in the presence of mild pain frequently means neurological disease.

He was returned to the physician and investigated for neurological disease, most probably multiple sclerosis.

Lumbopelvic Case 11 Discussion

If you have manual therapy skills, a biomechanical examination may help you to narrow down the differential diagnosis further. If a specific segmental restriction implicating the articulation (pathomechanical or hard abnormal end feel) is found in one of the two lower lumbar levels, then cautious manual therapy aimed at mobilizing the joint hypomobility should be tried. If no articular hypomobility is found, then the possibility that the diagnosis is disk herniation is stronger. If an articular hypomobility is present, a disk herniation is not excluded as a diagnosis, because there is no reason why a biomechanical dysfunction should not coexist with a disk herniation, but the possibility is reduced. This patient did have evidence of articular hypomobility, in that the end feel was jammed into flexion.

In the absence of a biomechanical examination, or even in conjunction with it, an assessment to evaluate the condition's response to repeated exercises could be undertaken. Extension would be the obvious movement to test but bilateral extension was full range, so prior to testing repeated movements, assess unilateral extension. In this case, extension and right-side flexion was limited to about 50% of the combined movement to the left and was painful in the right low back and buttock. This extra information allows us to move to unilateral extension (that is extension and left-side flexion), if bilateral extension fails to improve the patient. In this patient, repeated (40 times) bilateral extension in prone lying improved both his range of flexion and the straight leg raise.

Treatment

The patient was advised to avoid prolonged sitting, bending, and lifting and to use a lumbar support when he did sit and to get up as frequently as possible (before the time required for symptoms to be provoked) if he did have to sit for any length of time.

Given the possibility that a disk herniation was present, it was decided not to treat the articular hypomobility at this time but to see how extension exercises affected his signs and symptoms. The patient was instructed to do prone extension (half push-ups) exercises in sets of 10 every half hour at home and when at work to bend backward 10 times every 30 minutes.

On reassessment the next day, he claimed to be feeling better although there was little objective improvement to see. The straight leg raise may have increased by a few degrees but that was all. However, because he was feeling better, he was asked to continue the program for another 2 days and to return for further assessment. When he did, there was definite improvement in his signs—the straight leg raise was full range with slight low-back pain. On flexion he was able to reach his ankles and experienced only an ache across the right low back. He had not felt any thigh pain for 2 days. On examining his intervertebral movements, it appeared that the biomechanical flexion dysfunction was still present. Another couple of days of the same program was prescribed, but on return, he had not improved and complained of mild aching during sitting if he did not use the support.

Because there was no further improvement, the treatment had to be changed. One direction of change would have been to move the extension exercises from bilateral to unilateral, by having the patient extend and right-side flex. This would be a good direction to take if manual therapy is not an option. It was decided to manipulate the lumbosacral joint to increase right joint flexion. After this, flexion increased to full range and was painfree. Non-weight bearing flexion exercises were added. The patient was seen a week later when he was at full function, with full ranges, and painfree. After advising him to start a regular exercise activity, he was discharged.

Lumbopelvic Case 12 Discussion

Diagnosis

The patient is suffering from a posterior instability of L4/5, regardless of the results of the manual biomechanical tests of stability. We have no idea of how sensitive these tests are, nor can we be too sure of their validity. In fact, the biomechanical tests were not really necessary to the diagnosis. Given the factors in the subjective examination that indicated instability and the minimal articular signs on gross movement testing, instability is the only reasonable diagnosis. The posteroanterior pressure suggests one of the two lower segments. The painful extension and extension activities indicate a posterior instability. The positive biomechanical tests demonstrating extension hypermobility at L4/5 also confirms and localizes the diagnosis and the fact that the test reproduced the patient's pain increases its significance.

Treatment

The patient was advised that treatment of stability therapy could take considerable time and could not be started until he was out of the painful phase. He was treated for 6 weeks with generalized and segmental stability therapy until he fully understood the exercises and was able to do them correctly.

During the next 6 months he had three episodes of back pain, none of which lasted more than a week. The following year he had only two episodes.

Lumbopelvic Case 13 Discussion

Diagnosis

Diagnosis is inferior anterior tibiofibular ligament grade 2 sprain (pain and movement on the stress test) or first sacral nerve palsy with motor deficit probably due to a small disk protrusion or contained herniation compressing the nerve. Presumably gradual compression may not cause pain.

Treatment

Heel raises were put into both shoes to limit dorsiflexion during walking. This immediately eliminated his walking pain. When he stopped stretching the calf muscles, he was painfree, and continuing stress and increasing instability were prevented. However, to correct the problem, at least as far as it was correctable, the lumbar spine had to be addressed.

The problem was in trying to reduce the disk protrusion. This calls for exercises into the limited quadrant of motion and the risk of increasing the palsy. However, if this is done in prone lying, the patient's weight is removed from the equation. There is a chance that motion can be increased while sparing the nerve from further pressure. In addition, progressive and very gradual strengthening exercises were given to the patient to increase the strength of the plantar flexors, although whether this will help is another matter, but it can't hurt.

Over a period of 12 weeks, the strength of the plantar flexors increased very slowly, whereas the range of motion in the left extension quadrant increased. On examination of the ankle at 10 weeks, the dorsiflexion hypermobility was absent but the tibiofibular instability was still present. The patient experienced no pain provided that he wore the heel lifts.

Lumbopelvic Case 14 Discussion

Diagnosis

It would appear from the neurological tests that at least two roots are being compressed bilaterally with the more severe compression on the right. These are L5 and S1, as evidenced by the weakness and reflex loss of the extensor hallucis brevis, tibialis posterior and peroneus longus for L5, and the plantar flexors and hamstrings for S1. However, more likely L4 and S2 are also being compressed as indicated by weakness of the dorsiflexors and gluteals and sensation loss over the dorsum of the foot. This combination of bilateral signs and symptoms almost certainly affecting more than two spinal nerves is very indicative of cauda equina compression, even though the S3 and S4 roots seem unaffected as yet.

Treatment

This is potentially a very serious situation for the patient. Any increase in pressure could cause the disk to herniate further posteriorly, rupture the posterior longitudinal ligament, and cause irreversible damage particularly to the genitourinary system of the patient. The physician must be informed of the examination findings and be advised that he should try to speed up the orthopedic consult. This was done, and the patient was set to see the orthopedic surgeon in a week.

Prognosis

Prognosis is poor. This is a large disk lesion. The chances are that it will get worse rather than better. If it does improve, it is unlikely to be due to treatment, and more than likely, it will recur sooner rather than later.

He was treated with mechanical traction in the line of the deformity and with the lumbar spine in neutral while waiting for his consultation. He was also put into a lumbar support to prevent him from flexing and to keep him more comfortable. No exercises were given. He was advised to keep himself as comfortable as possible. During the few days he had treatment, the patient was continuously asked about genitourinary signs or symptoms and perineal pain or paresthesia. On the third treatment, the patient described pain in the left calf and plantar aspect of the foot with paresthesia in the left great toe. The left straight leg raise had decreased to 30° and caused left calf pain. He was due to see the orthopedic surgeon the day after this. The orthopedic surgeon ordered an MRI that demonstrated a large central disk prolapse. He had successful surgery 2 days later.

Although this case was missing some of the classical signs of the cauda equina syndrome, it had enough. Bilateral multisegmental neurological deficits indicate that the cauda equina is under threat and if the disk herniation should worsen, a frank cauda equina compression could easily occur. This patient was heading that way when his signs and symptoms worsened.

Lumbopelvic Case 15 Discussion

An easy diagnosis to arrive at having heard the mechanism of injury is an iliac upslip (cranial subluxation of the sacroiliac joint). But the only thing in common with this problem is the fall onto the buttocks being classical for an upslip. However, an upslip is not as severely painful or disabling as this patient's problem.

The severity of the immediate pain and loss of range indicates profound tissue damage. The most likely pathologies following this type of compression injury are fractures and disk herniations. A fracture large enough to cause this degree of disability and pain would almost certainly show up on x-ray, so a disk herniation is more likely. But if it is herniation, it is not compressing neural tissues. The absence of pain demonstrates that fact. Nor is it compressing dural tissues, because the dural tests were also negative.

Diagnosis

This only leaves one possibility—the disk herniation was vertical, fracturing the end plate. The very positive compression tends to support the diagnosis. The end plate fracture might not show up on plain radiographs except much later as Schmorl's node.

Treatment

The patient must be kept as comfortable as possible through the acute stages using pain and anti-inflammatory modalities and then mobilized with exercises. The patient gradually improved over the following 4 weeks and returned to work as a medical lab technician.

If treatment had not improved him, an MRI should demonstrate the vertical prolapse. If not, other objective tests should be carried out to determine if there are any other serious pathologies present.

Lumbopelvic Case 16 Discussion

Clearly the two pains are not associated anatomically. The apparent neuromeningeal signs are exactly that, apparent. If there was compromise of neuromeningeal mobility, the next question has to be by what? Certainly not a disk prolapse. The minor articular signs do support the contention that this is a posterolateral disk herniation. The symptoms are the wrong type for a far lateral herniation; there is neither lancinating pain nor any paresthesia. Generally, a far lateral herniation will miss the dural sleeve of the spinal nerve. The inability to extend the knee in lying could be due to compromise of the dural sleeve, but the Lesague's test tends to contradict this thought. If the limitation of the knee extension with the hip relatively extended was 20°, you would expect the limitation to be much greater with the hip flexed. Because it was the same, the possibility that this is a calf, knee, or ankle problem must be considered.

Objective Examination Continued

The lower limb was examined and the following was found. Passive and active knee extension was limited to 160° with severe calf pain and spasm on passive overpressure. Active and passive ankle dorsiflexion was limited to the point that the dorsiflexion range could not be reached and passive testing caused strong spasm. All other movements of the knee and ankle were negative. Light palpation was not tender.

This is obviously a calf and/or ankle problem. There is no history of trauma, which tends to rule out joint dysfunction and gastrocnemius tear. The latter is also unlikely in the face of painfree light palpation. Deep palpation was not attempted because of the probability that the patient had a deep vein thrombosis, which turned out to be the case.

Although not a condition commonly associated with this type of onset, it is far from unheard of. Prolonged sitting in conditions where the legs cannot easily be moved around may cause thrombosis. A long airplane trip is one of the activities that causes this condition.

Lumbopelvic Case 17 Discussion

Many possible causal and contributive factors could have been involved in the destabilization of the lumbosacral junction. These include leg length discrepancy, foot and ankle dysfunctions, hip dysfunctions (particularly extension hypomobility), and sacroiliac joint biomechanical dysfunction.

The first place to look is within the functional unit of the symptomatic joint or segment—in this case, the lumbopelvic complex that includes the lumbar spine, sacroiliac joint, and hip joint.

The right sacroiliac joint was jammed or subluxed into anterior rotation or extension. This was determined by passive movement testing and the assessment of the end feels from these mobility tests. This sacroiliac joint dysfunction is certainly a potential cause of the lumbosacral junction instability and is very treatable with manual therapy. But we have the same problem as earlier. We do not know what has caused it. The sacroiliac joint is an extremely stable articulation.

Although severe trauma may destabilize it by way of fracture, the ligaments do not rupture without avulsing bone, an incident likely to be remembered by the patient. However, from clinical experience, we know that instability with subsequent subluxation of this joint does occur. The question is what is putting prolonged stress through this joint in the direction that would allow it to sublux into anterior rotation (extension)?

Any of the conditions mentioned above are capable of doing this. A long leg will cause the hip to flex by way of the innominate rotating anteriorly. (Paradoxically, anteriorly rotating or extending the innominate in non-weight bearing will lengthen the leg.) Prolonged exposure to this kind of stress may cause the sacroiliac joint to sublux. The long leg may be caused by a number of nonstructural events, including anterior subluxation of the talus.

The first thing to check within the lumbopelvic complex is the hip. In this patient, as is common, the hip was found to have an extension hypomobility. This makes sense as a cause of right sacroiliac and lumbosacral joint dysfunction.[1] The lack of extension will cause a dynamic long leg when the stride during walking is decreased as well as put dynamic increased stress through the two joints when they try to compensate for the decreased stride length by hypermobilizing and in the sacroiliac joint's case, by subluxing.

We can go still further. What is causing the decreased extension at the hip? Often this joint seems to be one of those joints that is simply vulnerable to osteoarthrosis. If so, what is commonly found is that the inner flexion quadrant (flexion, medial rotation, and adduction) is often painful and limited. If not, a cause for isolated extension hypomobility must be sought. A possible source of this is the upper lumbar spine. If there is segmental facilitation with significant hypertonicity of the psoas, this could limit hip extension.

In this case, the upper lumbar spine was normally mobile and the inner flexion quadrant of the hip was somewhat painful.

Diagnosis

- ❏ Asymptomatic osteoarthrosis of the right hip
- ❏ Anterior subluxation of the right sacroiliac joint
- ❏ Right torsional instability of the lumbosacral junction

Treatment

- ❏ Stretch the hip to gain full extension
- ❏ Use quadrant scouring to relieve the inner flexion quadrant pain

---

1. Hurwitz DE, et al. Gait compensations in patients with osteoarthritis of the hip and their relationship to pain and passive hip motion. *J Orthop Res.* 1997; 15(4):629–635.

- ❏ Manipulate or mobilize the right sacroiliac joint
- ❏ Stability therapy for the lumbosacral instability
- ❏ Alter and/or limit activities until the hip and sacroiliac joint are mobile and the patient has sufficient functional control of his lumbosacral instability

Prognosis

The mobilization aspect of this condition is simple. It is the ability of the patient to stabilize the spine that will be critical. If he can do this, then there is an excellent chance that he will be able to resume full activities with minimal chances of serious relapse within 6 to 8 weeks. In this case, this is what happened. The patient checked back 3 months later to say that he was running his normal distances without problems. Although it was no longer the season for cross-country skiing, he felt confident that he would be able to get back to it for the next winter.

Lumbopelvic Case 18 Discussion

A number of things should be considered in this case. First is the traumatic onset. I realize that the classical manner to cause an upslip (cranial subluxation) of the sacroiliac joint is to fall onto the buttock. But this should not be the first consideration. The threat here is a sacral fracture. The immediate onset of strong pain tends to support something a little more profound than a biomechanical sacroiliac joint dysfunction, especially because it was ongoing for a good deal longer than would be expected from a simple bruise. The negative x-ray does not exclude the possibility of a fracture especially in the pelvis where they can be extremely difficult to visualize (nearly half of fractures without neurological involvement being missed on first readings[2]).

Testing of the hip revealed that hip flexion was limited by pain to about 70°, whereas medial and lateral rotation with the hip in neutral were full range and painfree. Isometric extension was painful and weak. The patient demonstrated the sign of the buttock, one of the causes of which is a fractured sacrum.

Diagnosis

Diagnosis is a fractured sacrum. This was confirmed when the x-rays were re-read as a low left Zone 1 fracture; that is, the fracture is lateral to the sacral foraminae. In this case, it did not produce neurological deficit.

---

2. Lenke LG. Fractures and dislocations of the spine. In: Perry CR, et al. *Handbook of fractures.* New York: McGraw-Hill; 1995:194–197.

Treatment

The initial bed rest was serendipitously the correct treatment. However, the patient returned to full activities much too quickly. Treatment of this type of injury is based on pain relief initially, and then gradual increase in activity. This was done with this patient with a graduated and progressive exercise and activity program. He returned to full activities in 7 weeks after the injury date.

Lumbopelvic Case 19 Discussion

Other Clinical Tests

1. Ask about other joint involvement. However, if this is ankylosing spondylitis, it is a very early case and other joints are not likely to be symptomatic.

2. Definitively exclude the lumbar spine by doing a biomechanical examination.

3. Examine rib excursion during maximal respirations.

4. Examine rib springing (it should be elastic and resilient). Look for little movement and a much harder end feel.

5. Examine the joint glides of the costotransverse articulations.

6. Assess distraction at the sternoclavicular joint for mobility.

7. Make sure that the lumbar spine is moving by using Schober's test.

8. Assess the mobility of the hips. If the ipsilateral hip is hypomobile, particularly into extension, then it may be contributing or causing the sacroiliitis.

9. Carry out secondary stability testing for the sacroiliac joint.

Diagnosis

He denied any other joint pain apart from minor aches and pains after playing contact sports. The lumbar spine seemed to be moving reasonably, and rib expansion and springing also appeared to be normal. There did seem to be some stiffness of the upper half of the costotransverse-costovertebral joints, although this was marginal. The hips were equally mobile, although both seemed to be less mobile than would be expected in somebody of his age.

The secondary stability tests were negative, in that though they did reproduce his pain. No instability was detected. The negative secondary stability tests suggest that the sacroiliitis is not due to cumulative stress destabilizing the joint. Because there is no history of trauma that would allow a diagnosis of posttraumatic sacroiliitis, it makes ankylosing spondylitis a front runner.

This patient was put into a sacroiliac belt and sent back to the physician for further investigations. After he was found to have an elevated erythrocyte sedimentation rate, he eventually had a CT scan, which showed change at the sacroiliac joints.

Lumbopelvic Case 20 Discussion

The leg pain is not likely to be neurological as it is to be somatic in nature. The cause of the pain is unlikely to be a disk herniation, because, with the exception of flexion, the lumbar movements are full range and painfree. Additionally, sitting is not a problem.

The straight leg raise and the slump test give indications about what is happening. The reproduction of somatic sciatica would suggest some compromise of the dura between L4 and S2. The absence of neurological symptoms associated with the straight leg raise would suggest that the neura is not likely to be involved. The fact that slumping while holding the painful straight leg raise did not increase the pain suggests two things. One, the amount of extra stretch that flexing the lumbar spine applies to the neuromeninges is insufficient to produce symptoms. And two, the increased compression force that slumping causes had no effect, so the cause is probably not disk herniation.

The relief of the leg pain with neck flexion during straight leg raising and the slump test would suggest that pulling the neuromeningeal tube cranially actually relieved pressure or stretch on the tissue. I have already discussed in Chapter 12 how relief of pain during straight leg raising with neck flexion suggests to me a medial prolapse. However, in this case, it seems very unlikely that a prolapse is present. Another possibility suggested by Pettman[3] is that the cranial pull of the neuromeninges relieves the stretch from adhesions, if they are orientated inferiorly as they might be if their formation was influenced by walking.

Diagnosis

I partly agree with the referring physician's diagnosis. There are adhesions present but they are dural not neural and were caused either by the disk herniation or by the surgery.

Treatment

If there is adverse tension of the neuromeninges caused by adhesions, stretching is the treatment of choice. However, it is important to ensure that there is no mechanical impediment to movement. In this case, it

---

3. Pettman, Erl. Personal communication.

seems unlikely that there is any other reason for these symptoms, but a biomechanical examination of the lumbar spine and sacroiliac joint must be carried out before stretching.

With this patient, the biomechanical tests were clear. She was treated with careful, graduated, and progressive stretching of the lumbosacral dural sleeves. The slump position, without neck flexion, was used and, except for one incident in which the patient decided she would stretch or rather than overstretch at home, there was gradual improvement during 10 treatments over 3 weeks. At the end of the program, which also included exercises to reeducate movement and beneficially stress the segmental structures, the patient still had the same paresthesia in the lateral toes of the left foot and very mild aching in the left leg on prolonged flexion.

Lumbopelvic Case 21 Discussion

It is possible that the fall disturbed the fusion. She should probably be x-rayed before treatment is undertaken. However, mobility testing of the L4/5 segment did not produce pain or spasm. It seems more likely that the back pain is arising from the L5/S1 segment because testing here did reproduce her back pain.

Diagnosis

❏ Neural (possibly neuromeningeal) of the L4/5 spinal nerves and/or roots
❏ Irritable extension hypermobility of the L5/S1 segment

Treatment

The acute lumbar pain was settled with modalities and a lumbar support as a temporary measure. Then once the pain was under control, stabilization therapy was initiated.

For the leg pain, the slump test was used to stretch the nerve root adhesions.

Lumbopelvic Case 22 Discussion

The reproduction of the back and leg pain and spasm and the production of paresthesia would suggest that manual correction of the shift at this time was unlikely to work. An alternative method is to lay the patient on the left hip so that the deviated shoulder is down on the bed. A muscle stimulator is connected to the left-side side flexors and a hot pack applied over the electrodes. The contraction should be strong enough to be seen. Fifteen to thirty minutes of this is given. The patient is taught symptom-free shift correction exercises and is asked to come back the next day.

Traction can be used, but the positioning of the patient must be done very carefully. The traction must be given through the line of the deformity and must not try to correct the deformity because this usually results in the patient suffering a lot of pain when the traction lets off.

Diagnosis

Diagnosis is L4/5 disk herniation with L4 dural and neural compression. The straight leg raise and the paresthesia attest to this probability.

Treatment

This patient was treated with gradual shift correction as outlined above. When he was capable of lumbar extension, passive extension exercises were added. The patient improved gradually over the 6-week period.

Lumbopelvic Case 23 Discussion

Everything about the history suggests instability. If we look at the other common pathologies that can cause back pain, we can exclude each one. An uncontained disk herniation is extremely unlikely. There are no dural or neural signs; he has full range of motion and is able to sit without discomfort. A contained herniation is also improbable; sitting is painfree and all other movements are full range and, with the exception of flexion, painless. The patient's ability to walk and stand for prolonged periods tends to eliminate stenosis as a diagnosis. A zygopophyseal joint dysfunction is also doubtful as a diagnosis because it tends to painfully affect more ranges especially in reducing motion. Other conditions such as discitis and systemic arthritis would limit range, and neoplastic disease should have made itself known after all of these years.

Reasons to include instability as a diagnosis are the full range of motion in the back, pain on returning from flexion rather than going toward it, and pain with minimal provocation such as turning in bed (the other major cause of this is sacroiliitis, which was excluded by the negative Fortin finger test and pain provocation tests).

Biomechanical tests are necessary. The tests most likely to confirm this diagnosis are, of course, the segmental stability tests. In this patient's case, there was an extension hypermobility at the lumbosacral junction with an anterior instability.

Diagnosis is anterior instability L5/S1. Treatment should be stability therapy.

Lumbopelvic Case 24 Discussion

Given the fact that the lumbosacral hypermobility was painless plus all of the other considerations give above, it is probable that the pain was caused by an extension hypermobility.

If we are looking at long-term management, we must look for causes other than the obvious, which when you think about it is not obvious at all. It is not a reasonable assumption that running was a direct cause. This patient had been running for many years without lumbar problems. It is possible that other causes had moved the joint closer to its anteriorly rotated (extended) position, so this particular run had sparked her symptoms. One possibility is a long leg on that side. This may cause the ilium to rotate so that the hip is flexed and the leg shortened.

Commonly dynamic long legs may be caused by a plantar flexed ankle (anterior talus subluxation), hip extension hypomobility, or an anteriorly rotated innominate (extension subluxation).

We know that the patient has an extension subluxation, but this is symptomatic and likely a result rather than the cause of a long leg. This would be supported by the extension hypermobility found at the lumbosacral junction, which also probably results from the leg length discrepancy. We have to check the hip and ankle.

On examination, the ankle was found to have an anterior talar subluxation, probably remaining from the ankle sprain earlier. The hip was slightly hypomobile into extension.

Diagnosis is an extension subluxation of the left sacroiliac joint. Treatment should include manipulation or mobilization of the sacroiliac joint as well as the ankle and mobilization of the hip extension.

The patient was painfree on examination after the sacroiliac joint manipulation. He was advised not run for a week or two. He resumed normal activity in a week and had no recurrence when he was checked a month later.

Index

ISBN 0-07-041235-9

90000

9 780070 412354